Principles and Practice of Renal Nursing

Edited by

Paul Challinor

School of Nursing Studies
St Cadoc's Hospital
University of Wales College of Medicine
Cardiff

and

John Sedgewick

Faculty of Nursing
Institute of Health Sciences
Muscat Nursing Institute
Muscat, Sultanate of Oman

First published in 1998 by Stanley Thornes (Publishers) Ltd

Reprinted in 2001 by:
Nelson Thornes Ltd
Delta Place
27 Bath Road
CHELTENHAM
GL53 7TH
United Kingdom

04 05 / 10 9 8 7 6 5 4

A catalogue record for this book is available from the British Library

ISBN 0 7487 3331 0

Typeset by WestKey Ltd

Printed and bound by Antony Rowe Ltd, Eastbourne

Contents

Contributors

Pam Buckley, Senior Transplant Co-ordinator
Freeman Hospital, High Heaton, Newcastle-upon-Tyne.
Chapter 17

Paul Challinor, Lecturer
School of Nursing Studies, St Cadoc's Hospital, University of Wales College of Medicine, Cardiff.
Chapters 2, 5, 6 and 8

Debra Coupe, Nurse Practitioner
Renal and Urology Directorate, University Hospital Birmingham NHS Trust, Edgbaston, Birmingham.
Royal College of Nursing, RCN Dialysis and Transplant Nursing Forum, European Dialysis and Transplant Nurses Association.
Chapter 4

Josie Digioa, Renal Nurse Co-ordinator
Renal Unit, City Hospital, Hucknall Road, Nottingham.
Chapter 15

Liz Ford, Clinical Nurse Specialist
Fresenius Medical Centre, Nunn Brook Road, Huthwaite, Sutton-in-Ashfield, Nottinghamshire.
Chapter 13

Anne Frankton, Transplant Sister
Renal Outpatients, City Hospital, Hucknall Road, Nottingham.
Chapter 15

Coral Graham, Clinical Nurse Specialist
Fresenius Medical Centre, Nunn Brook Road, Huthwaite, Sutton-in-Ashfield, Nottinghamshire.
Chapter 10

Lesley Russell, Senior Dietician
Department of Nutrition and Dietetics, City General Hospital, Newcastle Road, Stoke-on-Trent, Staffordshire.
Chapter 12

John Sedgewick, Lecturer
Faculty of Nursing, Institute of Health Science, Muscat Nursing Institute, Muscat, Oman.
Chapters 1, 3 and 7

Alison Shakeshaft, Renal Dietician SRD
Department of Nutrition and Dietetics, University Hospital of Wales, Health Care NHS Trust, Heath Park, Cardiff.
British Dietetic Association.
Chapter 9

Marcelle de Sousa, Adolescent Project Manager
Middlesex Hospital, Mortimer Street, London.
Chapter 18

Nicola Thomas, Lecturer in Renal Nursing
St. Bartholomew School of Nursing and Midwifery, City University, Bartholomew Close, London.
Chapter 16

Jane Torrington, Renal Dietician SRD
Department of Nutrition and Dietetics, University Hospital of Wales, Health Care NHS Trust, Heath Park, Cardiff.
British Dietetics Association.
Meetings organiser of Renal Dialysis Group.
Chapter 9

Krys Turner, Lecturer Practitioner
Renal Unit, Manchester Royal Infirmary, Oxford Road, Manchester.
Chapter 11

Geraldine Ward, Paediatric Chronic Renal Failure Sister
Department of Paediatric Nephrology, Guys Hospital, St. Thomas Street, London.
Chapter 18

Victoria Warmington, Community Sister
Baxter Training Centre, Tooting, London.
Chapter 14

Foreword

Principles and Practice of Renal Nursing takes renal care forward in developing nursing whilst retaining the renal patient as the focus of care.

This book is written for nurses but provides education for all members of the multiprofessional team. It is a comprehensive guide to learning all the exciting aspects of nephrology nursing. The use of learning objectives and review questions at the end of each chapter reinforces the process of learning. It gives a tour through the processes required to achieve a level of post-basic education for nurses, enhancing their contribution to excellence in practice.

In the fifteen years I have been caring for renal patients, I have not had the opportunity to benefit from such a comprehensive 'package of knowledge'. There has previously been a lack of good reference literature for nephrology care, but nursing in particular, and this book redresses the balance. It provides support for nurses new to this stimulating field of care and challenges experts already practising within nephrology. It is a book to read and re-read, providing stimulation and growth.

Principles and Practice of Renal Nursing will be welcomed by all English speaking Health Care professionals across Europe and throughout the World.

Julie Hartley-Jones
President
The European Dialysis and Transplant Nurses Association/
European Renal Care Association 1997/1998

Acknowledgements

The editors wish to extend their thanks to the contributors to this book. Without their enthusiasm and hard work this book would have not been possible. Special thanks to numerous clinical staff who have commented upon the various chapters in the book and offered their constructive comments. To Julie Hartley-Jones for her contribution to the Foreword of the book and to her vision that she has provided and continues to provide for renal nursing.

We are indebted to numerous people who have shared with us their thoughts on this book. Past students who we have taught on the Renal Nursing courses as well as colleagues in clinical practice and education.

The editors would like to thank Rosemary Morris formerly of Chapman & Hall who provided guidance and support during the early part of the project and latterly to the Publishers, Stanley Thornes, for their commitment to this project. Thank you to Tony Wayte, Commissioning Editor for his guidance on the technical aspects of the book. The editors would like to pay special attention to the patients and families who we have cared for and have come to learn so much from. Through them we have learnt to understand the nature of living with renal impairment and the unique contribution of renal nursing to their lives.

To the following very special people we owe so much; our wives Gill and Karen, children Sam, Faye and Nia, whose encouragement, time and space to complete this book was never ending.

Fundamentals of nephrology nursing

John Sedgewick

LEARNING OBJECTIVES

At the end of this chapter the reader should be able to:

- Identify the importance of nephrology nursing, establishing its research base.
- Describe the concept of advocacy and its implications for nephrology nursing practice.
- Examine educational issues shaping renal nursing practice at a professional level.
- Discuss the impact of ethical issues in renal nursing practice.
- Examine the nature of multidisciplinary practice and its impact upon renal care.

INTRODUCTION

Nephrology nursing is shaped by health policy and economics as well as by social trends. Importantly, the care of patients with renal failure must be a collaborative activity and one that draws upon the unique contribution of every member of the multidisciplinary team. Nephrology nursing as a distinct speciality has made significant advances in the development of the role of the renal nurse as a central member of the health-care team.

IMPACT OF CHRONIC ILLNESS ON HEALTH-CARE DELIVERY

Lindsey (1995) suggests that chronic illness and disabilities are the leading health problems globally, representing one of the major health challenges of this era. The traditional Western illness care model, which has profoundly influenced health-care and nursing practice, is viewed as oppressive,

Health-care delivery should:

- reduce stress on the family
- evolve with the individual and the family
- maintain the patient's quality of life
- focus on the patient's needs

inappropriate and inadequate to meet the needs of individuals living with chronic conditions. Lindsey (1995) argues that health-care staff should increasingly employ research of a phenomenological nature when studying patients living with different chronic conditions. Newby (1996) discusses the impact of chronic illness, suggesting that it creates increased family stress, requires constant adaptation by family members and poses a challenge to nurses in understanding individuals and families.

There is at present an almost exclusive dependence on the diagnostic disease model, which is an obstacle to dealing with the burden of illness and disability typically seen in primary medical care. With ageing populations and an increasing prevalence of chronic disease and disability, new approaches to patient assessment and intervention are needed. Consideration must be given to promoting function and maintaining patients' quality of life. On an individual level, this includes modifying impairments, increasing patient motivation and encouraging helpful attitudes, teaching coping strategies, educating family members and employers and providing support (Mechanic, 1995).

> **Key reference:** Mechanic, D. (1995) Sociological dimensions of illness behavior. *Social Science & Medicine* 41(9): 1207–16.

Chronic illness results in:

- individual and family stress
- disruption to daily living
- feelings of powerlessness and hopelessness
- need for constant adaptation

The role of the spiritual wellbeing of patients and how their beliefs and faith assist them in adjustment to chronic illness have been long been recognized. Chronic illness brings about disorganization and disruption in a patient's life and may result in spiritual distress. Renal nurses require the personal resources to provide effective spiritual care as part of their attention to quality of care for patients (Narayanasamy, 1996).

FAMILY CARE AND SOCIAL SUPPORT

Patients are not the only ones who suffer when they have a chronic illness: significant others and family members also suffer. As the number of elderly individuals increases, the number of chronically ill patients joining maintenance renal care programmes is also increasing. This makes significant demands upon hospital resources in delivering care to a particularly vulnerable group of patients who already have a co-morbid illness that further limits their quality of life.

Individual personal factors (both environmental and those related to the illness) create feelings of powerlessness among family members and significant others (Davidhizar, 1994). Chronic illness causes increased family stress, requires constant adaptation by family members and challenges nurses to better understand and meet the needs of the family as well as the patient. Rena *et al.* (1996) examined the role of 'sense of coherence' (SOC) in the experience of managing stressful life events. SOC was significantly related to disability adjustment in both patients with disability and their spouses, suggesting that SOC is a personality factor that may explain individual differences in coping with disability, regardless of its level of severity. As renal nurses and the health-care team work to assist patients with end-stage renal disease (ESRD) and their families, increasing attention should be focused upon developing commitment, coherence and control within care, all of which have been identified as the major components of SOC.

Family support is a primary source of patient support and the impact of illness on families can be substantial. Social support research highlights the problems of support in families who are collectively coping with illness and disability (Ell, 1996). The need to work with the family unit, mobilizing resources to assist them, is important. As increasing numbers of elderly patients are being nursed in the community, the impact of community care services on service delivery is increasing in importance. Increasing numbers of elderly patients with ESRD may be cared for in residential care homes and at this level the renal unit team need to work within community agencies to support patients.

PATIENT EDUCATION AND THE ROLE OF THE HEALTH-CARE TEAM

Within nephrology, patient education forms one of the principle cornerstones of practice and one that draws upon all members of the renal multidisciplinary team. A significant volume of research has been undertaken on factors thought to influence an individual's ability to learn. When one considers the salient features of living with renal replacement it is evident that, throughout all phases of a patient's career on dialysis, understanding and managing complex life-sustaining skills is vital.

As nursing continues to strive to develop its theoretical base to support practice, nurses have began to examine the usefulness of a number of nursing models (Diffey, 1996; Neff, 1993). Nursing models are attempts to create explicit frameworks for the concept of nursing, and are usually derived from a theory (Chinn and Jacobs, 1979). One particular conceptual model that has received intense attention among nephrology nurses is Orem's model of self-care (Michos, 1985; Montenegro *et al.*, 1994). Orem advocates: 'Nursing has as its special concern man's need for self-care action and the provision and management of it on a continuous basis in order to sustain life and health, recover from disease or injury, and cope with their effects' (Orem, 1991, p. 1). Orem believes that people require nursing care when their needs for care exceed their own ability to meet these needs. Orem calls needs 'self-care requisites' and ability 'self-care agency'. When individuals' self-care needs exceed their ability, this situation is called a self-care deficit (Orem, 1991).

For renal nursing, one of the attractions of Orem's model is its emphasis upon the individual's need for self-care action and the provision and management of it on a continuous basis in order to sustain life and health, recover from disease or injury and cope with their effects. Miller (1992) argues that the concept of self-care is an important concept for individuals adjusting to and managing a chronic illness. End-stage renal disease presents individuals with the need to learn complex life-sustaining skills while balancing the demands of treatment with its integration into their lives (Stapleton, 1992).

Key reference: Miller, J. (1992) *Coping with Chronic Illness: Overcoming Powerlessness* (2nd edn). F.A. Davis Company, Philadelphia.

The demands imposed upon patients and families living with ESRD include gaining knowledge and understanding on how to manage the illness and complex treatment regimens. Education of patients is a central function of the renal-care team, where life skills and competencies are developed. 'Self-care', a philosophy firmly embedded within the speciality of renal care, aims to reduce the feeling of powerlessness experienced by patients undergoing dialysis.

Dines (1994) considers that when addressing how patients view their health and their health behaviours it is important to understand the differences between 'public' and 'private' accounts of health, the 'taken-for-grantedness' of health, its emotive nature and the difficulty of accessing 'unpolluted' lay views of health. Sociological research concerning health beliefs and illness can develop nurses' understanding of the difficulties renal patients encounter in adhering to health behaviours. Non-compliance with therapeutic regimens is a recognized problem among renal patients and is a complex process influenced by many factors. Gaining an understanding of patients' beliefs about their health provides the nurse with information that can be developed within health education programmes.

Hayslip and Suttle (1995) argue that the education of patients with renal disease focuses on the inevitability of reaching end-stage renal disease and requiring renal replacement therapy. Established education programmes begin the process during the late stages of renal disease progression or after the patient reaches ESRD. Uraemic symptoms negatively influence the patients' ability to learn and make decisions about their health care. Early education for the pre-ESRD patient has the potential to improve the quality of patient satisfaction, delay the onset of dialytic treatment and increase cost-effectiveness. Despite more than 20 years experience in the treatment of ESRD patients, there are relatively few reports in the literature about early education or pre-ESRD education.

Health problems and disease have changed during the last century, with an increase in the numbers of people with chronic illness. Literature reveals patients changing from a passive role to active participation in care management. A study of factors influencing self-management, using both quantitative and qualitative methods, revealed that it is more important than ever before that individuals be actively involved in self-care activities and that they and their families receive education and support to help them cope with chronic illness (Coates and Boore, 1995).

Fealy (1995) believes that increased attention should be directed towards examining the precise nature of caring. Where cultural diversity is evident, as in many centres, it is important that members of the health-care team embrace the principles of transcultural care and provide culturally sensitive and appropriate care during all phases of the patient's renal career. Leininger (1996) contends that in today's health-care settings nurses are almost forced to use transcultural nursing theories and practices in order to care for people of diverse cultures.

QUALITY ASSURANCE AND ECONOMICS FACING RENAL NURSING

Health-care organizations committed to developing quality care use new measuring and reporting mechanisms that underpin the principles of total quality management. Organizations involved in the provision of renal replacement therapies are looking for quality initiatives that enable routine care delivery to be measured. Nephrology nurses must become more informed about the changes taking place, participate in the learning curve and become 'active players' in judging organizational quality (Biddle, 1995). The development of contracts for services between purchasers and providers, as provided for by the National Health Service reforms, have promoted the development of a better-quality, customer-focused health service.

> **Key reference:** Biddle, G. (1995) Quality improvement in the ESRD program: implications for nephrology nurses. *Advances in Renal Replacement Therapies* 2(2): 112–20.

DEMOGRAPHIC AND EPIDEMIOLOGICAL INFLUENCES SHAPING NEPHROLOGY NURSING

The scope and practice of renal nursing continues to be shaped by a multitude of factors, not least the emerging demographic trends identified by the European Dialysis and Transplantation Registry (Valderrábano *et al.*, 1996). The incidence of treated end-stage renal disease has been increasing at a similar rate in most countries that record counts of new ESRD patients per year. Port (1995) identifies data from the United States Renal Data System that suggest an exponential growth for both incidence and prevalence rates. The number of new patients per year doubled over a recent 8½ year period and this interval was even shorter for older patients, Asians, Native Americans and patients with ESRD caused by diabetes or hypertension. Reasons for this growth in incidence include acceptance to therapy of more older and sicker patients, reduced mortality from other conditions and possibly an increase in the incidence of kidney disease. A recent reduction in mortality rates for ESRD patients in the USA has added to the growth in prevalence.

> **Key reference:** Valderrábano, F., Berthoux, F.C., Jones, E.H.P. and Mehls, O. (1996) Report on management of renal failure in Europe, XXV, 1994 End stage renal disease and dialysis report. *Nephrology Dial Transplant* 11(Suppl. 1): 2–21.

Molzahn (1996) has provided figures indicating that the overall incidence of new patients will rise to 300 per million population per year, with the prevalence of patients on treatment exceeding 1000 per million population in some European countries, Japan and the USA. The increasing number of elderly patients requiring dialysis represents a significant demand on services. This group often have co-morbid conditions that further exacerbate their renal problems, the most notable being diabetes mellitus. The long-term effects of haemodialysis in diabetic patients with ESRD may appear minor, but further examination reveals their impact upon every aspect of patients' lives. Such long-term effects range from vascular access problems and complications such as limb amputation, to feelings of loss of control, hopelessness and powerlessness.

> **Key reference:** Molzahn, M. (1996) Future evolution of the ESRD patient population – a perspective for the year 2000: *Nephrology Dialysis Transplantation* 11: (8) 59–62.

QUALITY OF LIFE ISSUES

Quality of life (QoL) has become an increasing concern for staff caring for renal patients, with voluminous research devoted to this topic. Gudex (1995) examined the health-related quality of life (HRQoL) of patients on different forms of treatment for ESRD in such a way that the data could be used in a cost-utility analysis of renal failure treatment in the UK. Compared to the general population, patients with ESRD experienced a lower quality of life. Various factors contributed to this, but uncertainty about the future and lack of energy emerged as key components. Transplant patients reported better HRQoL than dialysis patients, and had fewer problems with physical mobility, self-care, social and personal relationships and usual activities. They also experienced significantly less distress, while dialysis patients reported problems with depression, anxiety, pain and uncertainty about the future. It has been suggested that QoL is marginally better on continuous ambulatory peritoneal dialysis than on haemodialysis. Long-term results from studies in Italy by Valderrábano *et al.* (1996) has indicated that lack of help, loneliness and patient 'burnout' are important factors in patients' QoL.

Molzahn *et al.* (1996) study examined the perceived quality of life of 215 patients with ESRD. QoL was measured using the Self-Anchoring Striving Scale, the Index of Well-Being, and the Time Trade-Off Technique, examining patients' medical characteristics, health status, functional status, support and outlook. Outlook, functional status and treatment modality had significant direct effects on QoL. Support greatly influenced QoL and couples were able to adjust to disability within the family. Many patients with ESRD are functionally impaired in their ability to undertake routine aspects of daily living; the impact of fatigue is a particular distressing problem for many patients (Brunier and Graydon, 1996).

> **Key reference:** Molzahn, A.E., Northcott, H.C. and Hayduk, L. (1996) Quality of life of patients with end stage renal disease: a structural equation model. *Quality of Life Research* 5(4): 426–32.

Kimmel *et al.* (1995) argues that effectively measuring quality of life in chronically ill patients is difficult. Different measures may assess varied aspects of patients' experience, which may be interrelated in different ways. The relationship between quality-of-life measures including indices of psychological wellbeing, social support and severity of illness in ESRD patients treated with haemodialysis (HD) was prospectively assessed by Kimmel *et al.* (1995). This study sought to determine whether patients' assessment of quality of life was related to patient compliance. Social support scores correlated with perception of illness, depression and satisfaction with life, while adjustment to illness scores correlated with social support. This study identified that quality of life in patients treated with HD must be measured in several ways. Quality of life and perception of the effects of illness are not necessarily associated with functional ability.

Landis (1996) examined the importance of spiritual wellbeing in the psychological adjustment to chronic illness. Spiritual wellbeing was considered to buffer the effects of uncertainty on psychosocial adjustment to chronic illness, suggesting that it may be an important internal resource for persons forced to adjust to uncertainty about long-term health problems. During assessments, renal nurses should identify patients' principal coping methods and their individual support resources and enhance their use of these.

ETHICS IN NEPHROLOGY NURSING

As a result of rapid developments in medical technology, renal nurses and other staff are increasingly faced with decisions about prolongation of life and withdrawal of dialysis. Such decisions are complex and present moral dilemmas that are complicated by prevailing politicoeconomic, social and cultural influences. A knowledge and understanding of these factors will help renal nurses to examine moral issues surrounding life and death (Trnobranski, 1996).

The place of advance directives in the care of renal patients has received increasing attention. Perry *et al.* (1995) examined the attitudes of dialysis patients, their relatives/friends, primary nephrologists and nurses regarding advance directives. A high proportion of patients (84%) indicated the importance of a living will; interestingly, only 18% of these patients had actually left an advance directive. However, 52% of patients and relatives/friends believed that major treatment decisions should be left to the physician, a view that was not shared by medical staff or nurses. Patients, family/friends, nurses and medical staff held different views concerning advance directives. Health-care staff must realize that such differences exist and that further research must identify strategies to increase understanding of patient decisions in this area.

Advance directives are increasingly being considered as an option by patients suffering a long-term chronic illness. Colvin *et al.* (1993) suggest that nurses need to consider advance directives as a process of understanding, reflecting and discussing, and not just a written document. Further, health-care professionals must initiate the process of advance directive education in the outpatient setting. Renal nurses within the multidisciplinary team should consider the impact of advanced directives on care and practice, and support patients and families in their decisions.

Patients' perceptions of advanced directives in renal care, and situations that might predispose to the development of advance directives, were examined by Singer *et al.* (1995). In this study, 25% of patients wished to continue dialysis in case of severe stroke, 19% in severe dementia and 14% in permanent coma. Renal nurses may find it difficult when they are not convinced that advanced directive decisions have been made voluntarily and willingly. Webb (1996) suggests that literature concerning the care-and-cure dilemma puts forward the position that doctors do the curing and nurses do the caring, with patients rarely being included in discussions. The significance of ethics within the speciality of nephrology care has become an increasing focus for members of the health care team. The prolongation of life through life-sustaining therapies such as dialysis immerses staff in many controversies (McCormick, 1993).

End-stage renal disease (ESRD) patients can achieve a good death when care planning is combined with an ethic of care. Advance directives help to ensure that patients who want to participate in their treatment decisions may do so. An ethic of care ensures that the actual process of dying incorporates important factors such as readiness to die, appropriate interpretation of advance directives in terminal clinical situations, and proper timing of death. Campbell (1991) discusses terminal care of the ESRD patient foregoing life-sustaining dialysis therapy, suggesting that the care of patients who decide to do this constitutes a meaningful challenge.

Willard (1996) argues that, in order to secure professional standing, nursing has sought to discover and prove the value and uniqueness of its contribution to patient wellbeing. A prominent feature of this quest has been the assertion by nurses that the nurse has a specific and special function as patient advocate. Important concepts related to advocacy that renal nurses must explore include the patient's rights and interests in health-care, the moral status of patient autonomy and the obligations owed to patients by nurses.

NURSING STAFF AND THE ENVIRONMENT IN WHICH THEY PRACTISE

It is well known that caring for patients in a chronic care setting can be a source of stress for staff for a multitude of reasons. This issue was examined by Lewis *et al.* (1994), who examined possible relationships between personality types, personal and work-related stress, coping resources and sense of coherence among nephrology nurses. A positive relationship existed between perceived personal stress and work-related stress, particularly workload. A negative relationship emerged between personal/work-related stress and SOC, and between coping resources/ SOC and burnout. High levels of personal and work-related stress were related to inadequate coping resources. The main contributing factors to emotional exhaustion (a component of burnout) were low SOC, lack of staff support, personal stress and heavy workload. Renal nurses must recognize the impact upon themselves and co-workers that working within the setting of nephrology can have and work collaboratively to address known factors affecting staff performance and wellbeing. Staff support groups and peer support can greatly help staff in their roles.

NEPHROLOGY NURSING EDUCATION

In many countries, both within Europe and further afield, the need for nurses to maintain their continuing education (CE) as a prerequisite to relicensure is evident. Alongside the general expansion in educational opportunities for nurses wishing to pursue undergraduate and postgraduate studies, developments within the clinical specialism of nephrology nursing have emerged.

Given that continuing education is now mandatory within the UK, its value in promoting quality of nursing care merits serious consideration. Little research has been conducted into this, although Hogston's (1995) study revealed the importance that nurses attached to CE in supporting their professional status and the impact that CE and knowledge have on their professional competence. Therefore, the expanding opportunities for renal nurses to develop their professional competence in pursuit of patients' care are important. Educational developments within the field of nephrology nursing have included the emergence of a European core curriculum for nephrology nurses. This innovative and challenging project has focused on key themes and content areas seen as fundamental for nurses across Europe and has been instrumental in bringing about a number of changes. Nephrology nurses can now develop a common core of knowledge that can act as a catalyst for the development of standards and quality of care across Europe (Kuenzle and Thomas, 1995).

Attention has focused on the role of health-care assistants (HCAs) within nephrology. HCAs are integral members of the renal unit team and can assist in providing quality care through their developing clinical skills and experience. Despite controversy surrounding their responsibilities and role, it is clear that they can enable qualified nursing staff to develop other aspects of care and practice that have not previously received attention, particularly in the areas of research, counselling and patient education. To deliver optimum patient care, renal nurses must consider appropriate utilization of skills and the HCA can provide a valuable addition to the skill mix within the unit.

NURSING RESEARCH

As the speciality of nephrology nursing continues to develop, there must be a greater focus on the development and application of research. Attention is being directed towards 'evidence-based practice' and how the nursing contribution to patient outcomes must be continuously scrutinized. Hoffart (1995) identified the importance of nursing research in a study involving a sample of 400 nephrology nurses, whose research topics were broad and multidisciplinary in scope. This study indicated that nephrology nurses were beginning to explore a variety of patient care and administrative problems; however, research on other topics that present challenges to practising nephrology nurses, including symptom management, care of diabetic and elderly renal patients, ethical issues and the cardiovascular complications of renal disease, were absent. Most nurses in Hoffart's (1995) study held a master's degree and had already completed one research study. The patients in the majority of studies were adults, and psychosocial phenomena and quality of life were the most frequently identified study foci. Further experimental research is still required to test nursing interventions aimed at alleviating common problems experienced by renal patients.

CONCLUSION

As renal nursing continues to expand and develop it must be seen to respond to a variety of factors. Epidemiological developments such as the emergence of the Human Immunodeficiency Virus (HIV) and the increasing number of Hepatitis C patients will affect clinical practice and service delivery. Central to practice is a broad understanding and application of knowledge from many care disciplines. Developing the research base must continue to be an aim for those all involved in nephrology. Renal nursing is a dynamic specialty, where the concept of true multidisciplinary practice can become a shared reality. Social workers, renal dietitians and counsellors, as well as nursing and medical staff, can all work towards providing care that reflects patients' needs.

REVIEW QUESTIONS

- Identify the philosophies which are central to nephrology nursing practice.
- What are the current social, political and economic forces which are shaping the practice of nephrology nursing?
- Consider the range of ethical dilemmas the 'renal care' team encounter and offer suggestions on how such dilemmas can be addressed.
- In what way could the philosophy of 'self care' be seen as problematic to both patients, carers and staff and suggest why problems are encountered with this philosophy?
- Identify priority areas for research as a way to improving the focus of nephrology nursing.

REFERENCES

Biddle, G. (1995) Quality improvement in the ESRD program: implications for nephrology nurses. *Advances in Renal Replacement Therapies*, **2**(2), 112–120.

Brunier, G. and Graydon, J. (1996) A comparison of two methods of measuring fatigue in patients on chronic haemodialysis: visual analogue vs. Likert scale. *International Journal of Nursing Studies*, **33**(3), 338–348.

Campbell, M. L. (1991) Terminal care in patients with end stage renal disease. *American Nephrology Nurses Association Journal*, **22**(3), 294–300.

Chinn, P. and Jacobs, J. K. (1979) A model for theory development in nursing. *Advances in Nursing Science*, **1**(1), 1.

Coates, V. E. and Boore, J. R. (1995) Self-management of chronic illness: implications for nursing. *International Journal of Nursing Studies*, **32**(6) 628–640.

Colvin, E. R., Myhre, M. J., Welch, J. and Hammes, B. J. (1993) Moving beyond the Patient Self-Determination Act: educating patients to be autonomous. *American Nephrology Nurses Association Journal*, **20**(5) 564–568.

Davidhizar, R. (1994) Powerlessness of caregivers in home care. *Journal of Clinical Nursing*, **3**(3), 155–158.

Diffey, M. (1996) Nursing models: a useful strategy for nephrology nursing practice? *Journal of the European Dialysis and Transplant Nurses Association–European Renal Care Association*, **22**(2), 38–40.

Dines, A. (1994) A review of lay health beliefs research: insights for nursing practice in health promotion. *Journal of Clinical Nursing*, **3**(6), 329–338.

Ell, K. (1996) Social networks, social support and coping with serious illness: the family connection. *Social Science and Medicine*, **42**(2), 173–183.

Fealy, G. M. (1995) Professional caring: the moral dimension? *Journal of Advanced Nursing*, **22**(6), 1135–1140.

Gudex, C. M. (1995) Health-related quality of life in end stage renal failure. *Quality of Life Research*, **4**(4), 359–366.

Hayslip, D. M. and Suttle, C. D. (1995) Pre-ESRD patient education: a review of the literature. *Advances in Renal Replacement Therapies*, **2**(3), 217–226.

Hoffart, N. (1995) Characteristics of nephrology nurse researchers and their research. *American Nephrology Nurses Association Journal*, **22**(1), 33–39.

Hogston, R. (1995) Nurses' perceptions of the impact of continuing professional education on the quality of nursing care. *Journal of Advanced Nursing*, **22**(3), 586–593.

Kimmel, P. L., Peterson, R. A., Weihs, K. L. *et al.* (1995) Aspects of quality of life in hemodialysis patients. *Journal of the American Society of Nephrology*, **6**(5), 1418–1426.

Kuentzle, W. and Thomas, N. (1995) *European Curriculum for Nephrology Nursing*. F-Twee, Ghent.

Landis, B. J. (1996) Uncertainty, spiritual well-being, and psychosocial adjustment to chronic illness. *Issues in Mental Health Nursing*, **17**(3), 217–231.

Leininger, M. (1996) Culture care theory, research, and practice. *Nursing Science Quarterly*, **9**(2), 71–78.

Lewis, S. L., Bonner, P. N., Campbell, M. A. *et al.* (1994) Personality, stress, coping, and sense of coherence among nephrology nurses in dialysis settings. *American Nephrology Nurses Association Journal*, **21**(6), 325–335.

Lindsey, E. (1995) The gift of healing in chronic illness/disability. *Journal of Holistic Nursing*, **13**(4), 287–305.

McCormick, T. R. (1993) Ethical issues in caring for patients with renal failure. *American Nephrology Nurses Association Journal*, **20**(5), 549–555.

Mechanic, D. (1995) Sociological dimensions of illness behavior. *Social Science and Medicine*, **41**(9), 1207–1216.

Michos, M. S. (1985) The application of Orem's conceptual framework to enhance self-care in a dialysis program. *American Nephrology Nurses Association Journal*, **12**(1), 21–24.

Miller, J. F. (1992) *Coping with Chronic Illness: Overcoming Powerlessness*, 2nd edn, F. A. Davis, Philadelphia, PA.

Molzahn, M. (1996) Future evolution of the ESRD patient population – a perspective for the year 2000. *Nephrology Dialysis Transplantation*, **11**(8) 59–62.

Molzahn, A. E., Northcott, H. C. and Hayduk, L. (1996) Quality of life of patients with end stage renal disease: a structural equation model. *Quality of Life Research*, **5**(4) 426–432.

Montenegro, L., Dasi, M. J. and Carulla, M. T. (1994) Making the theory of nursing care more practical: a challenge to advance. *Journal of the European Dialysis and Transplant Nurses Association–European Renal Care Association*, **20**(4) 2–5.

Narayanasamy, A. (1996) Spiritual care of chronically ill patients. *Journal of Clinical Nursing*, **4**(6), 397–398.

Neff, M. L. (1993) Conceptual models in nephrology nursing practice. *Journal of the European Dialysis and Transplant Nurses Association–European Renal Care Association*, **21**(1) 26–27.

Newby, N. M. (1996) Chronic illness and the family life-cycle. *Journal of Advanced Nursing*, **23**(4), 786–791.

Orem, D. (1991) *Nursing: Concepts of Practice*, McGraw-Hill, New York.

Perry, L. D., Nicholas, D., Molzahn, A. E. and Dossetor, J. B. (1995) Attitudes of dialysis patients and caregivers regarding advance directives. *American Nephrology Nurses Association Journal*, **22**(5), 457–463; 481.

Port, F. K. (1995) End-stage renal disease: magnitude of the problem, prognosis of future trends and possible solutions. *Kidney International Supplement*, **50**, 3–6.

Rena, F., Moshe, S. and Abraham, O. (1996) Couples' adjustment to one partner's disability: the relationship between sense of coherence and adjustment. *Social Science and Medicine*, **43**(2), 163–171.

Singer, P. A., Thiel, E. C., Naylor, C. D. *et al.* (1995) Life-sustaining treatment preferences of hemodialysis patients: implications for advance directives. *Journal of the American Society of Nephrology*, **6**(5), 410–417.

Stapleton, S. (1992) Etiologies and indicators of powerlessness in persons with end-stage renal disease, in *Coping with Chronic Illness: Overcoming Powerlessness*, (ed. J. J. Miller), F. A. Davis, Philadelphia, PA.

Trnobranski, P. H. (1996) The decision to prolong life: ethical perspectives of a clinical dilemma. *Journal of Clinical Nursing*, **5**(4), 233–240.

Valderrábano, F., Berthoux, F. C., Jones, E. H. P. and Mehls, O. (1996) Report on management of renal failure in Europe, XXV, 1994. End stage renal disease and dialysis report. *Nephrology Dialysis Transplantation*, **11**(Suppl. 1), 2–21.

Webb, C. (1996) Caring, curing, coping: towards an integrated model. *Journal of Advanced Nursing*, **23**(5), 960–968.

Willard, C. (1996) The nurse's role as patient advocate: obligation or imposition? *Journal of Advanced Nursing*, **24**(1), 60–66.

2 Renal physiology

Paul Challinor

LEARNING OBJECTIVES

At the end of this chapter the reader should be able to:

- Describe the process by which urine is formed.
- List the functions of the kidneys.
- Describe the implications of end-stage renal failure on body function, relating these to symptomology associated with renal failure.
- Describe the effects of diuretics on the kidneys.
- Identify other drugs that affect the renal system and know their modes of action.

INTRODUCTION

Renal physiology presents a daunting image to a number of nurses. The complexity of the physiological systems involved in renal homoeostasis unfortunately prevents many renal nurses from fully exploring the issues that, if understood, could explain many of the symptoms patients present with. In order to give full care, and explain that care to patients and relatives, it is important that the fundamentals of renal physiology are understood. This chapter will attempt to explain relatively easily the way in which urine is formed and how some drugs affect the renal system, and show that renal failure is in truth a systemic disease, explaining the myriad of symptoms experienced by patients. This should enhance the nurse's knowledge and aid in planning appropriate care to improve patients' quality of life.

ANATOMY

The kidney is classically described as being a similar shape to a lima bean. In the adult it measures approximately 10–12 cm in length, and 5–7 cm in width. It is covered by three layers. The renal fascia is a fibrous connective tissue that anchors the kidney to surrounding structures. Within this is a mass of fatty tissue called the adipose capsule that acts as a protective layer. The renal capsule, the innermost layer, protects the kidney from trauma and infection.

When viewed in cross-section (Figure 2.1) distinct areas within the kidney can be identified: the outer cortex, the inner medulla and the renal pelvis. The medulla can be further divided into a number of triangular regions called renal (medullary) pyramids. These areas are formed by straight tubules and blood vessels. The renal pelvis contains extensions called major and minor calyces. Each minor calyx (of which there are between eight and 18) collects urine from the collecting tubules in the pyramids. The major calyces (two or three in number) drain the urine into the renal pelvis and from there into the ureter.

The functional unit of the kidney is the nephron. Each kidney contains about 1–2 million nephrons. The nephron can also be subdivided into distinct sections (Figure 2.2), each of which has distinct functions (these will be discussed later in this chapter). The Bowman's capsule consists of a cup-like structure that surrounds the glomerulus, a network of capillaries. Together these two structures constitute the renal corpuscle, which acts to filter out large cells, creating the urinary filtrate, which then enters the

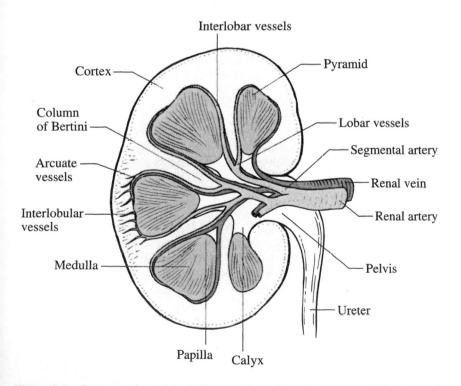

Figure 2.1 Cross-section of the kidney to show the main areas and blood vessels. The upper part of the pelvis is cut open to show the insides of the calyces. (Source: redrawn from Hubbard and Mechan, 1997, with permission.)

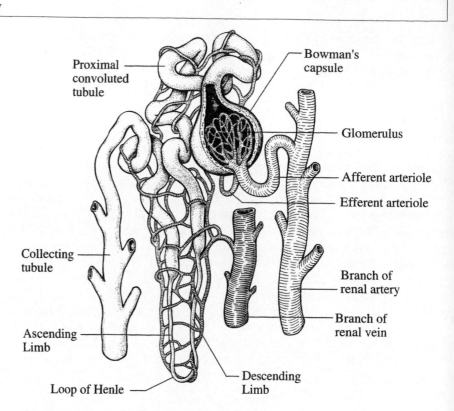

Proximal convoluted tubule

Bowman's capsule

Glomerulus

Afferent arteriole

Efferent arteriole

Collecting tubule

Branch of renal artery

Branch of renal vein

Ascending Limb

Loop of Henle

Descending Limb

Figure 2.2 Diagrammatic structure of the nephron, illustrating the peritubular capillary network. (Source: adapted from Bunker Rosdahl, 1995)

proximal tubule. The proximal convoluted tubule, like the renal corpuscle, lies in the cortex of the kidney. The cells of the proximal tubule actively reabsorb solutes, nutrients, electrolytes and proteins as the filtrate flows along its length. Many, though not all, nephrons have a long loop into the medullary area of the kidney. This section is known as the loop of Henle. Its main function is to facilitate the reabsorption of water and thus to concentrate the urine before it enters the distal convoluted tubule. The distal tubule is again situated in the cortex. It too has an important part to play in reabsorbing solutes, but substances are also secreted into the filtrate in this section. The filtrate then drains into the collecting tubules, which in turn are drained by collecting ducts, before entering the calyces.

Renal blood supply is delivered by the renal artery (Figure 2.3), which divides immediately into two main branches that further subsequently subdivide into lobar arteries and then interlobar arteries. The interlobar arteries become the arcuate arteries at the cortex–medulla junction. Small interlobar arteries then give off numerous afferent arterioles leading to the capillaries (glomeruli) entering the Bowman's capsule. The capillary network leaving the glomerulus *via* the efferent arterioles is unusual because it gives rise initially to a second set of arterioles, which supply the peritubular capillaries. Blood then flows into stellate veins, and then into interlobular

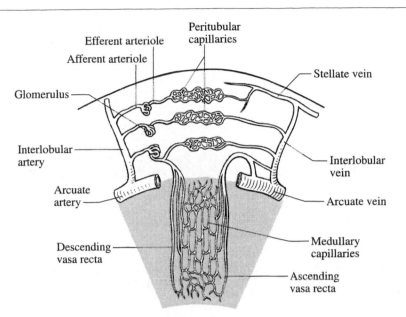

Afferent arteriole
Efferent arteriole
Peritubular capillaries
Glomerulus
Stellate vein
Interlobular artery
Interlobular vein
Arcuate artery
Arcuate vein
Descending vasa recta
Medullary capillaries
Ascending vasa recta

Figure 2.3 Blood supply within the kidney from the arcuate artery through to the arcuate vein, illustrating the intermediate blood circulation. (Source: redrawn from Hubbard and Mechan, 1997, with permission.)

veins. Not all blood passes through this system: most blood flows directly into the interlobular veins, then drains into the arcuate veins before entering the interlobar veins and leaving the kidney *via* the renal vein.

GLOMERULAR FILTRATION

Glomerular filtration rate

The volume of fluid filtered by the kidneys per unit of time is known as the glomerular filtration rate (GFR). The glomerular capillaries are more permeable to fluid than other capillaries; so much so that a net filtration pressure of 10 mmHg causes massive filtration. In a 70 kg person, the average amount filtered by the kidneys is 180 l/d (litres per day). This huge amount contrasts with only 4 l/d passing through all the other capillaries in the body.

In order for the kidneys to form such a large volume of filtrate, they must receive a large share of the cardiac output – about 20–25%. This means that the entire plasma volume is filtered about 60 times a day.

Composition of the filtrate

The fluid within the Bowman's capsule is essentially protein-free but contains all the other substances present in the plasma in virtually the same concentrations. The only exceptions to this are certain low-molecular-weight substances that are bound to plasma proteins and therefore cannot be filtered. Half the calcium and virtually all the fatty acids in the plasma are bound to plasma proteins. In reality, there is a very small amount of protein in the filtrate, as the glomerular membranes are not perfect sieves for protein. Normally this protein is completely removed by the tubules so that virtually no protein appears in the urine. However, in diseased kidneys, the glomerular membranes may become damaged and therefore become more permeable to protein, and/or the tubules may lose their ability to reabsorb protein from the filtrate. In either case protein will appear in the urine.

Forces involved in filtration

Glomerular filtration takes place by 'bulk flow'. The amount of filtrate is determined by opposing forces (Figure 2.4): hydrostatic forces favour filtration while osmotic forces created by the plasma proteins oppose filtration.

The pressure of the blood in the glomerular capillaries averages 55 mmHg, higher than in other capillaries of the body, because the afferent arterioles have relatively large diameters and offer less resistance to blood flow than most arterioles. This results in more of the arterial pressure being transmitted to the capillaries. The subsequent increase in hydrostatic pressure favours filtration across the membranes into the Bowman's capsule.

The fluid in the Bowman's capsule exerts a hydrostatic pressure of 15 mmHg, and this opposes pressure in the capsule. The presence of protein in the glomerular capillary plasma creates a second opposing force. This unequal distribution of protein favours an osmotic flow of fluid from the capsule into the capillary, equivalent to a pressure difference of 30 mmHg.

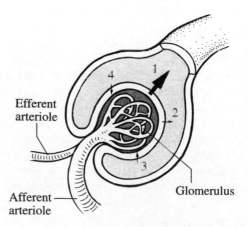

Efferent arteriole

Afferent arteriole

Glomerulus

Figure 2.4 Forces acting across the glomerular membrane. 1 = glomerular blood pressure (hydrostatic); 2 = net filtration pressure; 3 = capsular hydrostatic pressure; 4 = osmotic pressure created by the blood.

The net glomerular filtration pressure is approximately 10 mmHg. This pressure initiates urine formation by forcing an essentially protein-free filtrate of plasma through the glomerular membranes into the capsule. The glomerular membranes serve only as a filtration barrier and have no active (i.e. energy-requiring) function.

TUBULAR REABSORPTION

Many filterable plasma components are either absent from the urine or present in smaller amounts than when initially filtered in the glomerulus. This gives an idea of the magnitude and importance of the reabsorptive mechanisms. Table 2.1 shows the values for a normal person on an average diet.

Reabsorption of waste products is relatively incomplete. For example, only 44% of the urea filtered is actually reabsorbed, so large amounts are excreted in the urine. Reabsorption of most useful plasma components, such as water, inorganic ions and organic nutrients, is relatively complete, so that the amounts excreted in the urine are very small fractions of the total filtered load.

The reabsorption rates of many, but not all, organic nutrients such as glucose are always very high, and are not physiologically regulated. As such, the filtered loads of these nutrients are normally completely reabsorbed, with none appearing in the urine. The kidneys merely maintain whatever plasma concentrations already exist, which are generally the result of hormonal regulation of nutrient metabolism. In contrast, the reabsorptive rates for water and many inorganic ions, although also very high, are under physiological regulation.

Two-thirds of the filtered load of sodium is reabsorbed by active transport; in association with this two-thirds of the water is also reabsorbed. Sodium diffuses into the luminal wall, along with chloride and also in co-transport with glucose and amino-acids or in exchange with hydrogen ions.

The next short section briefly covers some of the substances dealt with by the kidneys.

- **Glucose** is freely filtered by the glomerulus and is completely reabsorbed, so its clearance = 0. If the concentration of plasma glucose rises, the transport mechanism in some tubules may become saturated, and glucose may appear in the urine. When the transport mechanisms in all tubules are saturated the transport maximum (Tm) is said to be reached.

Table 2.1 Comparative values for filtration and reabsorption

Substance	Amount filtered per day	Amount excreted per day	% reabsorbed
Water (litres)	180	1.8	99
Sodium (g)	630	3.2	99.5
Glucose (g)	180	0	100
Urea (g)	54	30	44

In man, with a glomerular filtration rate of 125 ml/min, the threshold plasma concentration required for glucose to appear is 10–20 mmol/l. The Tm for glucose is 15–20 mmol/l. A total of 98% of the filtered glucose is reabsorbed in the first part of the proximal tubule and is co-transported with sodium.

- **Amino acids** are completely reabsorbed: the plasma threshold is so high that the Tm is never reached. There are different transport mechanisms for different amino acids, but amino-aciduria can generally result from defects in these mechanisms. The most common type is genetically inherited cystinuria. Cystine has a low solubility in water, resulting in renal stones at an early age.
- **Urea** is fat-soluble, so it crosses cell membranes easily. It is freely filtered, but up to 40% is reabsorbed in the proximal tubule by diffusion down the concentration gradient caused by water reabsorption. Also, 95% of the filtered inorganic phosphate is reabsorbed in the proximal tubule.
- Many **drugs and environmental pollutants** are fat-soluble, making renal excretion difficult. The liver transforms them, usually by conjugation, into a water-soluble form, thereby aiding excretion.

Tubular reabsorption is a process fundamentally different from glomerular filtration. The latter occurs by bulk flow, with water and all low-molecular-weight solutes moving together. In contrast, in the tubules there is relatively little bulk flow; rather, reabsorption of some substances is by diffusion while that of others requires more or less specific mediated transport.

Reabsorption by diffusion

Many substances are also reabsorbed passively by diffusion. Urea reabsorption provides an example of this process. Initially, the urea concentration within the Bowman's capsule is the same as that in the plasma but, as the filtrate flows through the proximal tubule, water is reabsorbed, increasing the urea concentration within the tubule. As the tubular urea concentration increases in comparison with that in the interstitial fluid surrounding the tubule, urea diffuses down the concentration gradient created, into the interstitial fluid and then into the peritubular capillaries.

Reabsorption by diffusion is also important for many foreign chemicals. Many drugs and environmental pollutants are also reabsorbed by diffusion because, like urea, they are fat-soluble, which makes their excretion *via* the urine difficult.

TUBULAR SECRETION

Substances move from the peritubular capillaries into the tubular lumen by secretion. Hydrogen ions (H^+) and potassium (K^+) are among the most important substances that fall within this category. The kidney is also able to secrete a large number of inorganic ions, some of which are normally occurring metabolites such as chlorine and creatinine, while others are foreign chemicals such as penicillin. These substances move from the peritubular capillaries into the interstitial fluid around the tubular epithelial cells. They are then actively transported into the tubule.

RENAL SODIUM CONTROL

In the individual with normally functioning kidneys, urinary sodium excretion is reflexly increased when there is a sodium excess in the body and reflexly decreased when there is a sodium deficit. Both the amount filtered and the amount reabsorbed can be altered by reflexes initiated by various cardiovascular system (CVS) baroreceptors. These receptors respond to pressures within the CVS, which reflect changes in total body plasma volume and interstitial fluid volume. Low Na^+ levels cause low cardiovascular pressures, which, by means of baroreceptors, initiate reflexes that restore the cardiovascular pressures *via* direct actions on the CVS, and simultaneously lower GFR and increase Na^+ reabsorption. Increases in body Na^+ have the opposite effect.

Control of GFR

A reduced body Na^+ level elicits a decrease in GFR through a reduced glomerular capillary pressure. This occurs both as a direct consequence of a lowered arterial pressure in the kidneys and as a result of baroreceptor reflexes acting on the afferent arterioles, resulting in vasoconstriction.

Control of Na^+ reabsorption: aldosterone and the renin–angiotensin system

The major controller of Na^+ reabsorption is the adrenal cortical hormone aldosterone, which stimulates Na^+ reabsorption in the late distal tubules and the collecting duct. Aldosterone secretion is controlled by the renin–angiotensin system. Renin, the rate-limiting factor in the renin–angiotensin system, is secreted by the granular cells of the juxtaglomerular apparatus. When extracellular fluid volume decreases, renin secretion is stimulated by three inputs:

- stimulation of the renal sympathetic nerves to the granular cells by baroreceptor reflexes;
- pressure decreases sensed by the granular cells themselves;
- a signal generated by low sodium or chloride concentration in the lumen of the macula densa.

When renin is released into the bloodstream it catalyses with angiotensinogen to form angiotensin I (Figure 2.5). This is then converted to angiotensin II by angiotensin-converting enzyme (ACE), which is found in the capillary endothelial cells of the lung. Angiotensin II is a potent stimulator of aldosterone secretion. Captopril, an ACE inhibitor, works by obstructing the conversion of angiotensin I, preventing vasoconstriction.

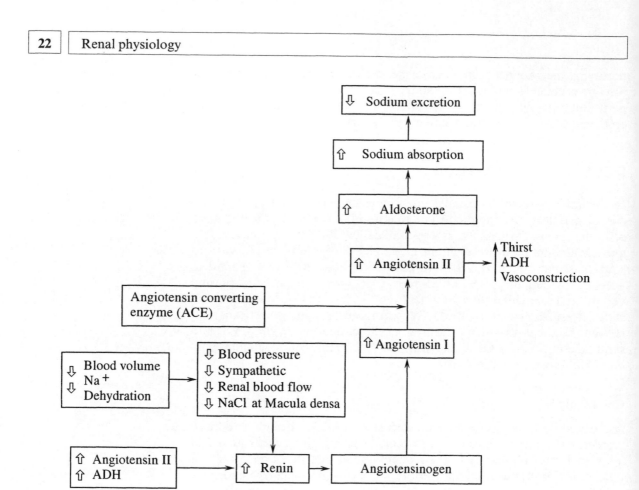

Figure 2.5 Sodium control *via* the renin–angiotensin system, identifying the link with renal water control *via* antidiuretic hormone (ADH).

Aldosterone acts by inducing an increase in the activity of the Na^+ pumps of the renal tubules, but also stimulates Na^+ transport from the intestine. In this manner less Na^+ is lost in faeces.

Atrial natriuretic factor

Atrial natriuretic factor (ANF) is synthesized and secreted by cells in the cardiac atria. It acts on the kidneys, inhibiting Na^+ reabsorption. It also inhibits secretion of both renin and aldosterone. The secretion of ANF is increased when there is an excess of Na^+ in the body, the stimulus being an increase in atrial distension.

RENAL WATER REGULATION

The baroreceptor-initiated GFR-controlling reflexes tend to have the same effect on water as on Na^+. The major determinant of water excretion is antidiuretic hormone (ADH), so water is regulated mainly by reflexes that alter the secretion of this hormone.

Baroreceptor control of ADH

A decreased extracellular fluid volume triggers an increase in ADH secretion. This increases the water permeability of the late distal tubules and collecting ducts, so more water is reabsorbed and less excreted. This reflex is mediated by several groups of baroreceptors, particularly those in the left atrium. When the atrial blood pressure increases, the baroreceptors increase firing impulses, resulting in a decrease in ADH secretion (Figure 2.6).

Osmoreceptor control of ADH

Osmoreceptors responsive to changes in osmolarity are located in the hypothalamus. If a person drinks 2 litres of fluid, the excess fluid lowers the body osmolarity, which inhibits the secretion of ADH *via* the hypothalamus osmoreceptors. As a result, water permeability of the distal tubules and the collecting ducts becomes very low and a large amount of dilute urine is excreted (Figure 2.6).

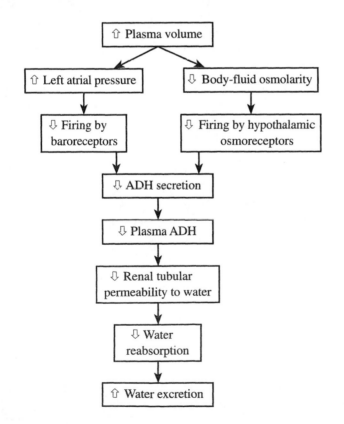

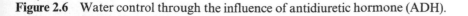

Figure 2.6 Water control through the influence of antidiuretic hormone (ADH).

Urine concentration

The ability of the kidney to produce a concentrated urine is a major determinant of the body's ability to survive without water. There are three mechanisms involved in this process:

- countercurrent multiplication (loop of Henle);
- countercurrent exchange (vasa recta);
- osmotic exchange (distal and collecting duct).

Countercurrent multiplication

To understand these processes, refer to Figure 2.7, which shows the hairpin bend of the loop of Henle bringing the descending limb in close apposition with the ascending arm. The tubular fluid is flowing in opposite directions (countercurrent flow) in the two arms.

There are variations in the permeability to water and ion in different parts of the loop. These are listed below:

- thin descending limb – permeable to water, but relatively impermeable to Na^+ and Cl^-;
- thin ascending limb – impermeable to water, but permeable to Na^+, Cl^- and urea;
- thick ascending limb and first part of the distal tubule – impermeable to water, and actively pumps Na^+ and Cl^- into the interstitium.

Normally the concentration of glomerular filtrate entering the proximal tubule is approximately 300 mosmol/l body water – at this concentration

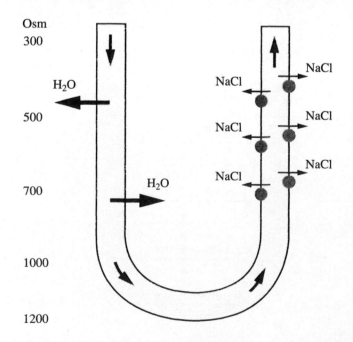

Figure 2.7 The loop of Henle and the concept of countercurrent multiplication, showing the relative osmolality of the extratubular tissue.

glomerular filtrate is isotonic with body fluids. A milliosmole represents the concentration of substances in the filtrate – mainly NaCl. The above diagram shows that the concentration of the interstitial fluid increases from 300 mosmol/l in the cortex to about 1200 mosmol/l in the medulla. To understand these changes, the most convenient point to start is in the thick ascending limb. Here Na^+ and Cl^- are actively pumped from the filtrate into the interstitial fluid – this limb is impermeable to water.

The thin descending limb is permeable to water, but relatively impermeable to Na^+ and Cl^-. Water moves passively out of the descending limb into the more concentrated interstitium created by the ascending limb, until the osmolarities at any point are equal. Fluid is progressively concentrated as it flows down the ascending limb until it reaches a maximum concentration of around 1200 mosmol/l at the tip of the loop (hypertonic in respect to body fluid).

Fluid moving into the thin ascending limb is more concentrated than the fluid in the interstitium. This limb is impermeable to water but permeable to NaCl and urea. NaCl moves passively from the concentrated lumen into the interstitium, leaving water behind. On moving into the thick ascending limb, NaCl is once more actively pumped out, leaving water behind. The fluid entering the distal and collecting duct is consequently hypotonic (100 mosmol/l) with respect to body fluids (300 mosmol/l).

Countercurrent exchange

The high concentration of sodium chloride in the interstitium is also the result of the countercurrent flow of blood in the vasa recta (Figure 2.8). As

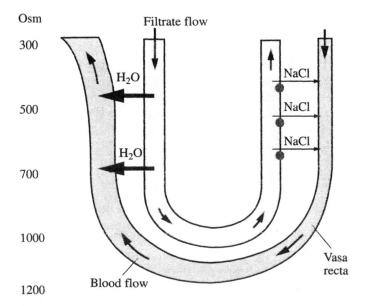

Figure 2.8 The loop of Henle and the vasa recta, illustrating the concept of countercurrent exchange and showing the relative osmolality of the extratubular

Table 2.2 Drugs and their effects on the kidney

Groups	Drugs	Action
Osmotically active substances	Mannitol, glucose	Diuresis produced by osmosis
Xanthines	Caffeine, theophylline	Diuresis possibly induced by decreasing Na^+ reabsorption and increasing GFR
Diuretic	Metalazone	Inhibits Cl^- reabsorption in loop of Henle and distal tubule, increasing osmotic effect
Diuretic	Frusemide	Inhibits Cl^- reabsorption in the loop of Henle
Diuretic	Spironolactone, amiloride	Inhibits action of aldosterone, thereby affecting Na^+/K^+ exchange in distal tubule (spironolactone) or preventing K^+ secretion (amiloride)

blood flows down through the descending arm of the blood vessel, Na^+ and Cl^- ions diffuse passively (from high to low concentrations) into it from the interstitium of the medulla. The concentration of the blood may reach 1200 mosmol/l at the tip of the vessel. As blood flows back towards the cortex, almost all the NaCl picked up on the way diffuses passively back into the interstitium of the medulla. Blood leaving the vasa recta is only slightly more concentrated than it was when it entered the medulla. Thus the countercurrent flow through the vasa recta permits most of the NaCl to remain in the interstitial fluid of the medulla.

Osmotic exchange

Fluid delivered to the distal tubule is hypotonic (100 mosmol/l) with respect to the body fluids. The permeability of the remaining part of the nephron, the distal tubule and collecting ducts is under the influence of ADH. In the absence of ADH this region of the nephron is impermeable to water and therefore no water is reabsorbed from the filtrate. The hypotonic fluid empties into the papillary ducts, calyces and renal pelvis, and from there into the bladder. The urine is therefore very dilute and, in the absence of ADH, may only be a quarter as concentrated as the plasma and the glomerular filtrate.

In the presence of ADH, the epithelial cells of the distal tubule and collecting duct become permeable to water. As the hypertonic filtrate from the ascending limb of the loop of Henle passes through, water is reabsorbed by osmosis. In the distal tubule the loss of water increases the filtrate concentration from 100–300 mosmol/l. As this isotonic fluid passes down into the medulla region through the collecting duct, it is exposed to the hypertonic interstitial fluid. As a result, large amounts of water can be reabsorbed by osmosis into the interstitium from the collecting duct. With maximum ADH secretion, the concentration of fluid in the collecting duct approaches 1200 mosmol/l. The fluid entering the bladder may be four times more concentrated than the plasma and the original glomerular filtrate.

Urea also contributes to the hypertonicity of the medullary interstitium. In the presence of ADH, urea diffuses passively out of the collecting duct into the interstitium and back into the ascending limb, where it recirculates back to the convoluted tubule.

A summary of drugs and their effects on the kidney is given in Table 2.2.

RENAL POTASSIUM CONTROL

Potassium is the most abundant intracellular ion, with only 2% of the total body potassium (K^+) in the extracellular fluid. Correct concentration of potassium in extracellular fluid is critical for the correct function of excitable tissues, notably nerve and muscle. Total body potassium balance is maintained in the normal person by daily excreting an amount of K^+ in the urine equal to the amounts ingested, minus the amounts eliminated in the faeces and sweat. Potassium losses *via* sweat and the GI tract are normally quite small, although large quantities can be lost through vomiting and diarrhoea. The control of renal function is the major mechanism by which body potassium is regulated.

Renal regulation of potassium

Potassium, like all electrolytes, is freely filtered at the glomerulus, but only a small amount of the filtered load is excreted. However, under certain conditions the amount excreted can be greater than the amount filtered, indicating that potassium can also be secreted by the tubules. Most of the potassium is reabsorbed regardless of the changes in the body potassium levels – potassium reabsorption does not seem to be controlled. Changes in excretion seem to depend upon the amount secreted in the late distal tubules and the collecting ducts.

Potassium secretion is linked to the active transport mechanisms, by Na^+ pumps, across the basolateral membrane into the tubular epithelial cells. In the late distal tubules and collecting ducts, there are potassium channels in the cell walls and therefore much of the potassium diffuses down its concentration gradient into the lumen to complete the secretory process. There are no potassium channels in the proximal tubule, so the potassium pumped into the epithelial cells just diffuses back out into the interstitial fluid.

Potassium excretion is controlled by aldosterone (Figure 2.9), which, by stimulating sodium reabsorption, increases potassium secretion. The potassium control of aldosterone production is different from the reflexes initiated by changes in extracellular volume. The aldosterone-secreting cells of the adrenal cortex are sensitive to the potassium concentration of

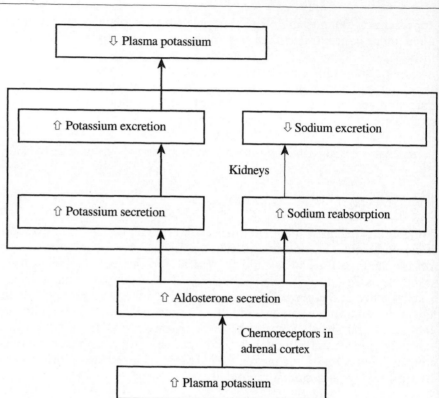

Figure 2.9 The effect of aldosterone on the urinary excretion of potassium and sodium.

the extracellular fluid bathing them. An increase in this concentration leads to an increase in the secretion of aldosterone; this leads to an increase in potassium secretion and sodium reabsorption, thereby excreting excess potassium from the body. Conversely, a low potassium level decreases aldosterone production, in turn reducing potassium secretion. Less potassium than usual is excreted in the urine, helping to restore the normal extracellular concentration.

The fact that aldosterone regulates excretion of both sodium and potassium can cause conflict. If a person is sodium deficient and therefore excreting large amounts of aldosterone, the potassium-secreting effects of this hormone tend to cause some potassium loss, even though the potassium balance was normal to start with. Normally such conflicts may cause only minor imbalances, because there are a variety of other counterbalancing controls of sodium and potassium excretion.

RENAL CALCIUM REGULATION

Extracellular calcium (Ca^{2+}) concentration must be kept relatively constant because of the effects of Ca^{2+} on neuromuscular excitability. A low Ca^{2+} increases the excitability of nerve and muscle, resulting in tetany.

Hypercalcaemia can also be life-threatening, causing cardiac arrhythmias and depressing neuromuscular excitability.

Approximately 99% of the total body Ca^{2+} is contained in bone, laid down as calcium phosphate. Bone is not a fixed unchanging tissue but is constantly being remodelled, and can either withdraw Ca^{2+} from extracellular fluid or deposit it there depending upon physiological needs. Under normal conditions a considerable amount of Ca^{2+} is not absorbed from the intestine and simply leaves with the faeces. Ca^{2+} is absorbed by active transport, and as such the amount absorbed can be increased or decreased in large amounts.

The direct role of the kidneys in Ca^{2+} homoeostasis is through filtration and reabsorption (Figure 2.10), but they also have an indirect, but very important, role in absorbing Ca^{2+} from the gut, and through their handling of phosphate the kidneys also control the extracellular fluid concentration of Ca^{2+}. The main hormonal control of Ca^{2+}, however, is through the release of parathormone.

Parathormone, either directly or indirectly, affects the bone, gastrointestinal tract or kidneys in respect to Ca^{2+} handling. The release of parathormone (produced by the parathyroid glands) is directly subject to the concentration of plasma Ca^{2+}. A decrease in Ca^{2+} stimulates parathormone production, and *vice versa*. Parathormone has at least four effects that influence Ca^{2+} homoeostasis (Figure 2.10).

- It increases the movement of Ca^{2+} from bone into extracellular fluid, making available this large store of calcium for the regulation of extracellular Ca^{2+} concentration.

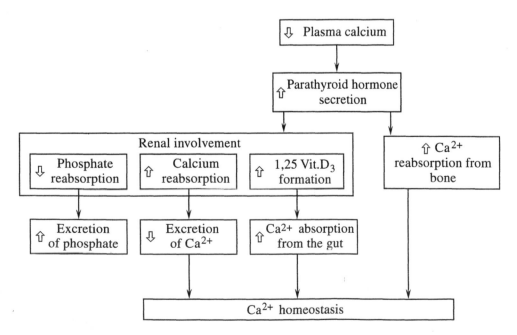

Figure 2.10 Calcium homoeostasis.

- It stimulates the activation of vitamin D, which increases intestinal absorption of calcium.
- It increases renal tubular Ca^{2+} reabsorption, thus decreasing urinary Ca^{2+} excretion.
- It reduces tubular reabsorption of phosphate, lowering its extracellular concentration.

The first three all tend to increase Ca^{2+} concentration, compensating for the decreased levels that originally stimulated parathormone production. Parathormone causes both calcium and phosphate to be released from the bone. If extracellular phosphate concentration were to increase as a result, further movement of Ca^{2+} from the bone would be retarded because a high phosphate level causes Ca^{2+} and phosphate to be deposited in bone and other tissues.

Vitamin D

Vitamin D_3 is formed by the action of ultraviolet radiation on a substance (7-dehydrocholesterol) found in the skin. A second form of vitamin D can be absorbed from the gut. Vitamin D_3 is first metabolized by the liver and then by the kidney to form 1,25 dihydroxyvitamin D_3. This is the active form of vitamin D_3. Because it is made in the body, it is really a hormone, not a vitamin.

The major action of vitamin D_3 is to stimulate the intestine to actively absorb calcium from the gut. A deficiency of vitamin D_3 reduces calcium absorption and lowers extracellular calcium concentration. In children, this causes rickets, and in chronic renal failure, renal bone disease. Vitamin D_3 metabolism is physiologically controlled by the action of parathormone of the kidneys.

RENAL INVOLVEMENT IN ERYTHROPOIESIS

Control of erythropoiesis

In health the rate of production of red blood cells (RBCs) equals the rate of destruction; this is controlled by erythropoietin (EPO) and stimulated by hypoxia. EPO increases mitosis in the committed cells. Approximately 10–15% of the circulating EPO can be produced by the liver and as such may be the source in anephric patients. The underlying cause of anaemia associated with chronic renal failure is EPO deficiency. EPO is present in the blood and urine in other anaemias, and its production can be suppressed by overtransfusion.

Other hormones that can have an effect on erythropoiesis include corticosteroids, androgens (e.g. testosterone), growth hormone and thyroxine. They may act by increasing the sensitivity of the RBC precursor to EPO.

Factors required for normal erythropoiesis

Very little is known about factors associated with the very early stages, from the stem cell to the proerythroblast. But if arrested development occurs this leads to the aplastic anaemias caused by irradiation and drugs. The cells are normocytic. Many of the contributing factors are important parts of the diet, and as diet is an integral part of renal care they are outlined below.

Folic acid

This vitamin is found in large amounts in leafy plants, yeast and liver. It is absorbed from the duodenum and jejunum. Folic acid stores can be exhausted after 2–3 months. It is involved in the synthesis of DNA and hence is necessary for cell division. When this vitamin is not present in adequate amounts, impairment of cell division occurs throughout the body, but is most striking in rapidly proliferating cells, including erythrocyte precursors. Thus fewer RBCs are produced when folic acid is absent.

Vitamin B$_{12}$

Production of normal RBCs also requires extremely small amounts (1 millionth of a gram per day) of vitamin B$_{12}$. Its action is closely linked to that of folic acid. Vitamin B$_{12}$ is not synthesized in the body, so its supply depends upon dietary intake. It is found only in animal products and strictly vegetarian diets may be deficient in it. Unlike folic acid, vitamin B$_{12}$ is also required for myelin formation, so a variety of neurological symptoms may also occur in vitamin B$_{12}$ deficiency.

Vitamin B$_{12}$ is a large molecule, and as such it requires an intrinsic factor to bind with in order to be absorbed. The intrinsic factor is produced by the parietal cells in the stomach. Once vitamin B$_{12}$ is taken into the mucosa of the ileum, it is absorbed and the intrinsic factor is destroyed. Being a protein the intrinsic factor has to be destroyed before it enters the bloodstream, otherwise antibodies could be produced against it.

The body store of vitamin B$_{12}$ in the liver will last 2–3 years without dietary intake. Deficiency is almost always due to impaired absorption, e.g. lack of intrinsic factor following gastrectomy, following ileal resection or through competition for vitamin B$_{12}$ from intestinal parasites.

Iron

Iron is the element to which oxygen binds. Small amounts of iron are lost every day *via* urine, faeces, sweat and cells sloughing off from the skin. In addition, women also lose a similar amount in menstrual blood. In order to remain in balance, the amount lost must be replaced by ingesting iron-containing foods such as meat, shellfish, beans, nuts and cereals.

The homoeostatic control of iron balance resides primarily in the intestinal epithelium, which actively absorbs iron from ingested foods. Only a small fraction of what is eaten is absorbed, but this fraction is increased or decreased according to need. These fluctuations are mediated by changes in the iron content of the intestinal epithelium: the more iron in the body, the more there is in the intestinal epithelium and the less new iron will be absorbed.

A buffer against iron deficiency is the body's considerable iron stores, mainly in the liver, bound up in a protein called ferritin. As old RBCs are destroyed in the spleen, their iron is released into the plasma and bound to the iron transport protein called transferritin. Almost all this iron is delivered to the bone marrow to be used again.

Iron-deficiency anaemia produces microcytic, hypochromic RBCs. It can be caused by increased physiological demand during, for instance, pregnancy or rapid periods of growth, by inadequate absorption as a result of gastrectomy or malabsorption syndrome, by inadequate intake or by chronic blood loss.

RENAL REGULATION OF pH

Body pH regulation

H^+ ions are constantly being produced as a result of metabolism and constantly being eliminated *via* the lungs and kidneys. The rate of H^+ production is not constant. We take in different amounts of acid in food and increase the acid production through exercise. Drugs, hormones and disease also influence H^+ production.

H^+ concentration can influence the concentrations of other plasma ions. If the H^+ concentration increases, some will displace K^+. This can lead to hyperkalaemia. If H^+ concentration is reduced, some of the free Ca^{2+} in the plasma will bind to the negatively charged protein, reducing free Ca^{2+}, which can lead to tetany.

The blood buffers

Plasma proteins and haemoglobin act as important buffering agents, binding or releasing H^+ as the pH falls or rises. Another important buffer in the plasma is bicarbonate (HCO_3^-). The addition of H^+ to HCO_3^- forms carbonic acid. Carbonic acid, unlike other acids, can be broken down by an enzyme, carbonic anhydrase, to CO_2 and H_2O. The CO_2 can then be excreted *via* the lungs. The concentration of HCO_3^- is slightly higher in venous blood than arterial blood, because of the addition of CO_2 from the tissues. If H^+ ions are added to the blood, the HCO_3^- concentration will drop, and more CO_2 and H_2O will then be produced.

The respiratory system

The respiratory centre is responsive to H^+ and CO_2 concentrations. Increases in H^+ and CO_2 lead to increased respiratory activity and the removal of CO_2. If there is an increased H^+ concentration there will be an increased respiratory rate and the reaction series will go in the direction of CO_2 and H_2O formation. The excess CO_2 will then be exhaled.

$$H^+ + HCO_3^- \rightarrow H_2CO_3 \rightarrow CO_2 + H_2O.$$

Renal control

The kidneys play an important role in H^+ regulation. They are able to secrete H^+ and they either decrease or increase their reabsorption of HCO_3^-. Renal regulation is not as rapid as respiratory control, but it is important in long-term control.

Both H^+ secretion and HCO_3^- reabsorption are controlled homeostatically so as to compensate for changes in body fluid pH. If the pH falls, because of increased H^+ production, the kidneys will excrete the additional H^+ and reabsorb more HCO_3^-. In contrast, if the pH rises, because of persistent vomiting, the kidneys excrete little H^+ and simultaneously reduce HCO_3^- reabsorption.

H+ secretion and HCO_3^- reabsorption are both achieved through a single mechanism – tubular secretion of H^+ (Figure 2.11). Virtually all the

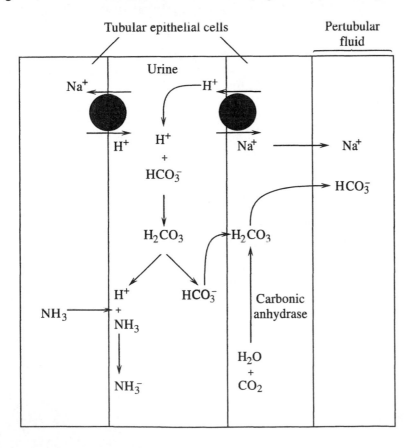

Figure 2.11 Tubular pH regulation.

H^+ excreted in the urine enters the tubule by secretion, which occurs in most nephron segments. The H^+ to be secreted is generated inside the tubular cells rather than in the blood. In the cells CO_2 and H_2O combine and are then catalysed by carbonic anhydrase. The resulting H^+ is actively transported into the lumen, while the resulting HCO_3^- enters the blood *via* the peritubular fluid. The net result is the same as if the secreted H^+ had come from the blood.

Once in the lumen, the H^+ to be excreted combines with one of several buffers and is then excreted. One of the major buffers is ammonia (NH_3). The ammonia is formed in the tubular cells by the deamination of certain amino acids supplied by the blood. From the cells the ammonia diffuses into the lumen, where it combines with H^+ to form NH_4^+. Other buffers are filtered phosphate or bicarbonate.

An important feature of this system is that an increased extracellular H^+ concentration lasting more than 1–2 days stimulates the rate of tubular cell ammonia production. This extra ammonia provides the additional luminal buffer required for combination with and excretion of the larger number of secreted H^+ ions.

CONCLUSION

When renal failure occurs it leads to systemic symptoms. These can be devastating, impairing the quality of life of those who suffer from chronic renal failure. The symptoms associated with acute renal failure are no less serious, and often lead to life-threatening situations. Renal physiology is complex, but an understanding of it underpins an understanding of the nursing care required for these patients.

REVIEW QUESTIONS

- Describe the mode of action of common diuretics and relate these to patient care.
- Describe the symptoms associated with renal bone disease, with reference to renal physiology.
- Describe why a patient in renal failure may be acidotic.
- Describe why glucose appears in the urine in diabetic patients, with reference to transport maximum systems.
- Describe the role that the renin–angiotensin system plays in controlling blood pressure.

REFERENCES

Bunker Rosdahl, C. (ed.) (1995) *Textbook of Basic Nursing*, 6th edn, J. B. Lippincott, Philadelphia, PA.

Hubbard, J. and Mechan, D. (1997) *The Physiology of Health and Illness: With Related Anatomy*, Stanley Thornes, Cheltenham.

FURTHER READING

Ganog, W. F. (1983) *Review of Medical Physiology*, 11th edn, Lange, Norwalk, CT.

Tortora, G. J. and Anagnostakis, N. P. (1990) *Principles of Anatomy and Physiology*, 6th edn, Harper Collins, New York.

Vander, A. J., Sherman, J. H. and Luciano, D. S. (1990) *Human Physiology*, 5th edn, McGraw–Hill, New York.

3 Psychological issues in renal failure

John Sedgewick

LEARNING OBJECTIVES

At the end of this chapter the reader should be able to:

- Discuss the process of psychological adaptation to renal replacement therapy.
- Identify the difficulties facing the health-care team in assisting patients and families to adjust to renal replacement therapy.
- Describe the importance of rehabilitation as it relates to individuals undergoing renal replacement therapy.
- Examine the phenomenon of loss, hope, powerlessness and risk-taking in chronic illness, specifically in relation to renal replacement therapy.
- Discuss the concept of stress in chronic illness and how this manifests itself in patients undergoing renal replacement.

INTRODUCTION

Health-care staff are increasingly faced with assisting patients and families to adjust to the demands imposed by end-stage renal disease. ESRD imposes major life changes upon patients and families, who are required to cope with a new way of living. Patients and their carers can testify to the overwhelming and devastating impact of ESRD physiologically, psychologically and socially. Patients face multiple threats to their existence while attempting to adapt to the demands of dialysis; this process of adjustment is often one of turmoil and anguish and for some patients a continual struggle to accept the inevitable changes. Where the onset of renal failure has been an insidious process, patients may have had time to prepare for the inevitability of life on dialysis.

Understanding the psychological impact renal failure has upon patients and their families is an important task for the renal care team. DiMatteo and DiNicola (1982) argue that professional nursing practice requires nurses to consider the meaning attached to the illness by the patient. The development of holistic care planning to achieve realistic therapeutic outcomes that reflect individual needs of patients is an important goal of care. Research has identified factors thought to affect successful coping, including illness and treatment stressors, treatment modality, social support and compliance with prescribed treatments.

Quality of life and ethical dilemmas in renal care have become areas of growing interest among staff working within the renal care setting. Cameron and Gregor (1987, p. 672) suggest that chronic illness is a lived experience involving loss or dysfunction; it is contended that chronic illness has a reality all of its own (Benner and Wrubel, 1989). The need to depend upon life-sustaining machinery (dialysis) perpetuates the feeling of vulnerability experienced by renal patients. The dehumanizing effects of dialysis technology result in additional stress for patients, who attempt to make sense of it for themselves and for those involved closely within their care.

Key reference: Benner, P. and Wrubel, J. (1989) *The Primacy of caring.* Addison Wesley, Menlo Park, California.

THE IMPORTANCE OF COPING WITH RENAL FAILURE

The term 'coping' has multiple meanings depending on which perspective is examined. Research has examined the role of psychological variables thought to influence coping, particularly stress mediators, locus of control, hardiness and stress adaptation. The notion of 'illness careers' is discussed by Price (1996), who contends that chronic illness is dynamic and complex and that motivating factors influencing patients' behaviour are based upon assessment of goals, needs, resources and priorities.

Coping has been defined as those constantly changing cognitive and behavioural efforts, both action-oriented and intrapsychic, to manage (master, tolerate, reduce, minimize) specific external and/or internal demands (stress) that are appraised as taxing or exceeding the resources of the person. Coping can be defined as efforts to manage, which allows the word to include any of the person's thoughts, regardless of how well or badly they work. In relation to stress it is important to understanding the process of cognitive appraisal, which determines how patients perceive their immediate environment. Individuals with renal failure are likely to appraise aspects of their environment as damaging or potentially threatening. Thus, renal patients faced with the environment of a dialysis unit and the demands of learning complex life-sustaining skills may experience feelings of overwhelming stress. This must be borne in mind by renal care staff who are required to support patients and families through the transition process to dialysis care.

ADAPTATION MODELS

Where the onset of ESRD has been gradual, the patient and family may have had time to adjust to the idea of dialysis and make an informed choice about treatment modalities. Patients may initially feel relief at starting dialysis when symptoms of uraemia have been troublesome. If the onset of dialysis has been sudden an acute crisis phase of adjustment may be experienced, with feelings of shock, disbelief, desperation and depression. A number of stages have been identified that patients may experience as they come to terms (or not, as the case may be) with their situation. The first stage, often referred to as 'the honeymoon stage', may last from a few weeks to months. During this stage patients appear positive and hopeful, their confidence being high. Reduced feelings of confidence and hope mark the 'stage of disenchantment and discouragement'. The limitations imposed by dialysis become evident during this stage and there are feelings of sadness and helplessness. Arriving at some level of acceptance is associated with periods of contentment, often alternating with periods of depression (Fricchione *et al.*, 1992). Returning to some previously meaningful activity may often facilitate the adaptation process. Many patients experience feelings of intense helplessness in their attempts to adapt to the illness. On one hand patients wish to be passive and dependent while being 'expected' by the health-care team to be active and independent, and this promotes a feeling of being 'trapped' (Reischman and Levy, 1972).

It is important to understand that such a process is not always clear-cut and that individuals respond differently to the realities of ESRD (Levy, 1981; De-Nour, 1981).

Renal nurses must assess the feelings expressed by patients and recognize that they may be representative of the stage the patient has reached in acceptance of his/her illness. Supporting patients who are expressing intense emotions, which may fluctuate between the various states highlighted, is a challenge for renal care staff. A close supportive relationship between the nurse and patient is vital to create a climate of trust and support. Patients and families benefit from continuity in care during this phase and the appointing of a named nurse who can be responsible for coordinating care is an important way of enhancing the quality of care delivered. As time progresses the 'named nurse' can develop a thorough assessment of the patient, encompassing psychological and social factors that will influence the patient's adjustment to dialysis.

STRESS IN CHRONIC ILLNESS

ESRD results in multiple stressors being experienced by patients and family; the extent of stress varies depending on the patient's illness, his/her individual coping resources and the environment in which care is delivered. Multiple threats are felt by patients, relating to life, physical wellbeing, self-concept, belief systems, social and occupational functioning and emotional wellbeing. It is not uncommon for patients to express fears about dying, since life itself is now thrown into question. For many patients the thought of death is not discussed and instead is suppressed, potentially as a coping method.

The environment of a dialysis unit presents vivid images of 'illness and sickness'. No matter how well a patient may feel, the presence of other sick patients is a constant reminder of how vulnerable his/her own life is. Through the close relationship that the unit staff develop with patients the prospect of dying may be addressed. For some patients it is important that the possibility of death should be openly acknowledged, and this should be considered, although it is an area that must be approached sensitively, openly and honestly. The moment to address such an issue is not always clear-cut; listen and watch intuitively for 'cues' from patients that might signal such concerns.

Uncertainty about the future is a threat for patients and carers when life's goals and values have been drastically altered. Patients are sometimes conscious of loss of autonomy and control, which imposes its own additional stress. Involving patients and families in the decisions concerning their care is important, as allowing them to maintain control must be a cornerstone of treatment. During the initial stages of dialysis, educational programmes should reflect the individual learning needs of the patient and family. A structured, well-developed educational programme supported by educational materials that the patient can read will assist him/her to acquire knowledge about his/her treatment. Patients should be encouraged to assume some level of self-care appropriate to their abilities although, because of cognitive and physical limitations, the level of self-care attainable will vary. Nurses play an important role in identifying the appropriate level of self-care to aim at for each patient. Working closely together through the continuous ambulatory peritoneal dialysis or haemodialysis training programme can be a rewarding experience for both patient and renal care staff.

Besides the physical pain and discomfort associated with renal replacement therapy, the integrity of the patient's body suffers multiple threats due to ESRD and treatment regimens. Within the renal care setting, palliative care is important, and the multidisciplinary team will help the patient and family with symptom control, pain relief and the attainment of a peaceful death where death is likely. When required, the renal care team should utilize additional resources and specialists to assist with palliative care, such as Macmillan nurses and district nurses, who also have a part to play in the care of the patient and family.

Having to adjust to unfamiliar surroundings of the dialysis unit may result in feelings of powerlessness and depersonalization. Threats to social roles may be experienced, particularly changes to family functioning, and separation from friends and other important support networks is often experienced. Nurses should identify within their assessments of patients those support networks that will play an important role in the patient's therapy and attempt to make use of them.

Eichel (1986) examined stressors and coping in a group of 30 continuous ambulatory peritoneal dialysis (CAPD) patients and compared their findings with studies of haemodialysis patients in the literature. Limitations in activity coupled with fatigue were seen as most stressful to the CAPD patients, a similar finding to HD patients. Eichel (1986) argues that renal nurses should avoid focusing solely on stressors related to the dialysis procedure since stressors identified in their study were generic to chronic renal failure. Further research undertaken by Bihl *et al.* (1988), which examined stressors experienced by CAPD and HD patients, identified uncertainty about the future as the greatest stressor to CAPD patients and fatigue and boredom with routine as the major stressor to the HD patients. This study supports the findings of Gurklis and Menke (1988), who identified that, in their sample of 68 patients, feeling tired was the most stressful factor, other stressors cited including restricted food and fluid intake and reduced physical activity.

Gurklis and Menke (1995) attempted to describe perceptions of stressors, coping methods and social support in a group of 129 chronic haemodialysis patients. Patients in this study used multiple coping methods such as acceptance, optimism, maintaining control, seeking support and staying active to handle 62 stressors, including physiological complications, psychosocial concerns about haemodialysis, and restrictions. Patients positively evaluated their support and discussed concerns for support persons and needs for more support. The importance of support cannot be underestimated, although the type and extent of support available to patients will vary. Attention must be focused on providing care for the support networks, who may often feel overwhelmed and burdened by the demands that face them.

The types of stressor and coping method and their impact upon quality of life was the focus of Lok's (1996) survey. This study revealed limitation of physical activity as the most troublesome stressor, followed by decrease in social life, uncertainty about the future, fatigue and muscle cramps. Problem-solving methods were considered to be more effective than affective measures in dealing with stressors. Quality of life was perceived as below average in both haemodialysis and continuous ambulatory peritoneal dialysis patients. However, CAPD patients experienced a higher quality of life than HD patients. The length of time on the dialysis programme was not related to coping behaviour. The findings of this study can further help renal nurses to provide support, information and alternative solutions and to assist patients to make better use of problem-solving methods to enhance their quality of life on dialysis.

HEALTH BELIEFS

The role that health beliefs play in understanding why some patients are able to adapt to renal failure and others are not offers an interesting area for research. The health belief model (HBM) developed by Rosenstock (1966) has been incorporated into many research studies. The HBM identifies factors within the individual and environment that may be applied to individuals coping with dialysis. The theory of locus of control (LOC; Rotter, 1954) suggests that individuals who believe they can control their life and events around them have an internal locus of control. This is in contrast to individuals who adopt a fatalistic belief that they are unable to shape what happen to them, who are said to have an external locus of control.

This is an important model to consider in relation to renal failure since it can enable health-care staff to focus on particular aspects known to be influencing the individual's locus of control. Oberle (1991) offers a cautionary note concerning the weaknesses of many studies that have attempted to link an individuals LOC to individual health actions. While volumes of research have been undertaken on LOC, Oberle (1991) argues that the majority of studies have suffered methodologically, particularly from validity and reliability problems. Many studies have also failed to address the multidimensional nature of the construct of LOC and instead have addressed the construct in a unidimensional way. Oberle (1991) cites Rock *et al.* (1987), whose work examined six clusters of LOC orientations based upon a combination of scores on internal, chance and powerful-others scales. Increasingly the need to consider the role of reinforcement of the individual and the psychological situation in LOC studies must be addressed (Rotter, 1975).

Renal nurses should continue to examine the impact of LOC upon patient health behaviours by adopting a more rigorous approach to research studies. The pressing need to use experimental and quasi-experimental research designs has been expressed by Oberle (1991), particularly in relation to the value of teaching programmes tailored to the individual. The need to address the role and value of 'reinforcement' in studies of LOC is vital. Oberle (1991) provides a number of interesting directions for future research that renal nurses should address if research into LOC is to offer anything meaningful to clinical practice. Antonovsky (1992) supports many of the points raised by Oberle (1991) but argues that the limitations of existing studies indicate that the construct of LOC itself may be problematic. Staff can evaluate patients LOC through the use of structured questionnaires and build upon the findings when planning patients' educational programmes. It is also worth considering regular assessment of patients' LOC and using the results to assess their overall coping and adjustment to treatment. In a number of renal units the support of a unit clinical psychologist has greatly assisted staff in their endeavours.

Within the field of nephrology health-care staff have continued to search for ways of understanding factors that potentially shape an individual's ability to adapt to prescribed treatment regimens (Christensen *et al.*, 1996). Research into locus of control has uncovered a complex relationship between perceived control and psychological adjustment. LOC has been suggested to be less important than the patient's overall sense of control over life (Bremer *et al.*, 1995). It has been suggested that interventions designed to increase an individual's perception of control are likely to have a positive impact on qualitative aspects of treatment. In order to improve a patient's potential quality of life the renal care team must consider his/her sense of agency. When patients see themselves as possessing control over non-health aspects of life such as employment and community issues they may respond better to treatment (Bremer *et al.*, 1995).

When attempting to apply LOC theory to renal nursing practice a number of important factors must be considered. Patients who are internally orientated often seek information, and need to feel that they are in control of treatment outcomes. It is essential to stress the reasons behind positive self-management of the treatment regimen, taking account of health information offered by the renal care team. It is valuable when working with such patients to draw their attention to how their behaviour influences important measurements such as potassium and phosphorus levels and interdialytic weight gains. Patients should be encouraged to discuss their views on the laboratory measurements and to suggest likely solutions to problems (Wilson, 1995).

> **Key reference:** Wilson, B.M. (1995) Promoting compliance: the patient–provider partnership. *Advances in renal Replacement Therapy* 2(3): 199–206.

Working with patients who display an external LOC presents challenges to staff. These patients benefit from being informed exactly what needs to be done and from the involvement of family members and others who influence the patient. Promoting an increase in internal orientation has been suggested, with the implementation of contingency contracting. This involves both patient and nurse agreeing upon mutual goals for behaviour change. Adopting such an approach, according to Wilson (1995), is a way to show externally orientated patients that their actions do affect outcomes; central to the contracting process is the provision of suitable rewards for behaviour changes. Patient involvement is increased when patients are the ones to select the reward, since different people find different things rewarding. The notion of providing scheduled 'cheat' times has been discussed, as well as making exceptions to the renal diet restrictions to help patients to adapt to them (Nix, 1993).

The importance of actively encouraging patients to participate in self-care activities in the management of their treatment has been discussed. Montemuro *et al.* (1994) found that both nurses and patients underestimated the amount of their participation in care. Patients rated their overall perceived and desired control as moderate; likewise, nurses' global score for desired control was rated as moderate. This study revealed that nurses overestimated the patients' desired control over the technical aspects of dialysis care but underestimated their desire for more control over non-technical aspects of care. This study has important implications for the planning and design of individualized education programmes where patients are intended to have different levels of involvement in the care programme. Overestimating the amount of involvement in certain aspects of the programme that a patient wishes to have may further exacerbate the felt stress experienced by that patient.

> **Key reference:** Montemuro, M., Mohide, E.A., Martin, L.S., Beecroft, M.L. and Jakobson, S. (1994) Participatory control in chronic hospital-based hemodialysis patients. *American Nephrology Nurses Association Journal* 17(1): 63–66.

Hardiness (Kobasa, 1979), a psychological resource that bolsters the stresses of illness, is also important in understanding the coping processes of individuals in ESRD. Many patients, no matter what they face, are able withstand major stresses. Personality factors are known to play a major role in psychological adjustment to dialysis therapy. The premorbid personality of the patient is thought to be a significant factor: how s/he coped with stress prior to the onset of renal failure and his/her general ability to adapt to alterations in lifestyle are important. Whichever view is taken of the complexities of adjusting to renal failure it is evident that multiple factors shape a patient's ability to manage and adapt to ESRD and treatment.

PATIENT EDUCATION AND ADAPTATION

Research has examined factors thought to predict adherence to dialysis treatment regimens. Weed-Collins and Hogan (1989) examined the role of health beliefs and knowledge in the taking of phosphate-binding medication and whether these were related to a more positive adherence to therapy. Results from questionnaires indicated that perceived barriers – forgetting and being away from home – were the most significant predictors of non-adherence. It is therefore suggested that nurses should plan interventions that minimize barriers to taking medication.

Educating patients is a major role of the renal care team, but opinions differ as to when is the most appropriate time to teach patients. During dialysis may not be the optimum time. Smith and Winslow (1990) examined the presence of cognitive changes in chronic renal patients during haemodialysis and found that renal patients may have decreased cognitive functioning at that time. As in many renal units the dialysis period appears to present the ideal time for teaching patients, further research is needed to substantiate the findings of this study as well as to help renal staff plan appropriate teaching strategies.

Patients from ethnic minority groups form a large part of the patient population in many renal units. In this situation the renal care team must ensure that educational materials are translated into the relevant language and that concerted attempts are made to minimize the communication difficulties experienced by both patient and staff. Cultural differences must be borne in mind when developing educational programmes. It is important to respond to patients' unique cultural needs and where possible the principles of transcultural nursing should be embraced. A misunderstanding of cultural beliefs can have negative consequences for patients, so staff should be familiar with the dietary needs, beliefs and values of the different cultures in the patient community with which they work. Staff should be appropriately supported and receive education and training where necessary to help them to provide culturally appropriate renal care.

Predialysis preparation of the individual and the family is significant for their overall adaptation to dialysis. This period enables questions to be answered, educational programmes to be commenced and a relationship between unit staff and family to be developed. The patient has opportunities to address concerns and an environment is created where patients and family can discuss renal replacement. Sharing information and knowledge with patients can help them to develop a sense of control over their illness and its treatment. Nursing staff can direct educational programmes according to patient needs and, based upon their nursing assessments, tailor programmes to individual patients and families.

NON-ADHERENCE TO THERAPEUTIC REGIMENS

A common question among members of the renal unit care team is: 'Why do patients knowingly take risks with their dialysis schedules and aspects of their management?' Patients may 'test out' prescribed dietary limits and gradually increase their risk-taking practices. They may fail to take prescribed medications or adjust doses to suit their particular requirements. Achieving compliance with prescribed dialysis regimens is an important factor in the patient's overall management and their general wellbeing. Various definitions of compliance have been posited and there is no real agreement between the authors as to the central criteria, various interpretations being offered. According to Barofsky and Lundwall (1975) compliance is the extent to which a person's behaviour (in terms of taking medication, following diets or executing other lifestyle changes) coincides with medical or health advice. Non-compliance is when a person's behaviour does not coincide with medical or health advice. Persistent self-induced fluid overload and dietary non-compliance are often an indication of the internal struggles the patient is facing.

The term 'compliance with' prescribed regimens brings with it images of patient subservience and lack of control. It seems more appropriate to consider patients' behaviour as a therapeutic alliance rather than compliance. The idea of therapeutic alliance is discussed by Barofsky and Lundwall (1975), who relate the concept of compliance along a social control continuum. 'Compliance' suggests coercion, 'adherence' suggests conformity and 'therapeutic alliance' suggests negotiation. Increasingly, the term 'self-management of treatment' appears the most appropriate term since the focus of care should be encouraging the self-management of behaviours that will maintain the patient in an optimum state of health and free from uraemic symptoms.

Renal nurses must foster the patient's role in the decision-making process and provide information so that s/he can make health choices. During the assessment of the patient guidelines should be established about keeping to the prescribed regimen. Advice and information given should always take into account the patient's individual lifestyle and social factors such as family and employment and where possible the goals set should be ones that the patient can realistically achieve. Failure to adhere to prescribed health advice is a major source of conflict between patient and staff: frustrations arise and tensions may surface within the nurse–patient relationship.

It is known that a patient's ability to follow health advice is strongly influenced by multiple factors such as LOC. Nursing assessments undertaken during the early stages of dialysis should indicate the patient's LOC and identify areas where difficulties may be experienced.

Dependency upon dialysis to remove excess fluid consumed may be evident; this sets up a cycle where the patient gradually sees dialysis as something that will effectively deal with their non-adherent practices. It is important that the patient is the main decision-maker about his/her lifestyle and staff need to be realistic about what they can achieve with patients. Over time uncooperative behaviour will need to be addressed sensitively by all members of the health-care team. In some situations it may be necessary to hold a case conference, which should involve the patient, family and care team. The establishment of a patient behavioural contract outlining what is expected from the patient is another option that has been employed in some units with varying degrees of success.

Lack of adherence with dialysis treatment regimens is a common problem in patients with ESRD and can mean that patients fail to receive the full benefit from therapy. Nurses can, through careful assessment and intervention, work to encourage self-management of patients' treatment. Viewing 'self-management' as a partnership between members of the renal multidisciplinary team and the patient may help resolve difficulties (Currier, 1993).

Cleary *et al.* (1995) examined medication knowledge and compliance among patients receiving long-term dialysis. Although 80% of the patients could recall the three target medications, only 39% of the haemodialysis patients and 57% of CAPD patients could recall all their medication. Significantly more patients knew the indication for their antihypertensive medication and calcitriol than for their phosphate-binder. Both sets of patients were more knowledgeable about and compliant with their antihypertensive and calcitriol regimens than their phosphate-binder regimens. It is important for renal nurses to consider how and through what means patients gain their knowledge and how they process this knowledge when making decisions about self-management.

Renal patients are often responsible for the self-administration of medication (SAM) although the relationship between self-administration and adherence to medication can not be determined. Furlong (1996) suggests that this relationship is a tentative one and that improvements in knowledge and compliance with medication regimens cannot be linked directly with a SAM programme. Self-administration of medication may improve patient knowledge but opportunities to obtain knowledge may not be unique to such programmes.

Developing creative teaching strategies is one means through which adherence to dietary advice can be encouraged. Lewis *et al.* (1990) developed and implemented a creative teaching strategy to stimulate patients' motivation to incorporate learned dietary concepts into their daily lifestyle. A total of 35 haemodialysis patients were given a pamphlet that described herbs and spices to enhance the flavour of specific foods and 25 sample seasoning packets to experiment with. Most patients stated that the pamphlet was helpful (82.9%) and that use of the spices made the diet palatable 75% or more of the time (93.4%). The importance of working with the unit dietitian in devising teaching programmes is important.

SELF-CARE AND AUTONOMY

Enabling patients and family members to assume a 'self-care role' is important. Patients experience enforced dependency, subjected to dialysis routines imposed by the health-care team. Not all patients are capable of assuming self-care or wish to do so, but it should form a component part of individual patient assessment during the early stages of dialysis. Whether the patient faces maintenance haemodialysis or peritoneal dialysis a well-structured and planned educational programme that reflects the individual learning needs of the patient can ease the feeling of powerlessness so evident among many renal patients.

Entry into hospital can have a dehumanizing effect on patients; enforced routines and roles heighten their feeling of dependency. Pressly (1995) attempted to ascertain whether a relationship existed between psychosocial characteristics of CAPD patients and the occurrence of infectious complications. The results highlighted a significant relationship between the incidence of peritonitis, time to the first episode of peritonitis, and total incidence of infectious complications.

The physiological changes associated with renal failure present reminders of how vulnerable their life is. Patients feel incapacitated by lethargy, vascular access difficulties or persistent itching, all reminders of their illness. Patients experience stigma emphasizing further how 'different' they are. Throughout their care and management the need to provide patients with as positive an outlook as is realistic is important.

The nature of the relationship that the multidisciplinary team establishes with the patient is critical to his/her satisfaction with treatment and also helps to create a forum where shared decision-making and partnership in care can become a reality. The renal unit health-care team should demonstrate 'unconditional positive regard' for patients and offer an environment where fears and concerns can be openly discussed. Through this relationship personal issues can be explored sensitively, particularly altered sexual functioning, which is a problem for patients and their partners (Zarifian, 1992). Referrals can be made to other agencies for support and strategies identified where possible that will enable the patient to deal with such problems (Hart *et al.*, 1995).

The patient scenario below identifies some of the issues that can be involved.

Patient scenario

Peter is a 26-year-old who has been receiving maintenance centre haemodialysis for 2 years. His primary renal disease is unknown and he presented in ESRD over a short span of time. He lives with his elderly patients, who are in good health, and recently ended a stable long-term relationship for 'sexual reasons', as he freely reveals. During the early days of dialysis Peter was interested in his therapy and took an active interest in his management. Over a period of 6 months he has persistently arrived at the unit grossly fluid-overloaded (6 kg) for each dialysis and has been rude to members of the nursing team. Peter lives for the weekend when his social life comes alive; he talks freely about his visits to nightclubs where his attempts to 'pick up' women are usually successful. Towards the end of the week Peter's mood state is fairly elevated as he looks forward to his weekend plans. Peter has had a consultation with the liaison psychiatrist concerning a failed suicide attempt when his relationship with his long-term girlfriend ended and is currently receiving antidepressant medication. Peter shows little interest in his treatment now and says he is controlled by the unit staff and 'the beast' (the dialysis machine).

Questions
- What options are open to the renal multidisciplinary team in the management of Peter's persistent non-adherence to his prescribed therapy?
- Discuss aspects of the nurse–patient relationship that may play a role in helping Peter with his difficulties.
- In view of Peter's history, identify possible reasons for his current lack of interest in his treatment.

FAMILY ROLE IN ESRD

It is well known that ESRD places significant demands not just upon the patient but also upon other family members, particularly spouse and children where they are present. The renal unit social worker is a vital member of the team and plays an important role in assessing home and family circumstances that may be important in the patients adjustment to dialysis. Patients who are self-caring in the community and are attended to by a family member need particular support: visits from the community dialysis nurse act as an important link between the hospital and the patient's home environment.

The family's role in managing chronic illness has been an area of ongoing research. ESRD impacts upon all members of the family, who have to adjust to the demands imposed upon them (Hartigan and Harris, 1991). Social support is an important factor in assisting patients to cope with their illness. How families manage the 'illness demands' must be an area of concern for all members of the renal multidisciplinary team.

Brock (1990) explored renal families' information needs, uncertainty level and perceived coping effectiveness in relation to living with chronic kidney failure and haemodialysis therapy. This study indicated that knowledge correlated negatively to uncertainty; that level of education positively correlated with coping effectiveness; and that neither knowledge nor uncertainty were significantly correlated to coping effectiveness. The renal care team should consider individual factors within the family that enhance their ability to cope.

The importance of carers, who are often the 'hidden army' in the whole process, has received limited attention. Richardson *et al.* (1989, p. 57) suggests that: 'Caring is a job with a difference. It has no fixed hours and no wages, no qualifying exams and no clear contract. It arrives through and takes place in a relationship.'

The effects upon family members assisting with home dialysis must be considered. Various psychological perspectives have provided descriptions of how spouses cope with the stresses associated with dialysis. However, important societal, gender and economic factors affecting patients with ESRD and their families have been overlooked. More comprehensive research would highlight the extent of the effects home dialysis has on the family (Brunier and McKeever, 1993).

Many patients are cared for at home by their spouse and research has identified the insidious position of spouses in the care-giving process. Quality of life experienced by spouses must be a concern since their support has a positive influence on the patient's ability to cope and adjust. Indeed, it would seem important that QoL studies be extended to renal families, since without their support and wellbeing the effects upon the patient can be devastating. This concern was addressed by Dunn *et al.* (1994) in their research into quality of life of spouses of continuous ambulatory peritoneal dialysis (CAPD) patients and what factors were the best predictors of the spouses' perceived QoL. This study indicated that 21% of the spouses perceived their QoL as high, 55% perceived their QoL as moderate and

24% perceived their QoL as fair to poor. The results indicated that the QoL for the spouse is similar to that of CAPD patients with the exception of the family domain. On the family domain, spouses scored significantly lower. Marital adjustment was the best predictor of QoL for the spouse. Income was the next best predictor.

Understanding the effect that a chronic illness has upon spouses enables renal nurses to provide quality care for both the patient and his/her spouse. It may be necessary for family therapy or family support groups to be established where mutual support can be gained from among the patients. Assistance with practical aspects concerning financial difficulties can be obtained through the unit social worker.

Renal staff should consider the coping style of families since this provides a window on their coping capabilities. A variety of family coping styles may exist, as identified by Flaherty and O'Brien (1992). This qualitative study of 50 families identified five predominant styles of family coping. A 'remote' family style exists where it is evident that the impact of ESRD has not 'touched the lives of family members'. In families where the effects of ESRD can be seen to have increased and strengthened the bonds between family members an 'enfolded' family style is present. Families demonstrating this characteristic have a tendency to approach the impact and effects of ESRD as a family affair. Many families coping with ESRD are required to undergo major changes in terms both of their structure and of their daily activities. This may mean changes in work and school patterns, family income, recreational activities and holidays; families making such changes display an 'altered' family style. In attempting to address the demands of living with ESRD it is not uncommon for a sense of loss and grief to be expressed within the family. Concern voiced for the individual member or ongoing negative responses to the illness highlights a family with a 'distressed' family style. Renal nurses often encounter families who accept the diagnosis and the inevitability of dependence upon dialysis and work together with health-care providers within the prescribed restrictions. Support from family members or religious beliefs is often a source of immense strength as a coping resource. Such families demonstrate a 'receptive' family style.

> **Key reference:** Flaherty, M.J. and O'Brien, M.E. (1992) Family styles of coping in end stage renal disease. *American Nephrology Nurses Association Journal*. 19(4): 345–9, 366.

Renal nurses should work towards individualizing care according to the predominant family style and, where possible, facilitate coping and adjustment according to their needs. This study has implications for renal nurses who work with families during the early stages of adjustment to the regimen. That renal nurses understand the significance of social support for the patient is crucial, especially where a family member may be demonstrating a remote family style. In such a case the unit staff may be perceived as the 'significant other' for the patient. Equally, a family member demonstrating a 'distressed' or 'altered' family style should signal the need for heightened levels of support to explore and work through problem areas. Renal nurses must enter into the care of the patient taking full account of the needs of the family and how the family can influence an individual's adaptation to therapy. Interestingly, within the above study Flaherty and O'Brien (1992) found that the 'remote' family style was the most frequent. ESRD affects all age groups, which often bring with them their own particular difficulties, as is seen with paediatric and adolescent patients. Adolescent patients already face the stresses associated with their particular developmental stage, which are further compounded by the effects of their illness, and as a result struggle to cope: the demands of ESRD may often conflict with adolescent needs (Gallo et al., 1992). As increasing numbers of elderly patients join maintenance renal programmes the need to assess quality of life in such patients becomes more important. Morgan (1990) examined the relationship between chronological age and perceived quality of life of haemodialysis patients, finding no significant relationship between patient age and how they perceived the quality of their lives.

How patients manage the daily requirements of their illness and its interpretation is an important focus for renal care staff. Rittman (1993) identified three themes in their study of the experience of living with ESRD, including 'taking on a new understanding of Being', 'maintaining hope' and 'dwelling in dialysis'. The central pattern that guided living with ESRD was that of 'control and the meaning of technology'. The study illuminates the meaning of technology in the lives of renal patients and highlights the need for nurses to develop meaningful supportive relationships with them. The feeling of kinship among patients in a renal unit emerged: shared suffering and social attachment were important. The renal unit became an important source of social contact, being seen by many as 'home'. These findings should encourage the renal care team to consider the levels of attachment that develop within their patient group and how the experience of shared suffering can be significant. This is particularly important when a fellow patient dies and the renal care team are required to support the associated feelings of loss and pain.

QUALITY OF LIFE AND ADJUSTMENT TO ESRD

Quality of life is a multidimensional concept and difficult to measure, and has attracted increasing interest among researchers working within nephrology. Health-care staff are increasingly concerned about the quality of life of patients undergoing dialysis therapy (Bradley and McGee, 1994). The environment in which renal care is delivered is one dominated by technology, where patients strive for 'normality' within the confines of their illness. Altered physiological functioning coupled with uraemic symptoms impose their own restrictions upon patients. Lethargy, bone pain, sickness and nausea are common features of the illness and, despite dialysis partly alleviating them, for many patients the symptoms of renal failure still restrict their activities. The requirement to be dependent upon dialysis for survival does not automatically equate with a satisfactory quality of life for patients; this area increasingly causes professional dilemmas for health-care staff caring for particularly vulnerable patients. Where concerns about quality of life are evident all parties involved should address the issues with the patient and family. When questions arise as to whether the will to live a machine-dependent existence exists the renal unit team should respect the psychological state of the patient as a true reflection of their perceived quality of life and not base judgments solely on objective measures of quality of life (De Nour, 1995).

Key reference: Bradley, C. and McGee, H. (1994) Improving quality of life in renal failure: ways forward. In *Quality of Life Following Renal Failure* (eds.) H. McGee and C. Bradley. Harwood Academic Publishers, Chur, Switzerland.

Key reference: De Nour, K. (1995) Psychological, social and vocational impact of renal failure. In *Quality of Life Following Renal Failure*. (eds.) H. McGee and C. Bradley. Harwood Academic Publishers, Chur, Switzerland.

Molzahn (1991) studied the QoL of 10 home haemodialysis patients, finding that patients were deprived of factors influencing their quality of life, including health, vigour, pleasurable feelings, freedom of action and free time. Brunier and Graydon (1993) identified the influence of anaemia, non-specific symptoms and physical activity on fatigue in 43 patients with ESRD on chronic haemodialysis. Low levels of physical activity and frequent uraemic symptoms were related to high levels of fatigue felt by these patients. The provision of a planned programme of physical exercise for renal patients can have a positive effect upon a patient's QoL and general health. Rehabilitation exercises can be devised by a physiotherapist to help selected patients who wish to maintain some level of physical exercise. A full physical assessment prior to commencing such a programme is essential. Renal nurses should work with patients to develop appropriate health promotion activities within their limits, although many patients may be unable to participate. A steady programme of daily gentle exercises can greatly increase a patient's general level of fitness, within the restrictions imposed by their illness, and improve their QoL.

REHABILITATION IN END-STAGE RENAL DISEASE

Retaining employment has been identified as important in the quality of life of renal patients, but balancing work commitments with dialysis schedules can be problematic for many patients. Employers may require assistance to help them understand some of the difficulties patients may encounter. Progressive renal failure results in periods of protracted illness and symptoms of uraemia preventing the patient from continuing to hold down regular employment. Financial hardships due to diminished income place an added burden upon the family.

Peters *et al.* (1994) found that, in 248 work-eligible ESRD patients, relatively few significant differences existed between employed and unemployed patients in terms of demographics, physical function, psychosocial adaptation and vocational rehabilitation potential. However, unemployed patients reported lower energy levels, less stamina for working, greater benefits of not working and problems with vocational rehabilitation programmes. Unemployed patients also demonstrated more negative attitudes about achieving life goals and former job experiences.

Despite their difficulties, many patients are able to retain their employment, integrate renal dialysis into their lives and have an acceptable QoL, thus reducing the intrusive nature of dialysis. These patients may display a strong sense of personal worth and manage to cope with crises as they arise. The setting of realistic goals with patients and family members is an important function of the health-care team and can be used to assess progress in patients' adjustment. Renal unit staff can help patients overcome barriers to rehabilitation by focusing on the management of ESRD complications, assisting patients with support groups, connecting patients to rehabilitation resources early and encouraging employed patients to continue working as long as possible. The unit social worker can provide a critical link between the patient's desire to maintain employment and other agencies involved in this process.

HOPE AND ITS ROLE IN ADJUSTMENT TO RENAL FAILURE

Renal failure imposes many changes upon those involved, and a feeling of hopelessness is often expressed by patients. Carpenito (1989) suggests that hopelessness is a sustained emotional state where patients see no alternatives or choices and therefore cannot mobilize energy on their own behalf to set goals. The importance of hope to ESRD patients must be appreciated: hope enables patients to 'hang on' and not give up despite what they are faced with. Patients hope for release from the turmoil of dialysis, for a transplant, etc. Health-care staff can assess the level of hope displayed by patients while recognizing that hope may at times be counterproductive and unrealistic. Enabling patients to face their future and discussing their hopes and fears are important functions for the health-care team. It has been suggested that haemodialysis patients experience greater feelings of helplessness. Rydholm and Pauling (1991) compared the perceptions of helplessness in haemodialysis and peritoneal dialysis patients using the Learned Helplessness Scale. A greater sense of helplessness was reported by haemodialysis patients. The results of this study suggest the need for nursing interventions that improve the level of personal control in both groups of patients, although haemodialysis patients appeared to demonstrate a greater need.

CONCLUSION

Understanding the meaning that patients and families attach to their illness experience must be a goal for all members of the renal multidisciplinary team.

This point is addressed by Price (1996), who contends that nurses need to understand the patient's perspective of his/her illness. Indeed the need for the health-care team to understand the patient's definition of illness and his/her experiences is central to the planning of nursing care. Renal nurses should conduct ongoing assessments of patients' stressors, coping and social support so that they can assist them to alleviate stressors and attain or maintain effective coping methods and support resources (Ormandy, 1995). Research should focus on the development and testing of specific nursing interventions to help patients cope with stressors and increase their level of support. The importance of the renal multidisciplinary team working closely with families and patients can not be over-stated.

REVIEW QUESTIONS

- Identify factors responsible for non-adherence to prescribed therapeutic regimens.
- Discuss locus of control, hardiness and the health belief model in adaptation to ESRD.
- Examine how quality of life for both patients and carers is affected by ESRD
- Identify the main priorities when developing educational programmes for patients joining maintenance renal replacement.
- Discuss the role of the multidisciplinary team in facilitating a patient's adjustment to dialysis.
- Discuss nursing interventions to respond to a patient who expresses negative feelings regarding his therapy to unit staff.

REFERENCES

Antonovsky, A. (1992) Locus of control theory. *Journal of Advanced Nursing*, **17**, 1014–1015.

Barofsky, F. and Lundwall, L. (1975) Dropping out of treatment: a critical review. *Psychological Bulletin*, **82**(5), 738–783.

Benner, P. and Wrubel, J.(1989) *The Primacy of Caring*, Addison Wesley, Menlo Park, CA.

Bihl, M. A., Ferrans, C. E. and Powers, M. J. (1988) Comparing stressors and quality of life of dialysis patients. *American Nephrology Nurses Association Journal*, **15**, 27–34.

Bradley, C. and McGee, H. (1994) Improving quality of life in renal failure: ways forward, in *Quality of Life Following Renal Failure* (eds H. McGee and C. Bradley), Harwood Academic Publishers, Chur, Switzerland.

Bremer, A. B., Haffly, D., Foxx, R. M. and Weaver, A. (1995) Patients perceived control over their health care: an outcome assessment of their psychological adjustment to renal failure. *American Journal of Medical Quality*, **10**(3), 149–151

Brock, M. J. (1990) Uncertainty, information needs and coping effectiveness of renal families. *American Nephrology Nurses Association Journal*, **17**(3), 242–245; 267.

Brunier, G. M. and Graydon, J. (1993) The influence of physical activity on fatigue in patients with ESRD on hemodialysis. *American Nephrology Nurses Association Journal*, **20**(4), 457–461.

Brunier, G. M. and McKeever, P. T. (1993) The impact of home dialysis on the family: literature review. *American Nephrology Nurses Association Journal*, **20**(6), 653–659.

Cameron, K. and Gregor, F. (1987) Chronic illness and compliance. *Journal of Advanced Nursing*, **12**, 671–676.

Carpenito, L. J. (1989) *Nursing Diagnosis: Application to Clinical Practice*, 3rd edn, J. B. Lippincott, Philadelphia, PA.

Christensen, A., Wiebe, J., Benotsch, E. G. and Lawton, W. J. (1996) Perceived health competence, health locus of control, and patient adherence in renal dialysis. *Cognitive Therapy and Research*, **20**(4), 411–421.

Cleary, D. J., Matzke, G. R., Alexander, A. C. and Joy, M. S. (1995) Medication knowledge and compliance among patients receiving long-term dialysis. *American Journal of Health System Pharmacy*, **52**(17), 1895–900.

Currier, H. (1993) Case management of the anemic patient: epoetin alfa–focus on compliance. *American Nephrology Nurses Association Journal*, **20**(4), 470–473.

De Nour, K. (1995) Psychological, social and vocational impact of renal failure, in *Quality of Life Following Renal Failure* (eds H. McGee and C. Bradley), Harwood Academic Publishers, Chur, Switzerland.

DiMatteo, M. R. and DiNicola, D. D. (1982) *Achieving Patient Compliance*, Pergamon Press, New York.

Dunn, S. A., Lewis, S. L., Bonner, P. N. and Meize-Grochowski, R. (1994) Quality of life for spouses of CAPD patients. *American Nephrology Nurses Association Journal*, **21**(5), 237–246, 257.

Eichel, C. J. (1986) Stress and coping in patients on CAPD compared to hemodialysis patients. *American Nephrology Nurses Association Journal*, **13**, 9–13.

Flaherty, M. J. and O'Brien, M. E. (1992) Family styles of coping in end stage renal disease. *American Nephrology Nurses Association Journal*, **19**(4), 345–349; 366.

Fricchione, M. D., Howanitz, E., Jandorf, L. *et al.* (1992) Psychological adjustment to end-stage renal disease and the implications of denial. *Psychosomatics*, **33**(1), 85–91.

Furlong, S. (1996) Do programmes of medicine self-administration enhance patient knowledge, compliance and satisfaction? *Journal of Advanced Nursing*, **23**(6), 1254–1262.

Gallo, A. M., Schultz, V. A. and Breitmayer, B. J. (1992) Description of the illness experience by adolescents with chronic renal disease. *American Nephrology Nurses Association Journal*, **19**(2), 190–193, 214.

Gurklis, J. A. and Menke, E. M. (1988) Identification of stressors and use of coping methods in chronic hemodialysis patients. *Nursing Research*, **37**, 236–248.

Gurklis, J. A. and Menke, E. M. (1995) Chronic hemodialysis patients' perceptions of stress, coping and social support. *American Nephrology Nurses Association Journal*, **22**(4), 381–388.

Hart, K. L., Fearing, O. M., Milde, F. and Cox, D. M. (1995) Sexual dysfunction: the teaching of renal dialysis and transplant recipients. *Dialysis and Transplantation*, **24**(11), 621–632.

Hartigan, M. F. and Harris, C. H. (1991) Family involvement: help and frustration. *American Nephrology Nurses Association Journal*, **18**(1), 51–53.

Kaplan De-Nour, K. (1981) Prediction of adjustment to chronic hemodialysis, in *Psychonephrology: Psychological Factors in Hemodialysis and Transplantation*, (ed. N. Levy), Plenum Press, New York.

Kobasa, S. C. (1979) Stressful life events, personality and health. An inquiry into hardiness. *Journal of Personality and Social Psychology*, **37**(1), 1–11.

Levy, N. (1981) *Psychonephrology: Psychological Factors in Hemodialysis and Transplantation*, Plenum Press, New York.

Lewis, D. J., Robinson, J. A. and Robinson, K. (1990) Spice of life: a strategy to enhance dietary compliance. *American Nephrology Nurses Association Journal*, **17**(5), 387–389.

Lok, P. (1996) Stressors, coping mechanisms and quality of life among dialysis patients in Australia. *Journal of Advanced Nursing*, **23**(5), 873–881.

Molzahn, A. E. (1991) The reported quality of life of selected home hemodialysis patients. *American Nephrology Nurses Association Journal*, **18**(2), 73–80; 194.

Montemuro, M., Mohide, E. A., Martin, L. S. *et al.* (1994) Participatory control in chronic hospital-based hemodialysis patients. *American Nephrology Nurses Association Journal*, **21**(7), 429–438.

Morgan, B. W. (1990) The relationship between chronological age and perceived quality of life of hemodialysis patients. *American Nephrology Nurses Association Journal*, **17**(1), 63–66.

Nix, Z. (1993) Creative eating, creative cheating. *Journal of Renal Nutrition*, **3**, 100–102.

Oberle, K. (1991) A decade of research in locus of control: what have we learned? *Journal of Advanced Nursing*, **16**, 800–806.

Ormandy, P. (1995) Life with long term dialysis: the patient's perspective. *Journal of the European Dialysis and Transplant Nurses Association–European Renal Care Association*, **3**, 28–29.

Peters, V. J., Hazel, L. A., Finkel, P. and Colls, J. (1994) Rehabilitation experiences of patients receiving dialysis. *American Nephrology Nurses Association Journal*, **21**(7), 419–426, 457.

Pressly, K. B. (1995) Psychosocial characteristics of CAPD patients and the occurrence of infectious complications. *American Nephrology Nurses Association Journal*, **22**(6), 563–572.

Price, B. (1996) Illness careers: the chronic illness experience. *Journal of Advanced Nursing*, **24**, 275–279.

Reischman, F. and Levy, N. (1972). Problems in adaptation to maintenance dialysis. *Archives of Internal Medicine*, **130**, 859–865.

Richardson, A., Unell, J. and Ashton, B. (1989) *A New Deal for Carers*, Kings Fund Caring Support Unit, London.

Rittman, M., Northsea, C., Hausauer, N. *et al.* (1993) Living with renal failure. *American Nephrology Nurses Association Journal*, **20**(3), 327–331.

Rock, D. L., Meyerowitz, B. E., Maisto, S. A. and Wallston, K. A. (1987) The derivation and validation of six multidimensional health locus of control scale clusters. *Research in Nursing and Health*, **June**, 185–195.

Rosenstock, I. M. (1966) Why people use health services. *Milbank Memorial Fund Quarterly*, **44**, 94–127.

Rotter, J. B. (1954) *Social Learning and Clinical Psychology*, Prentice-Hall, Englewood Cliffs, NJ.

Rotter, J. B. (1975) Some problems and misconceptions related to the construct of internal versus external control of reinforcement. *Journal of Consulting and Clinical Psychology*, **34**, 56–67.

Rydholm, L. and Pauling, J. (1991) Contrasting feelings of helplessness in peritoneal and hemodialysis patients: a pilot study. *American Nephrology Nurses Association Journal*, **18**(2), 183–186, 200.

Smith, B. C. and Winslow, E. H. (1990) Cognitive changes in chronic renal patients during hemodialysis. *American Nephrology Nurses Association Journal*, **17**(4), 283–286.

Weed-Collins, M. and Hogan, R. (1989) Knowledge and health beliefs regarding phosphate-binding medication in predicting compliance. *American Nephrology Nurses Association Journal*, **16**(4), 278–282, 285.

Wilson, B. M. (1995) Promoting compliance: the patient–provider partnership. *Advances in Renal Replacement Therapy*, **2**(3), 199–206.

Zarifian, A. A. (1992) Sexual dysfunction in the male end stage renal disease patient. *American Nephrology Nurses Association Journal*, **19**(6), 527–532.

4 Predialysis management and education

Debra Coupe

LEARNING OBJECTIVES

At the end of this chapter the reader should be able to:

- Understand the management of the patient with chronic renal failure.
- Consider the response of the patient newly diagnosed with chronic renal failure and the role of the renal nurse in assessment with regard to renal replacement therapy options.
- Identify strategies to help inform patients and to support them in decision-making about renal replacement therapy modality.
- Examine the care pathway of the patient with chronic renal failure.

ISSUES IN PREDIALYSIS EDUCATION

Referral to the nephrology team

An individual with chronic renal failure can reach the nephrology team through a variety of different referral pathways and each year the number of new patients commencing renal replacement therapy (RRT) is increasing, with the ceiling as yet unclear. Areas of the UK with a large Asian or African-Caribbean population have a potentially higher take-on rate, partly because of the increased incidence of diabetes and hypertension in these ethnic groups.

Early detection of renal disease may be hindered because of the late development of any uraemic symptoms in relation to the degree of impairment (Walls, 1995). Many patients with progressive renal impairment will be identified before end-stage renal failure is reached and will find themselves under the care of the specialist team before they require RRT. However, a significant proportion of patients present at end-stage, which may have implications for their further management (Wolfson *et al.*, 1995). Table 4.1 identifies the most common causes of chronic renal failure.

Table 4.1 Most common causes of chronic renal failure (Source: from Walls, 1995)

Cause	% of patients
Glomerulonephritis	25
Diabetes mellitus	25
Hypertension	10
Chronic pyelonephritis/reflux	10
Polycystic kidney disease	10
Interstitial nephritis	5
Obstruction	3
Miscellaneous/unknown	12

Key reference: Walls, J. (1995) Chronic renal failure – causes and conservative management. *Medicine* 23(4), 144–148.

Investigations and monitoring of renal function

When a patient is first referred to the renal team, and the diagnosis of chronic renal failure is established, it is essential to spend time discussing the severity and progressive nature of the problem. If the patient is asymptomatic and there are no outward signs of ill-health, coming to terms with the diagnosis can be difficult and for some may take time.

Investigations (Table 4.2) are necessary to establish the level of renal function and to monitor the rate of progression to end-stage. Such investigations may also include admission to hospital for biopsy and/or intensive treatment of the underlying cause. Patients admitted to renal wards will be exposed to other individuals with renal disease, some of whom may be seriously ill. What is seen and what they hear from patients and staff may influence their longer-term decision-making about treatment modalities.

Health promotion and decline of renal function

Long-term monitoring of a patient at the renal clinic offers the potential for ongoing health education and support. This is particularly relevant in chronic renal failure because of the large amount of information (from a variety of health-care professionals) that needs to be imparted in order to

Table 4.2 Tests and functions included in the monitoring of renal function

Blood	Urine	Imaging
Serum chemistry	24-hour urine collection	X-ray (KUB and IVU)
Bone and liver profile	Midstream specimen of urine	Ultrasound of kidney
Haematology/full blood count		Isotope scan
Immunology screen		Renal biopsy
Screening for blood-borne viruses such as Hepatitis B and C		

help them adapt to their chronic ill-health and manage their treatment and any life changes. As with any health-care programme, there is an emphasis on self-care. The impact of chronic renal failure on an individual may have a significant psychological effect (Killingworth, 1995) and it is therefore important that time is clearly allocated to provide appropriate intervention and support to meet their needs. As renal function deteriorates, so the uraemic symptoms and complications become apparent and intervention is required.

Medication

As time progresses, patients may find themselves taking an increasing number of medications to help control symptoms, correct complications of renal failure and maintain general wellbeing. Repetition of information has been shown to help renal patients retain information and increase their knowledge with regard to medication and diet (Ramsdell and Annis, 1996). However, poor compliance can be a major factor affecting therapeutic response. Groups in which this can be particularly troublesome include the elderly and those on long-term therapy, especially when the disease itself produces few symptoms, e.g. hypertension (Turner *et al.*, 1986).

Patient medication cards with information about the name, description and reasons for taking a specific drug, and any special instructions, can reinforce any verbal information. Dispensers are also useful if a patient is having serious problems.

If a patient has insulin-dependent diabetes, intensive treatment and control may influence the rate of progression of the disease (Diabetes Control and Complications Research Group, 1995) as will the use of ACE inhibitors (Lewis *et al.*, 1993).

HYPERTENSION

Control of hypertension can influence the rate of deterioration of renal function (Klahr *et al.*, 1994) lengthening the time before renal replacement therapy is required. This should be made explicit to patients taking anti-hypertensive medication. The primary health-care team can be involved, using shared-care cards, and patients may also be taught to monitor their own blood pressure. Targets for blood pressure control have been suggested by the Renal Association (1995).

Renal osteodystrophy

Early initiation of treatment for renal bone disease with alphacalcidol and phosphate binders is recommended (Bourgoignie, 1992). Calcium-based phosphate binders can be unpalatable, and the patient will require specific advice and on-going monitoring in an effort to maintain levels within acceptable limits. However, the level of knowledge about phosphate control is not always associated with compliance (Uttley *et al.*, 1993).

Anaemia

Treatment of anaemia in predialysis patients with erythropoietin, aiming to restore haemoglobin levels to greater than 10 g/dl, is becoming an accepted standard of care. While hypertension may be exacerbated and require control, the patient's quality of life and exercise capacity can improve (Lim, 1991) without accelerating the rate of progression of the renal disease (Roth *et al.*, 1994) and there are possible long-term cardiovascular benefits.

Diet and fluids

Early dietary assessment and monitoring may help to prevent malnutrition and renal dietitians have an increasingly important role in patient management. Diet should be tailored to the individual's needs, be it potassium control, phosphate control or protein intake. The benefit of a low-protein diet in delaying progression of chronic renal disease is known to be limited (Klahr *et al.*, 1994) and may lead to the patient starting dialysis in a malnourished state. Fluid intake may need to be controlled to prevent fluid overload/pulmonary oedema, providing other symptoms and blood chemistry are acceptable. Diuretics are often prescribed to assist in the prevention of fluid retention. However, as renal function deteriorates fluid restriction may need to be introduced to prevent fluid accumulation. Sodium bicarbonate can help to maintain serum bicarbonate within acceptable limits if there is a systemic metabolic acidosis.

Criteria for referral to the dietitian should be developed to help maintain an optimal nutritional state. Patients requiring specific attention may include those with weight loss, poor appetite, albumin below 35 g/l, or protein intake less or greater than normal (0.8–1 g/kg body weight). If a patient is catabolic s/he will need to increase his/her calorie intake. Patients run the risk of becoming malnourished prior to commencing dialysis, and the associated links between low albumin, morbidity and mortality once on the dialysis programme are well documented (Bergstrom and Lindholm, 1993; Lowrie and Lew, 1990).

Pruritus

Pruritus can be difficult to control and is one of the more frustrating symptoms for the patient. It has been linked to uraemic toxins, but is not necessarily relieved by dialysis (Feinstein, 1994). Correction of calcium and phosphate balance may help alleviate this, but relief may require the prescribing of antipruritic agents. Patients may also obtain local relief from aqueous creams or lotions and oils.

Nausea and vomiting

Nausea and vomiting are notable symptoms as patients progress towards end-stage renal failure and may contribute to malnutrition and weight loss if uncontrolled. With such symptoms, dialysis must be considered.

Lifestyle

Patients should be encouraged to continue their activities and lifestyle as best they can. As with any individual, appropriate advice about smoking and alcohol consumption is recommended.

Employment is often a matter of concern and, depending on the nature of their work, patients should be encouraged to stay in employment (provided this is also their wish). A period of sickness is almost always necessary when RRT is first commenced and employers can be prepared for this if there is appropriate planning. It may also be useful for a member of the renal unit nursing staff or community team to go along with patients to their place of work to meet their employers or visit the personnel department to discuss any special needs they may have once they are receiving RRT. If the patient's work is manual or especially strenuous, it may be possible to negotiate a change of duties or role. Referral to the social worker is appropriate at this stage to allow an opportunity to discuss financial and other concerns.

LEARNING ABOUT CHRONIC RENAL FAILURE AND RENAL REPLACEMENT THERAPY

Education regarding chronic renal failure can begin when the patient first attends the renal clinic. More difficult to judge is when to begin dialogue about renal replacement therapy options. In most centres, providing there are no medical contraindications to one particular treatment, patients are able to make decisions about their choice of treatment modality; although complete freedom or range of choice can be limited because of resource implications.

Discussions about treatment modalities generally begin when the creatinine is in the region of 400–500 μmol/l and when progression to end-stage appears inevitable. It is impossible to put a precise figure on the length of time it takes to support an individual in the adaptation to the prospect of living with chronic renal failure (CRF) and provide them with enough information and time to make a decision about RRT options. Early referral is preferable and each patient should be individually assessed.

Response and coping

The impact of a particular illness on an individual and his/her family can be difficult to estimate and can only be assessed in the context of that person's life (Buckman, 1992). It is necessary for staff to recognize and objectively evaluate the numerous responses and coping mechanisms people can demonstrate in response to bad news or impending 'crisis'. In chronic renal failure, this response is often one of loss and grief, a process that has been described as stages through which the individual passes (Bowlby, 1980; Kubler-Ross, 1982; Parkes, 1986). However, the emotions displayed should tell the observer something about the person, not about the stage they are passing through (Buckman, 1992), and the various stages coexist with one another and are experienced simultaneously rather than serially. The crisis of illness can also be linked to life transitions (Wright, 1993), which may in turn affect a person's response to illness and care.

We all have 'power resources' to maintain our control over life and events, and these include physical strength, psychological stamina and social support, positive self-concept, knowledge and insight, energy and motivation, and a beliefs system (Miller, 1992). The more power resources that are compromised, the more nursing strategies will be needed to help the patient overcome any lack of control. Thus, an understanding of coping mechanisms and health beliefs is essential to help to manage the patient's initial response and behaviour when first told that s/he has a chronic illness that will require long-term treatment, and to develop strategies to inform, support and assist the patient towards a decision and plan of action for their longer term care.

Buckman (1992) suggests using a six-step protocol for breaking bad news, which may be useful to follow during the initial discussions with a patient about CRF and long-term treatment options:

1. getting started, i.e. the environment where discussions take place, who should be there;
2. finding out how much the patient knows;
3. finding out how much the patient wants to know;
4. sharing the information;
5. responding to the patient's feelings, i.e. identifying and acknowledging his/her reaction;
6. planning and follow-through.

Sharing information and changing behaviour

Information-giving and education is best spread over time. Binges are not the solution and 'something told does not mean something heard, remembered or understood' (Nichols, 1984). Information-giving is clearly suitable for most people who can process and use this information towards decision-making, although different levels of information will be required. People who are 'vigilant focussers' will require minute details and up-to-the-minute information to help them regain some sense of control. On the other hand, bombarding the 'avoider' with information may diminish his/her ability to cope (Miller, 1992). The avoider needs information, and the skill is getting the right balance and giving information at the appropriate time and in an appropriate manner. By giving information, worry is not banished but the anxiety generated by needless uncertainty should be (Nichols, 1984).

After the initial shock of diagnosis, the majority of people will begin to adapt to the prospect of life on dialysis. With information and support they can begin considering the options for making a choice of treatment and preparing for a change of life. There will be others who, for what ever reason, are unable to do so. Patients who appear to adapt and cope well can reassure us that we have done our job well, but our strategies to support those who do not immediately adapt are possibly underdeveloped.

Patient-led change

In chronic illness a patient-led model for care may help people work through ambivalence about behaviour change or decision-making. A model using negotiating skills (Rollnick *et al.*, 1992; Stott *et al.*, 1995) has been demonstrated in diabetes care and is a framework that has the potential to be applicable to aspects of renal care. This method encourages patients to make judgments about what particular aspects (of diabetes) they wish to discuss and identify targets for change that can be achieved by the next review (Stott *et al.*, 1995). The readiness for change is measured by the patient using a 'readiness to change ruler' and the agenda is set by asking patients to select topics for discussion from a pictorial chart. Patients are then encouraged to go through a process of weighing up their values surrounding the behaviour in question. The pace should be led by the patient and s/he should not be pushed in the desirable direction. It is, however, a model that should be used for all patients and not just those we consider non-compliant or who are having difficulty in making decisions and changing behaviour.

Key reference: Rollnick, S., Heather, N. and Bell, A. (1992) Negotiating behaviour change in medical settings: The development of brief motivational interviewing. *Journal of Mental Health* (1): 25–37.

We also need to decide if we are aiming for compliance or informed choice as this may influence our approach. Being healthy means different things to different people and we have to consider how people with renal problems fit into the health education framework. Because of the complex nature of renal disease and RRT, all three categories of health education – primary, secondary and tertiary – often have to be tackled simultaneously.

Education programmes to support and prepare people for dialysis

There should be an identified person to take basic responsibility for providing and maintaining the level of information. This does not mean that s/he gives all the information, but his/her role is to check, clarify and make up deficits. The renal community team are in an ideal position to take on this role as they will be providing follow-up and continued care and support after the patient has commenced dialysis. Moreover, the patient should begin to develop a confidence in the staff that s/he meets and when information is given, it is vital that the messages are the same and consistent (see Patient scenario below). Effective communication is essential and time should be allocated in the unit multidisciplinary meetings to discuss new patients about to join the programme.

Patient scenario

Tom, a 46-year-old toolmaker, attended an 'MOT' day at his work and was discovered to be hypertensive. He was referred to his GP, who found his creatinine to be 570 μmol/l, and he was subsequently referred to the nephrology clinic. Over the past 6 months he has had three clinic appointments and a 3-day stay in hospital for BP control and investigation into the cause of his renal failure.

Tom feels physically well and he is asymptomatic, although he does get tired at the end of a long working day. His work can be physical and at times strenuous and he admits to finding it difficult to accept that there is anything wrong with him. He is willing to be visited at home to talk about dialysis, but at the moment feels unable to visit either unit. He has seen CAPD while an inpatient and was disillusioned by some of the problems he saw the patients having to deal with. From the literature he has read thus far, he has decided he wants home haemodialysis.

A nursing standard for a predialysis education programme should be set, audited and evaluated to identify any necessary developments or changes in the programme.

Giving and receiving information

Assessment of knowledge and expectations both prior to and after communications is vital. A nursing assessment provides a good basis for evaluation of the patient's current knowledge and understanding, from which an individualized plan of care and education can be formed (Chambers and Boggs, 1993).

It is important to identify and discuss early what are patients' main concerns or feelings about dialysis. Very often the answer is 'everything' and they may need help to direct their thoughts and focus on specific issues. Information-giving should be broken down into manageable packages. Staff may be unsure about how much to give patients; this must be assessed on an individual basis and can be patient-led using specific models or tools such as the one discussed earlier.

While predialysis education is not wholly 'counselling', counselling interventions are required along with listening and attending skills. It is important to be able to pick up non-verbals, recognize when a patient is saturated and be aware of manipulation of questions and answers and selective listening on the patient's part. The problem for the patient is how to make sense of what is happening and how to build up knowledge and information to gain an accurate appraisal of the immediate future with its various possibilities (Nichols, 1984). The challenge for the renal team is to support him/her through this process.

Formal education programmes

Digioia (1992) identified a need to develop more formal programmes of predialysis education in the UK. Evaluation of such education programmes in North America proves them to be beneficial to patient well-being and in helping to make informed decisions about choice of dialysis treatment (Grumke and King, 1994; Stephenson and Vilano, 1993). They have the potential to influence hospitalization rates and urgent initiation

Table 4.3 Suggested topics for inclusion in a formal patient education programme

- Normal kidney function
- What happens when the kidneys do not work
- Medication and symptom control
- Principles of haemodialysis
- Transplantation
- Diet and renal failure
- Social Services/social worker
- Living with renal failure and RRT/psychologist
- Support groups/Kidney Patient Association
- Meet with other patients
- Visit dialysis and transplant units and meet other members of staff

of dialysis and it has been proposed that they can delay the need to initiate dialysis in end-stage renal disease (Binik *et al.*, 1993), possibly because of changes in dietary compliance and increased knowledge and expectation.

The teaching methods reported from the USA appear to be relatively didactic. Patients attend classes on a voluntary basis and their knowledge is formally assessed, usually by questionnaire or multiple choice (Brundage and Swearengen, 1994; Devins *et al.*, 1990). In following this line, there is a danger of becoming too focused on behavioural objectives and assessment, and a caring element must be maintained (Molzahn, 1996).

How such a programme is run will be dependent on what works best for the patients and the unit. Trying to cover everything in one day will be too much and it may be best to run it over a number of days or weeks. Table 4.3 identifies suggested topics for inclusion into an education programme. The venue and timing of the programme should aim to increase the potential attendance, taking into consideration the elderly, who may not want to leave their homes on a dark winter's night, people who work and people with young children. If attendance is voluntary, alternative plans must be made for those who do not.

Learning aids and resources

Written literature is essential to support any verbal information. The presentation of such documents should be clear, concise, with illustrations, and available in a number of languages as appropriate to the region. Illiteracy in an individual is not always immediately obvious but needs to be ascertained before continuing with any education programme so that learning material can be presented appropriately. A translation service may need to be used.

Video-tapes that can be loaned out to individuals to watch at home are often helpful. While they may be expensive to produce at a local level, there are a number of video-tapes concerning general aspects of RRT produced by the renal care industries.

Audio-tapes can be produced quite cheaply and may serve a purpose for people with learning or visual difficulties. They can also be produced to contain information specific to your particular unit and in a variety of languages.

Posters, or a selection of leaflets, can be displayed in the clinic or ward area. Leaflets should not only contain information about RRT but cover underlying diseases, control of blood pressure, anaemia, etc. These can be produced locally or commercially and are also available from patient organizations.

Computer or more interactive learning is an area that has not yet been developed to its full potential (Luker and Caress, 1992) but will probably be of value in the future.

Home assessment

Visiting patients at home is invaluable and an essential part of any predialysis programme. Meeting people on their own territory increases our understanding of their lifestyle, and gives us the opportunity to meet other family members and to begin discussing some of the more practical issues, especially if home dialysis is being considered. More importantly, it gives the patient and his/her family opportunity to discuss concerns and ask questions in an environment where they feel comfortable, where they may find it easier to show their emotion, and where they have one-to-one contact with a nurse. Caring for patients in their own homes may help diminish some of the feelings of powerlessness (Stapleton, 1992; Turton and Orr, 1985).

> **Key reference:** Stapelton, S. (1992) Nursing strategies to decrease powerlessness. In: Miller, J.F. *Coping with chronic illness: overcoming powerlessness* (2nd edition). F.A. Davies Co, Philadelphia.

If information is primarily given in the format of patient information days, the visit to the home is a way of making it more individual and more real to the patient. Discussions about lifestyle can be more relaxed, and looking around the room at photographs, books or trophies can give cues to initiate comments about holidays and hobbies and how dialysis can be adapted to fit around daily activities.

Family involvement

The impact of chronic ill-health and dialysis on family dynamics is well recognized and preparing the family for dialysis is as important as preparing the patient. Everyone can get involved in the discussions and preparations, although tact and sensitivity need to be demonstrated to ensure that this is what the family wants and that it is appropriate to their own dynamics. If a family is not used to discussing problems or crises in an open forum, they are more likely to find it threatening or alien. Discover how the family usually handles or tackles problems and work from that position.

Making decisions about dialysis

Carlsson and Ahlmen (1992) described how patients who received adequate information about treatment options were likely to feel satisfied with their choice, with possibly more patients choosing peritoneal dialysis in favour of haemodialysis (Ahlmen and Carlsson, 1993). Kochavi (1990) also indicated an increase in the CAPD programme following structured predialysis education, although it must be noted that these studies took place in the USA, which has a relatively smaller CAPD programme than the UK.

When making decisions and deciding which treatment modality will best suit their lifestyle, patients are forced to review their lives and decide which aspects of their lifestyle are of greatest importance. Values and threats are considered and alternatives weighed up (Whitaker and Albee, 1996). No two pathways towards a decision will be the same. Some will very quickly make their decision and find it relatively easy, others agonize over it for months and swap and change. This can simply be down to personality and how we normally make decisions in life. For some, delaying the decision may be part of their coping mechanism: in making a decision about dialysis modality, they are acknowledging that it is going to happen.

> **Key reference:** Whittaker, A.A. and Albee, B.J. (1996) Factors influencing patient selection of dialysis treatment modality. *ANNA Journal* 23(4); 369–375.

What can help with decision-making?

Any number of things may influence a patient's decision about choice of treatment modality. A need for autonomy and control will influence a patient's decision-making, as will what s/he has learned from the renal team and the education programme. Nurses and social workers have been described as the most informative in helping people make decisions about RRT (Holley and Barrington, 1991) although staff may unwittingly or unintentionally be biased in the way they talk about a treatment (Campbell, 1991).

> **Key reference:** Campbell, A. (1991) Strategies for improving dialysis decision making. *Peritoneal Dialysis International* 11: 173–178.

Other influences may include prior knowledge and experience (Whitaker and Albee, 1996) and information or accounts from other patients and friends. Information from such sources can become distorted and it may be necessary to spend some time clarifying misconceptions.

Family influence will be important, and seeing the treatment for themselves is also very helpful. Patients (and the carer/family) should be encouraged to visit both dialysis units to see the mechanics of the treatment and to meet other staff and patients.

The media can also be influential. Coverage of transplantation in particular has been ritualized and given very positive exposure (Karpf, 1988).

New developments in treatment may be the subject of daytime TV/radio debate. However, care needs to be taken when considering these sources: the general or sweeping statements made on these programmes to 'make good viewing' may be grasped by patients and interpreted by them with little relevance to their own circumstances.

Choosing not to commence dialysis

Renal replacement therapy is a treatment, not a cure, for end-stage renal disease. With the treatment follows an endless regimen of dialysis, medication and clinic appointments. Discussions and debate about the withdrawal or stopping of dialysis often leave us with no precise or definite answers to the dilemmas faced in clinical practice, and the final decision relies on human judgment (Auer, 1997).

In the USA, guidelines for acceptance of individuals on to a RRT programme have been suggested (Price, 1992; Moss *et al.*, 1993), although they are not considered acceptable to all in the nephrology field. Here in the UK, access to treatment for CRF is generally considered to be open to everyone in need of it, with an increasing number of elderly and people with concurrent problems such as diabetes now receiving treatment that had not previously been available to them.

Decisions about not commencing dialysis are made on an individual basis rather than following any specific criteria. Adapting successfully to chronic illness includes a conception that the quality and quantity of life are worth the struggle (Lubkin, 1990). Hence, there are some patients who feel they are not, can acknowledge that they are approaching the end of their lives and have no desire to extend it with RRT.

Three broad issues emerge during discussions about stopping dialysis (Auer, 1997), which can equally be applied to discussions about not commencing dialysis:

- protecting the rights of the patient able to make his/her own decision;
- protecting the dignity and best interests of the patient unable to make his/her own decision;
- helping those who are left come to terms with the consequences (Auer, 1997).

In practice, this option is not openly discussed with every patient, although some may spontaneously ask 'What happens if I don't have dialysis?' When considering this option, careful thought needs to be given to the types of question that need to be asked to understand this response, but finding the answers may not be easy. What information have we given the patient and their family? How can we assess if we have given them enough information and in a format they have been able to understand? Have they any immediate fears about dialysis that have the potential to be overcome? If they appear depressed, is this exacerbated by the uraemia? How can we assess if they are making an informed decision? Listening to patients' thoughts and concerns can help them clarify their reasons for their decision.

Discussions and decisions about whether or not to commence treatment should include the patient and family and members of the renal multidisciplinary team and primary health-care team, who may know the patient well. Ideally, everyone should be in agreement with regard to the course of action. This issue becomes a problem when the patient's request conflicts with medical or nursing (or family) opinion and the justifiable limits of patient autonomy are challenged (Kerridge *et al.*, 1995).

If a decision not to commence dialysis is made, the patient should continue to be followed up by the renal team to continue support and care and help control symptoms. It has been suggested that renal teams could learn from palliative-care teams working in the community (Oreopoulus, 1995). While the involvement of the palliative-care team in patient management would appear to be quintessential care, in practice this may prove difficult (Andrews, 1995), although it could be a service for future development.

On-going support

Having made the decision about treatment modality, the patient will continue to be monitored until s/he reaches end-stage. Some patients describe this as being 'in limbo'. It has usually been an intensive few months learning about dialysis and preparing for change, but then life continues as before.

During this period, information and education can be repeated and reinforced to increase patients' level of understanding. Training in the dialysis modality can also begin. Follow-up visits should continue as needs dictate, but are sensible prior to significant events, i.e. before admission for access or to commence treatment or training.

Education programmes and discussions about CRF and dialysis must always be realistic. People value an honest and open approach when being given information and while it is important to stress positive aspects of dialysis, both short- and long-term complications and potential problems must be discussed.

Access

Early creation of vascular access can help smooth the transition on to dialysis. Having a functioning fistula at the time of commencing dialysis may avoid later admission to hospital and reduce the need for insertion of temporary access. Both haemodialysis and peritoneal access can be planned ahead and patients can be taught to care for their access until it is required. However, a large proportion of access is still not planned adequately, requiring emergency access to be created.

Predialysis transplantation

Assessment regarding suitability for transplantation can take place prior to commencing dialysis and there is an excellent opportunity to consider and begin the run-up for living-relative donation. Timing of placement on the list needs to be carefully assessed, as will the criteria for the kidney to be transplanted should one become available.

Commencing dialysis

When is the best time to commence RRT? This will vary between individuals and there should be judicious assessment of the patient's general condition, their symptoms and serum biochemistry to commence therapy at an appropriate time (Walls, 1995). The use of urea kinetics as a guide to when to commence dialysis has also been suggested (Tattersall *et al.*, 1995) and may result in patients commencing dialysis earlier than if decisions are made based solely on urea and creatinine levels.

SPECIAL GROUPS

Patients with a failing renal transplant

Transplantation is often seen as a light at the end of the tunnel by dialysis patients. Although graft survival rates are consistently good, when a transplant fails patients have to resume dialysis for a second or possibly third time. They obviously have insight into what living with dialysis involves and maintaining hope can be difficult. If it has been many years since their last dialysis treatment, there is every reason why they should go through the same education programme as new patients. Staff may presume that a patient knows more than s/he does and there is a risk that such patients will be perceived to need less support and information.

Patients who present at end-stage

Some 30–40% of people with CRF will present at end-stage or in urgent need of dialysis without prior assessment and they will have to make a transition from dealing with acute ill-health to dealing with chronic ill-health. Large chunks of information given during their initial illness are likely to be forgotten and here more than anywhere information should be given in short bursts. They are likely to need a period of adjustment, and decisions regarding long-term RRT options may be best withheld or at least reviewed when the patient has been on the programme for a period of time. Patients who present in such a way often undergo haemodialysis in the acute phase and may opt to stay with this form of RRT. This may be because of the perceived threat of additional surgery or fears of the unknown, which may outweigh other positive factors (Whitaker and Albee, 1996). Presentation at end-stage has also been advanced as an explanation for non-compliance (Wolfson *et al.*, 1995).

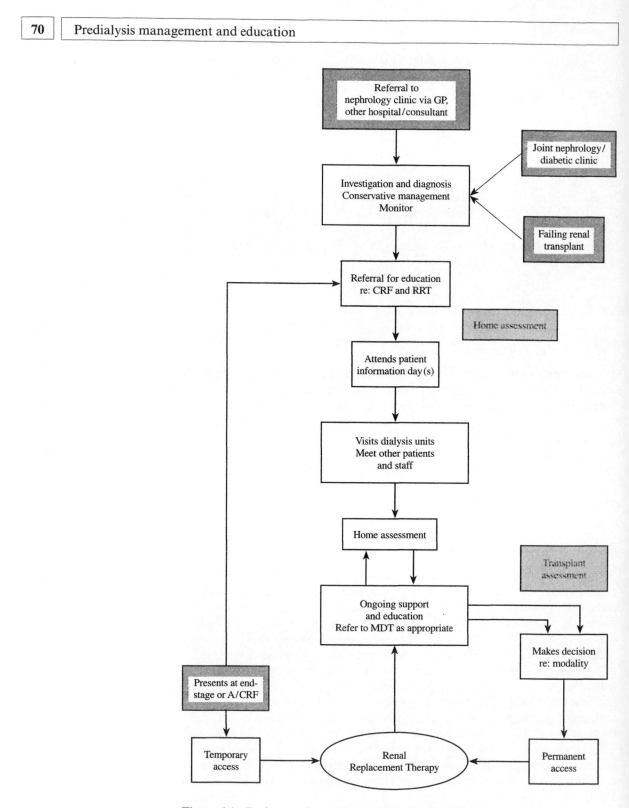

Figure 4.1 Patient pathways for predialysis education and support.

REVIEW QUESTIONS

- What strategies would you use to present information about renal replacement therapies to an individual like Tom?
- How best could you use the environment, facilities and resources you have?
- Who else could you involve in the support and education of the patient and his family during this stage?
- Thinking about a particular patient you have cared for, what was his/her reaction to new information and which issues needed greater priority?
- How can you assess a patient and ensure s/he is making an 'informed decision'?

REFERENCES

Ahlmen, J. and Carlsson, L. (1993) Well informed patients with end-stage renal failure prefer peritoneal dialysis to haemodialysis. *Peritoneal Dialysis International*, **13**(Suppl. 2), 196–198.

Andrews, P. (1995) Palliative care for patients with terminal renal failure (letter). *Lancet*, **346**, 506–507.

Auer, J. (1997) Dialysis withdrawal. *British Journal of Renal Medicine*, 2(1), 18–20.

Bergstrom, J. and Lindholm, B. (1993) Nutrition and adequacy of dialysis: how do haemodialysis and CAPD compare? *Kidney International*, **43**(Suppl. 40), S39–S50.

Binik, Y. M., Devins, G. M., Barre, P. E. *et al.* (1993) Live and learn: patient education delays the need to initiate renal replacement therapy in end-stage renal failure. *Journal of Nervous and Mental Diseases*, **181**(6), 371–376.

Bourgoignie, J. J. (1992) Progression of renal disease: current concepts and therapeutic approaches. *Kidney International*, **41**(Suppl. 36), S61–S65.

Bowlby, J. (1980) *Attachment and Loss 3: Loss, Sadness and Depression*, Penguin Books, Harmondsworth.

Brundage, D. and Swearengen, P. (1994) Chronic renal failure: evaluation and teaching tool. *American Nephrology Nurses Association Journal*, **21**(5), 265–270.

Buckman, R. (1992) *How to Break Bad News: A Guide for Health Care Professionals*, Pan Macmillan, London.

Campbell, A. (1991) Strategies for improving dialysis decision making. *Peritoneal Dialysis International*, **11**, 173–178.

Carlsson, L. and Ahlmen, J. (1992) Well informed patients with end-stage renal disease should be able to choose an appropriate mode of treatment. *European Dialysis and Transplant Nurses Association Journal*, **18**(3), 10–11.

Chambers, J. K. and Boggs, D. L. (1993) Development of an instrument to measure knowledge about kidney function, kidney failure and treatment options. *American Nephrology Nurses Association Journal*, **20**(6), 637–650.

Devins, G. M., Binik, M., Mandin, H. *et al.* (1990) The kidney disease questionnaire: a test for measuring patient knowledge about end-stage renal disease. *Journal of Clinical Epidemiology*, **43**(3), 297–307.

Diabetes Control and Complications Research Group (1995) The effect of intensive therapy on the development and progression of diabetic nephropathy in the Diabetes Control Complications Trial. *Kidney International*, **47**, 1703–1720.

Digioia, G. (1992) Do British renal units adequately prepare patients for treatment? *European Dialysis and Transplant Nurses Association Journal*, **18**(3), 8–9.

Feinstein, E. I. (1994) The skin, in *Handbook of Dialysis*, 2nd edn, (eds J. T. Daugirdas and T. S. Ing), Little, Brown & Co., Boston, MA.

Grumke, J. and King, K. (1994) Missouri kidney patient-education program: a 10 year review. *Dialysis and Transplantation*, **23**(12), 691–712.

Holley, J. L., Barrington, K. *et al.* (1991) Patient factors and the influence of nephrologists, social workers and nurses on patient decisions to choose Continuous Ambulatory Peritoneal Dialysis. *Advances in Peritoneal Dialysis*, **7**, 108–110.

Karpf, A. (1988) *Doctoring the Media*, Routledge, London.

Kerridge, I., Lowe, M. and Mitchell, K. (1995) Competent patients, incompetent decisions. *Annals of Internal Medicine*, **123**(11), 878–881.

Killingworth, A. (1995) Psychosocial impact of end-stage renal disease. *British Journal of Nursing*, **2**(18), 905–908.

Klahr, S., Levey, A., Beck, G. J. *et al.* (1994) The effects of dietary protein restriction and blood pressure control on the progression of chronic renal disease. *New England Journal of Medicine*, **330**(13), 877–884.

Kochavi, S. (1990) Implementing a pre-dialysis education programme for patients and families. *Dialysis and Transplantation*, **19**(10), 526–531.

Kubler-Ross, E. (1982) *Living with Death and Dying*, Souvenir Press, London.

Lewis, E. J., Hunsicker, L. G., Bain, R. P. and Rhode, R. D. (1993) The effect of angiotensin-converting inhibition on diabetic nephropathy. *New England Journal of Medicine*, **329**, 1456–1462.

Lim, V. (1991) Recombinant human erythropoietin in pre-dialysis patients. *American Journal of Kidney Diseases*, **4**, 34–37.

Lowrie, E. G. and Lew, N. (1990) Death risk in haemodialysis patients: the predictive value of commonly measured variables and an evaluation of death rate differences between facilities. *American Journal of Kidney Diseases*, **15**(5), 458–482.

Lubkin, I. (1990) *Chronic Illness: Impact and Interventions*, James Bartlett, London.

Luker, K. and Caress, A. L. (1992) Evaluating computer assisted learning for renal patients. *International Journal of Nursing Studies*, **29**(3), 237–250.

Miller, J. F. (1992) *Coping with Chronic Illness: Overcoming Powerlessness*, 2nd edn, F. A. Davis, Philadelphia, PA.

Molzahn, A. (1996) Changing to a caring paradigm for teaching and learning. *American Nephrology Nurses Association Journal*, **23**(1), 13–18.

Moss, A., Rettig, R. and Cassel, C. (1993) A proposal for guidelines for patient acceptance to and withdrawal from dialysis: a follow-up to the IOM report. *American Nephrology Nurses Association Journal*, **20**(5), 557–561.

Nichols, K. (1984) *Psychological Care in Physical Illness*, Chapman & Hall, London.

Oreopoulus, D. G. (1995) Withdrawal from dialysis: when letting die is better than helping live. *Lancet*, **346**(8966), 3–4.

Parkes, C. M. (1986) *Bereavement: Studies of Grief in Adult Life*, 2nd edn, Penguin Books, Harmondsworth.

Price, B. (1992) Is it time for patient selection criteria again? *Nephrology News and Issues*, **6**, 18–20.

Ramsdell, R. and Annis, C. (1996) Patient education: a continuing and repetitive process. *American Nephrology Nurses Association Journal*, **23**(2), 217–221.

Renal Association (1995) *Treatment of Adult Patients with Renal Failure: Recommended Standards and Audit Measure*, Royal College of Physicians of London, London.

Rollnick, S., Heather, N. and Bell, A. (1992) Negotiating behaviour change in medical settings: the development of brief motivational interviewing. *Journal of Mental Health*, 1, 25–37.

Roth, D., Smith, D., Schulman, G. *et al.* (1994) Effects of recombinant human erythropoietin on renal function in chronic renal failure pre-dialysis patients. *American Journal of Kidney Diseases*, **24**, 777–784.

Stapleton, S. (1992) Nursing strategies to decrease powerlessness, in *Coping with Chronic Illness: Overcoming Powerlessness*, 2nd edn, (ed. J. F. Miller), F. A. Davis, Philadelphia, PA.

Stephenson, K. and Vilano, G. (1993) Results of a pre-dialysis education program. *Dialysis and Transplantation*, **22**, 566–570.

Stott, N. C. H., Rollnick, S., Rees, M. R. and Pill, R. M. (1995) Innovation in clinical method: diabetes care and negotiating skills. *Family Practice*, **12**(4), 413–418.

Tattersall, J., Greenwood, R. and Farrington, K. (1995) Urea kinetics and when to commence dialysis. *American Journal of Nephrology*, **15**, 283–289.

Turner, P., Richens, A. and Routledge, P. (1986) *Clinical Pharmacology*, Churchill Livingstone, Edinburgh.

Turton, P. and Orr, J. (1985) *Learning to Care in the Community*, Hodder & Stoughton, London.

Uttley, L., Fawcett, J., Hutchinson, A. and Gokal, R. (1993) Phosphate control – what do our patients know? *European Dialysis and Transplant Nurses Association Journal*, **19**(4), 7–8.

Walls, J. (1995) Chronic renal failure – causes and conservative management. *Medicine*, **23**(4), 144–148.

Whittaker, A. A. and Albee, B. J. (1996) Factors influencing patient selection of dialysis treatment modality. *American Nephrology Nurses Association Journal*, **23**(4), 369–375.

Wolfson, M., Strong, C. and Hamel, K. (1995) Difficulty accepting lifestyle limitations after the abrupt onset of end-stage renal disease. *Advances in Renal Replacement Therapy*, **2**(3), 246–254.

Wright, B. (1993) *Caring in Crisis: A Handbook of Intervention Skills*, 2nd edn, Churchill Livingstone, Edinburgh.

5 | Acute renal failure

Paul Challinor

LEARNING OBJECTIVES

At the end of this chapter the reader should be able to:

- Identify those patients at risk of developing acute renal failure.
- Describe the nursing care of the patient in acute renal failure.
- Describe complications associated with acute renal failure, and discuss the nursing care involved.
- Describe the different forms of renal replacement therapy that may be used to treat a patient with acute renal failure.

INTRODUCTION

Acute renal failure (ARF) is often defined as a rapid and severe decline in renal function, with the consequent development of uraemia and hyperkalaemia due to the retention of substances normally excreted. It can occur over a number of days and is frequently associated with a specific cause; these are often categorized into three groups – prerenal, renal and postrenal. ARF is treatable, and often reversible unless the patient has some underlying renal dysfunction. However, it carries a high mortality rate of more than 50% despite the availability and development of dialysis treatments over recent decades (Abreo *et al.*, 1986; Kjellstrand and Solez, 1992). This high mortality rate may be influenced by the increased incidence of ARF in elderly patients undergoing more complicated surgical and medical treatments (Leblanc *et al.*, 1995).

Key reference: Leblanc, M., Tapolyai, M. and Paganini, E.P. (1995) What dialysis dose should be provided in acute renal failure? A review. *Advances in Renal Replacement Therapy* 2(3): 255–264.

An awareness of the risk factors and treatments involved in the nursing care of a patient with ARF could have a major impact on the mortality and morbidity associated with the disease. The nursing responsibility requires an understanding of the aetiologies and pathophysiology of ARF, and the potential clinical problems that may present when the patient is suffering from ARF.

CAUSES OF ACUTE RENAL FAILURE

The classification of the causes of ARF into the three groups of prerenal, renal and postrenal is to a certain extent artificial. There will be some crossover between groups with a number of causes. Prerenal refers to renal hypoperfusion resulting in oliguria but no parenchymal damage. Renal (intrinsic renal damage) refers to ARF associated with renal parenchymal damage, of which the most common cause is acute tubular necrosis (ATN) resulting from injury to glomerular capillaries and tubules. Postrenal refers to failure caused by obstruction distal to the tubules. Aetiology is important in deciding the appropriate management.

Prerenal acute renal failure

Prerenal failure results from a decreased renal blood flow and consequent reduced glomerular filtration rate, which is reversible and not associated with structural damage to the kidney (see Patient scenario below). Thus the patient is oliguric with a concentrated urine and an elevated plasma urea level, but responds to correction of the cause with a rapid reversal of the oliguria and uraemia.

Patient scenario

Mandy, a 23-year-old student, was admitted to the renal unit suffering from severe vomiting and diarrhoea, with resultant dehydration, following *Salmonella* poisoning. Her urine output had dropped below 400 ml/d and the plasma urea, creatinine and sodium levels were rising, although Mandy was suffering from hypokalaemia. A subclavian line was inserted and a CVP of -4 cmH$_2$O was recorded. Rehydration therapy was commenced and a positive CVP of 4–8 cmH$_2$O was maintained. Within 24 hours, renal function returned, with an associated increase in urine output. No dialysis was necessary. Six days after admission, Mandy was discharged when the diarrhoea and vomiting had subsided and her renal function was normal.

Intrarenal acute renal failure

This group is characterized by damage to the renal parenchyma resulting in a sudden deterioration of renal function. The most common cause of intrarenal damage is acute tubular necrosis following ischaemic damage or nephrotoxicity.

Severe and prolonged ischaemia results in necrotic changes to the glomerular basement membrane, as well as epithelial tubular damage (Brezis *et al.*, 1991). Unlike epithelial cells, basement membrane cells are unable to regenerate, which may result in irreversible damage. Patients at risk of developing ATN are those with hypotension, sepsis and trauma, but it is most common in patients combining sepsis and hypotension. This said, the sensitivity of patients to decreased renal perfusion is variable. Some tolerate hypotensive periods for hours without developing ATN, whereas others need only be hypotensive for minutes to develop it, although there is evidence that renal tissue damage will occur only if renal blood flow is less than 25–50% (Reubi, 1974; Meyrs *et al.*, 1984).

There are a large number of substances capable of causing nephrotoxic damage, not least drugs prescribed to combat infection or transplant rejection. The aminoglycoside antibiotics, the most common group to cause ATN, have nephrotoxicity as a major side-effect. ARF is a complication of between 10–16% of courses, even when monitoring of plasma levels is undertaken (Smith *et al.*, 1980). Nephrotoxic damage usually affects only the tubular epithelial cells, increasing the chance of the ATN being reversible.

Postrenal acute renal failure

Obstructive or postrenal failure accounts for less than 10% of all acute renal failure (Anderson and Schrier, 1988), but is easily diagnosed *via* ultrasound and is usually reversible. Causes include calculi, clots, bladder-neck obstruction, strictures and tumours. If obstruction is persistent, relief is obtained by insertion of a nephrostomy tube to bypass the obstruction until the cause can be cleared. Once the obstruction has been bypassed, a large diuresis may result. Care should be taken with fluid replacement and the electrolyte balance.

NURSING CARE

The nursing care of patients with established acute renal failure is primarily palliative in nature. Once renal failure is established, little can be done to restore function other than to treat the patient symptomatically until renal function returns. Nursing care can be divided into two main areas: established renal failure phase, or the oliguric stage; and the recovery phase or diuretic stage. The nursing care during each of these stages is slightly different, although in essence it is symptom management.

Established renal failure (oliguric) phase

Once a patient is in established renal failure, nursing care is aimed at preventing the complications of ARF from becoming potentially life-threatening, although the first line of treatment is always to treat the cause of the ARF.

The speed with which this phase is established depends upon the original cause of the ARF. It may become apparent suddenly, e.g. after a hypotensive episode, or may be more insidious following nephrotoxic damage by gentamicin. Urine output falls to below 400 ml/d, associated with an increase in serum creatinine, urea and potassium levels. The plasma urea increases daily, by approximately 3.6–8.9 mmol/l, and creatinine by 44–221 μmol/l (Rose, 1981). Hyperkalaemia (potassium levels greater than 5 mmol/l) and metabolic acidosis are also common during this phase. Clinical problems and nursing interventions are linked with these deranged physiological values and include symptoms of uraemia (nausea, vomiting, lethargy, pericarditis, coagulopathies), hyperkalaemia, fluid overload and increased susceptibility to infection.

Although ARF is associated with oliguria, between 30% and 60% of patients are non-oliguric and have a urine output in excess of 500 ml/d (Anderson *et al.*, 1977). Despite this, most patients in the early stages of acute renal failure are overhydrated, usually as a result of the delayed recognition of the onset of ARF, exacerbated by fluid challenges in an attempt to restore urine output (Hinds and Watson, 1996). The oliguric phase usually lasts 3–21 days. However, it is possible for this phase to last up to 3 months.

Diet

Dietary management plays an important role in the care of the patient with ARF. Tissue damage associated with ARF is often associated with catabolism, when the patient's energy requirements exceed the supply of available carbohydrates, resulting in the catabolism (breakdown) of the body's fats and protein stores.

Normally an individual requires around 2000 kcal of energy per day, but a patient in catabolic ARF requires considerably more, indicating that a calorie intake greater than 2000 kcal will be required to prevent deterioration in the patient's condition. As a general rule, the energy intake is based upon the patient's weight, and given as a ratio of 35 kcal/kg body weight. This should be reviewed regularly. If loss of body weight continues, then the energy intake should be increased. Energy is supplied in the form of carbohydrates and fats, and high-energy supplements are often required to meet the calorie target. Many supplements are in fluid form, and care must be taken not to exceed the fluid restriction while attempting to meet the calorie target.

Dietary protein intake in ARF has been undergoing review over recent years. Protein used to be restricted to 40 g per day. However, as most patients in ARF are given renal replacement therapy, protein intake is calculated at a rate of 1–1.2 g/kg body weight. This reduces the risk of malnourishment and catabolism during ARF. If peritoneal dialysis or haemofiltration are used as renal replacement therapies, protein intake may need to be increased. Protein losses *via* the peritoneum are widely recognized, but losses also occur *via* the haemofilter (Davies *et al.*, 1991).

Potassium is restricted to reduce the risk of hyperkalaemia and associated cardiac arrhythmias, although occasionally in non-oliguric ARF potassium restriction may not be required. Individual assessment of the patient's serum potassium is therefore recommended. Sodium may also be restricted, although most patients will be on a no-added-salt diet. If oedema is persistent despite fluid removal on dialysis, sodium may be restricted to

80–100 mmol/d. A high sodium intake can lead to thirst, making any fluid restriction difficult to maintain.

A number of authors in the past have advocated the use of parenteral nutrition to combat the effects of catabolism and negative nitrogen balances (Feinstein *et al.*, 1981; Baek *et al.*, 1975). However, the success of these studies have since been called into doubt, and recent authors have found no increase in the survival rates of patients treated with parenteral nutrition (Sponsel and Conger, 1995). In fact, the complications associated with parenteral nutrition, e.g. septicaemia, can exacerbate the already severe problems faced by the patient in acute renal failure.

> **Key reference:** Sponsel, H. and Conger, J.D. (1995) Is peritoneal nutrition therapy of value in acute renal failure patients? *American Journal of Kidney Diseases* 25(1): 96–102.

Fluid management

The fluid status of the patient in acute renal failure can be one of the most difficult areas to manage. The standard calculation for assessing daily requirements of fluid is 500 ml plus the equivalent amount of the previous day's urine output. The 500 ml is to replace that fluid lost by insensible loss: respiratory, faecal and perspiration loss. However, care must be taken: losses can be greatly increased if the patient is pyrexial, has diarrhoea, is vomiting or is losing large amounts of fluid following a burn. All fluid loss needs to be assessed and replaced.

Fluid balance monitoring is of utmost importance. An anuric patient may be restricted to a daily fluid allowance of 500 ml. This has to take into account oral fluids, as well as therapeutic fluids such as drugs and i.v. infusions. Fluid balance charts are the most common way of monitoring fluid balance. However, they are prone to inaccuracy – different nurses may chart differing volumes for the same cup size. Nor do they account for the ambulant patient who may be drinking from the bathroom tap. Fluid balance charts, however, have an important role in the monitoring of i.v. fluids and urinary output.

A more accurate method of fluid balance assessment is through daily weight – 1 kg equals 1000 ml, so any increases in weight should correspond to an increase in fluid retention. Weight should be recorded at the same time each day, with the patient wearing similar clothing. Inaccuracies can occur with weighing, especially if the scales are poorly maintained and calibrated but, in conjunction with fluid balance charts, accurate fluid balance assessment and trends can be identified.

Central venous pressure (CVP) monitoring provides the greatest accuracy when assessing fluid balance, although not every patient will require monitoring in this way. If CVP monitoring is being used then care must be taken to ensure that the zero is calibrated from the same place each time, either mid-sternum or mid-axilla, to prevent any errors occurring that may affect treatment. A CVP measurement of <0 cmH$_2$O is suggestive of volume depletion, and remedial action is required to replace the fluid. Pulmonary capillary wedge pressure (PCWP) measurement may also be indicated in acutely ill patients, especially those in cardiogenic shock. The risks associated with insertion of CVP and PCWP lines (haemorrhage, pneumothorax and infection) should be weighed against the value of the information gained and its influence on the treatment of the individual patient.

Oedema due to fluid overload may initially exhibit as left ventricular failure, especially if a fluid challenge has been given to reverse hypotension. Only later will dependent oedema present itself.

Control of infection

Infection presents problems for patients in ARF both as a causative factor and as a complication of ARF. Uraemia causes a reduction in the immune status of the patient (Schattner, 1994; Wardle, 1994), increasing the chance of serious infections such as septicaemia and pneumonia. This is further complicated by a reduction in core temperature, also due to uraemia. A patient may be harbouring a subacute infection initially, although it may not register as pyrexia. Other signs of infection must be taken into account when monitoring the patient.

Complications of acute renal failure

Hyperkalaemia

Hyperkalaemia presents as one of the most common complications of ARF, and one of the most dangerous. A serum potassium of more than 6 mmol/l greatly increases the chance of a cardiac arrest, although hyperkalaemia of less than this can also lead to cardiac arrhythmias. All renal patients are in danger, although those who are catabolic or suffering from rhabdomyolysis are at particular risk. However, patients with non-oliguric ARF are at less risk, and may even require potassium supplements.

Hyperkalaemia can be controlled in a number of ways. Calcium resonium may be given orally or rectally. It is important to check the patient's bowel actions regularly, as calcium resonium can cause severe constipation. If given rectally, calcium resonium should be mixed with methyl cellulose, reducing the chance of faecal impaction.

An infusion of 12 units of insulin and 50% dextrose (50 ml) will quickly reduce the plasma potassium by shifting potassium into the intracellular compartment. This is only a short-term effect: once the infusion is finished potassium will shift back into the vascular compartment, raising the serum concentration. The most effective way of controlling potassium is by renal replacement therapy.

Infection

Infection is a common complication associated with ARF, in part caused by the immunosuppression secondary to uraemia. Table 5.1 presents the infections most likely to be encountered.

Table 5.1 Common infections associated with acute renal failure (Source: adapted from Cumming and Winchester, 1994)

Infection	Cause	Prevention/treatment
Septicaemia	Cannulation Venous/arterial catheterization	Strict aseptic technique during insertion Observation Adequate dressing technique
Pneumonia	Pulmonary oedema Hypostasis Bedrest	Strict fluid balance monitoring Prevention of fluid overload Chest physiotherapy
Urinary tract infection	Urethral catheter Low urine output	Remove catheter if oliguric Strict aseptic technique during insertion and while *in situ*

With good nursing care infections should be avoided or identified at an early stage. Awareness of the risks should reduce the high mortality rate associated with infections and ARF.

Hypervolaemia

Electrolyte and water imbalances due to the ARF result in fluid retention. The oliguric patient is unable to excrete excess fluid, resulting in volume overload. In its less malignant form, fluid overload presents as dependent tissue oedema, associated with hyponatraemia due to sodium dilution by the excess fluid. Fluid overload in its malignant form results in pulmonary oedema and is often exacerbated by anaemia and any pre-existing cardiac disease. Pulmonary oedema as a complication of ARF carries a high mortality rate.

Initially fluid overload is treated with diuretics – especially frusemide, because of its renal vasodilatory effect – supported by dopamine in an attempt to convert oliguric ARF into non-oliguric ARF (Dolleris, 1992). If this is achieved, these patients are easier to manage and may require less dialysis. However, if the oliguric state persists, then fluid removal can only be achieved by dialysis or haemofiltration.

Haemorrhage

Coagulopathies associated with decreased platelet function due to the uraemic syndrome (Kjellstrand *et al.*, 1992) represent a real problem for patients with acute renal failure. This is further compounded by the use of anticoagulants during haemodialysis and haemofiltration, leading to an increase in the risk of gastric bleeding.

Uraemic pericarditis

If the patient complains of chest pain, especially on inspiration, uraemic pericarditis should be suspected. It is associated with a plasma urea in excess of 35 mmol/l, and frequently resolves once the urea levels have been reduced following dialysis. Because anticoagulation is usually used during dialysis or haemofiltration, care must be taken to prevent a cardiac tamponade. Clotting levels need to be closely monitored and the patient should be dialysed with a tight heparin regimen to reduce the risk of bleeding. Non-steroidal anti-inflammatories may also be prescribed if the patient remains symptomatic. If this is the case, the risk of gastric bleeding should be noted, as well as the fact that this group of drugs is also nephrotoxic. But the primary control of uraemic pericarditis remains dialysis.

Recovery (diuretic) phase

It is difficult to predict when the recovery phase will begin in individual patients. Factors that may influence the time spent in the established phase include the underlying cause of the ARF and the extent of the damage caused to the nephrons (ATN). The most common scenario is an increase in urine output on a daily basis, although not all patients experience diuresis as renal function improves. Diuresis can be large, in excess of 10 l/d. This is caused by loss of medullary concentration, fluid overload and a failure in tubular sodium and water reabsorption due to damage (Cumming and Winchester, 1994).

Care must be taken to ensure that fluid replacement keeps up with the urine output. Dehydration is a risk during this stage, but overhydration will perpetuate the large diuresis. However, the diuresis usually stabilizes within 5–8 days.

Sodium and potassium losses also increase, and the serum levels must be checked regularly with a view to relaxing the dietary restrictions and providing supplements if necessary. Protein intake should be monitored until renal function has recovered sufficiently to clear urea generation.

Following ATN there may be a time lag between the onset of diuresis and restoration of normal renal function. Dialysis therapy should therefore be given until renal function has recovered sufficiently.

RENAL REPLACEMENT THERAPY

There are three options for renal replacement therapy: haemodialysis, peritoneal dialysis and haemofiltration – continuous arteriovenous haemofiltration (CAVH), continuous venovenous haemofiltration (CVVH) and haemodiafiltration (CVVHD).

The decision to commence replacement therapy is influenced by a number of factors, usually associated with the symptomology and the care required. A urea greater than 35 mmol/l and/or a plasma creatinine greater than 500 μmol/l is usually indicative for the need for intervention, although lower levels may be consistent with severe symptomology requiring earlier intervention.

Hyperkalaemia can invariably be controlled by the means outlined above, but usually only in the short term. Uncontrollable hyperkalaemia requires dialysis for effective control. In the anuric–oliguric patient, dialysis will certainly be required to control fluid balance and to allow enough fluid space to deliver medication and dietary requirements.

Haemodialysis

Haemodialysis plays an important role in the care of the patient with ARF, despite an increase in the use of haemofiltration. Patients do not require nursing in the intensive care unit and are stable enough to be nursed within the renal ward, allowing for increased mobility and reducing the risks associated with prolonged bedrest. However, because haemodialysis is more aggressive than haemofiltration, it is a difficult procedure to undertake in hypotensive patients, which reduces the ability to create fluid space. The amount of fluid that can be removed is also less (around 0.5–2 litres) than the potential volumes that can be removed with haemofiltration.

Venous access is created via the use of a subclavian line (Chapter 7). The first haemodialysis session should be restricted to 1.5–2 hours, with the aim of reducing the plasma urea level by 30% to reduce the risk of disequilibrium syndrome, especially if the patient has a urea level in excess of 40 mmol/l. If the patient is catabolic, dialysis will probably need to be repeated daily for 3–4 hours per session, but as the catabolic stage passes this could be reduced to alternate days.

Bicarbonate concentrate should be used in all ARF patients to avoid the vasodilatory and acidotic effects of acetate dialysis. This is even more important in patients with liver dysfunction. Acetate is converted to bicarbonate in the liver; if conversion is delayed then increasing levels of acetate will exacerbate the acidotic state of the patient.

Peritoneal dialysis

The use of peritoneal dialysis (PD) as a first-line treatment in ARF has fallen out of fashion in recent years, being replaced by haemodialysis or haemofiltration. It does still retain a number of advantages over both haemodialysis and haemofiltration, but these tend to be outweighed by its disadvantages in respect to the other treatments. Peritoneal dialysis is simple and inexpensive to set up and run. If protocols are followed, relatively inexperienced nursing staff can provide an adequate dialysis. PD does not require the use of large doses of anticoagulants, which would be of benefit in patients already suffering from coagulopathies, although the risk of peritonitis and access site leaks restricts its effectiveness and it cannot be used following abdominal surgery or if there is a history of adhesions.

PD is usually well tolerated by acutely ill patients because of the continuous nature of the dialysis. However, patients being ventilated may experience increased respiratory pressures due to the fluid pressing on the diaphragm (Bargmann, 1990).

Adequate clearances are achieved by exchanges of 1.36% dialysate of 1500–2000 ml over short periods of time, around 60–90 minutes (Hutchinson and Gokal, 1995). If the patient cannot tolerate volumes of this size, smaller volumes and shorter cycles using a PD cycler will achieve good clearances. Many units build up to 2000 ml volumes over a 24–48-hour period to prevent leakage from the access site.

> **Key reference:** Hutchinson, A.J. and Gokal, R. (1995) Peritoneal dialysis in the ICU: What is its role? *Care of the Critically Ill* 11(3): 111–113.

Short PD cycles can cause hypokalaemia, so monitoring of the plasma potassium level is important. If hypokalaemia occurs, potassium can be added to the PD bags. Peritonitis remains the single greatest obstacle to the use of PD in the acute setting. Valeri *et al.* (1993) found that the incidence of peritonitis using closed-system PD was 1.7 per 100 patient days. This means that by day 15 of PD treatment the risk of developing peritonitis is 50%. This corresponds with a peritonitis rate among CAPD patients of less than 0.2 per 100 days.

Haemofiltration

The development of haemofiltration (HF) over the past decade has led to an increased number of clinical areas to care for ARF patients without the support of a renal unit on site. Continuous arteriovenous haemofiltration was first described by Henderson and colleagues in the 1960s. However, the equipment was cumbersome and complicated, and the treatment never caught on. This was taken further in 1976 by Silverstein, who, unlike Henderson, used haemofiltration in isolation from haemodialysis. However, the credit for the clinical application of haemofiltration as used today should go to Kramer, who was the first to use it as a treatment for acute fluid overload.

Haemofiltration has a number of **advantages over PD and haemodialysis**. The two main principles involved in HF are ultrafiltration and convection. Ultrafiltration (Figure 5.1(a)) is solely concerned with the movement of fluid across a membrane with the aid of a pressure gradient that acts as the driving force. This pressure can be altered in a number of ways, e.g. increasing the blood pump speed or altering the height difference between the filter and collection bag. Convection (Figure 5.1(b)) describes the movement of solute that occurs with the flow of fluid. This is different from the process of diffusion. As fluid moves across the filter it pulls solutes (urea, creatinine, sodium, potassium, etc.) with it. The rate of convection is dependent upon the size of the solute (the larger the molecule the slower the rate of convection), hydrostatic pressure, membrane permeability and ultimately the ultrafiltration rate.

Advantages over peritoneal dialysis

- Greater patient comfort
- Improved fluid balance management
- Can be used after abdominal surgery
- No risk of peritonitis

Advantages over haemodialysis

- Greater cardiovascular stability
- Reduced risk of disequilibrium
- Allows for greater fluid space

Continuous arteriovenous haemofiltration

Filtration is achieved by blood passing from an arterial catheter through a filter and returning *via* a venous catheter (Figure 5.2). Filtration is dependent upon the patient's blood pressure. Hypotensive patients are

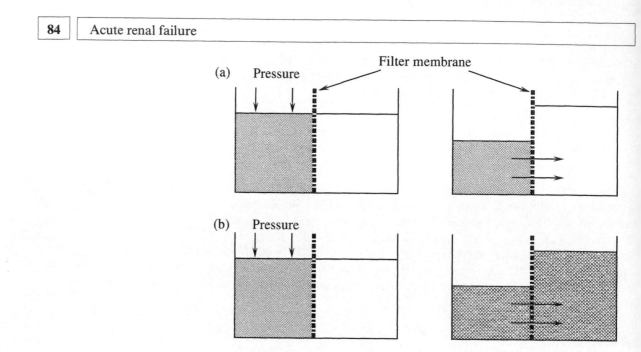

Figure 5.1 Ultrafiltration and convection. **(a)** Ultrafiltration: movement of water caused by a pressure gradient. **(b)** Convection: movement of solute dragged by fluid movement.

rarely able to provide enough arterial pressure to drive the blood through the system, often resulting in clotting of the lines and/or filter. With a cardiovascularly stable patient, an average filtrate of 10–15 l/24 h eliminates on average 18 mmol/l of urea in a patient with a concentration of 30 mmol/l, and is usually enough to maintain stasis. In a catabolic patient the system may have difficulty in achieving adequate clearances.

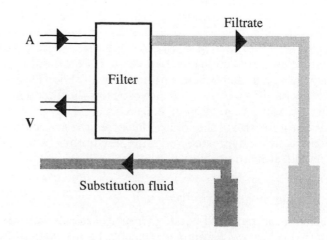

Figure 5.2 Continuous arteriovenous haemofiltration.

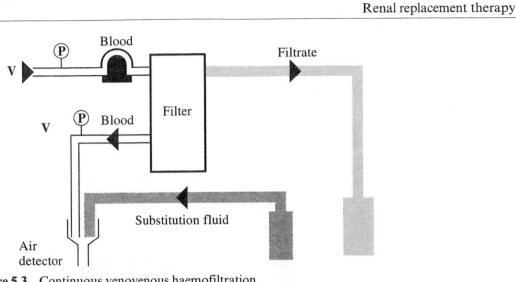

Figure 5.3   Continuous venovenous haemofiltration.

Continuous venovenous haemofiltration

The problems of relying upon blood pressure to drive the system are overcome by adding a blood pump to guarantee blood flow through the haemofilter (Figure 5.3). This in turn will increase the ultrafiltration rate and ultimately convection. Hypotension is no longer a limitation to the use of haemofiltration.

Continuous venovenous haemodiafiltration

This relies upon the use of a dialysis solution running through the filter to clear solutes *via* diffusion and fluid removal *via* osmosis (Figure 5.4). In this case, ultrafiltration and convection play a smaller role in clearance rates.

Nursing responsibilities when caring for a patient on haemofiltration

Haemofiltration is very effective at creating fluid space for nutritional (especially total parenteral nutrition) and other therapeutic fluids. Accurate input and output charting is therefore important as a tool in assessing the patient's fluid balance. Although this can only be part of the assessment, blood pressure, CVP and pulmonary wedge pressures are also important in this assessment process. Juggling with fluid volumes can be complicated by wound drainage, nasogastric drainage, urinary output, drugs, total parenteral nutrition (TPN) and changes in filtrate volume.

The filtration rate and its adjustment depends upon the requirement of a negative or positive fluid balance, which will vary depending upon the patient's condition and the original cause of the ARF. Filtration rates can be adjusted by altering the height differential between the filter and the collecting bag. The higher the filter the greater the siphoning effect, increasing the filtration rate, although if the patient is on CAVH, raising the height

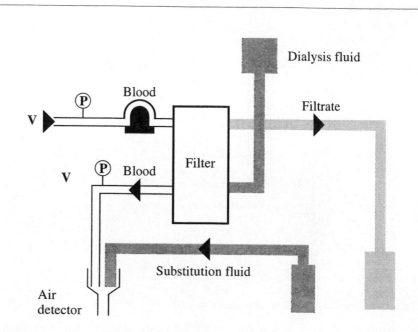

Figure 5.4 Continuous venovenous haemodiafiltration.

of the filter above the level of the patient's heart will reduce the flow and subsequently the filtration rate. Increasing or decreasing the blood pump speed can also affect the filtration rate.

Many units use volumetric pumps on the filtrate line to control the rate. Care must be taken with this system: many volumetric pumps are designed to pump fluid, not to act as a volumetric control, and inaccuracies can occur. Measuring the filtrate volume manually will prevent such inaccuracies.

Replacement fluid is given to prevent dehydration of the patient, to replace essential electrolytes lost in the filtrate and to provide a buffer to counteract the metabolic acidosis associated with ARF. It can be given either prefilter or postfilter. Prefilter fluid can help to prolong the life of the filter as it reduces the haematocrit, reducing the chance of clotting occurring in the filter. However, it does increase the cost of replacement fluid, as a certain amount of the replacement fluid will be filtered out, making it difficult to gain accurate fluid balance studies. Postfilter replacement fluid has the advantage of allowing greater accuracy in fluid balance studies, but in relation to prefilter replacement the clotting risk is increased.

Regular checks on the clotting status of the system is required if the filter is to remain efficient for any length of time. If heparin is to be used, then activated clotting times (ACT) should be checked regularly and kept at a level appropriate to the patient's condition. An ACT should be taken to identify a baseline level, and then anticoagulant should be given to keep the clotting time 20–30% longer. If there is a high risk of clotting low-molecular-weight heparin is given.

Clotting of the lines and filter is also affected by the pump speed. Below 75 ml/min, the risk of stasis within the filter increases the chance of clotting within individual fibres of the filter. However, blood pump speeds of greater than 150 ml/min for the protracted periods that are associated with haemofiltration damage red blood cells and platelets, thereby increasing the risk of coagulopathies. The presence of high plasma lipid levels increases the coagulability of the blood within the filter. This problem is associated with high-lipid TPN.

The use of a system such as haemofiltration requires that the integrity of connections are regularly checked to prevent the risk of air emboli or the introduction of infection. Most HF machines have fail-safe devices, so that if an alarm sounds the blood pump will stop automatically. The problem needs to be identified quickly to ensure patient safety and to limit blood stasis that might result in clot development.

CONCLUSION

ARF carries a high mortality rate, which has not improved over the past decade despite the increased complexity and success of treatments. This may be a reflection of the age and numbers of patients being treated. But that does not affect the fact that a number of cases can be prevented by identifying those at risk of developing ARF and taking remedial action. Good nursing care can prevent many of the complications associated with the condition.

REVIEW QUESTIONS

- Describe the nursing care required for a patient with prerenal acute renal failure.
- What special considerations must be taken when using peritoneal dialysis on a patient with acute renal failure?
- What advantages has haemofiltration over haemodialysis when used to treat a patient in acute renal failure?
- Describe the nursing care required during the diuretic phase of acute renal failure.
- Describe the dietary considerations for a patient with acute renal failure.

REFERENCES

Abreo, K., Moorthy, A. and Osborne. M. (1986) Changing patterns and outcome of acute renal failure requiring dialysis. *Archives of Internal Medicine*, **146**, 1338–1341.

Anderson, R. J. and Schrier, R. W. (1988) Acute tubular necrosis, in *Diseases of the Kidney*, (eds R. W. Schrier and C. W. Gottshalk), Little, Brown & Co., Boston, MA.

Anderson, R., Linus, S., Berns A. *et al.* (1977) Non-oliguric acute renal failure. *New England Journal of Medicine*, **296**, 1134–1138.

Baek, R., Makaboli, G., Bryan-Brown, C. *et al.* (1975) The influence of parenteral nutrition on the course of acute renal failure. *Surgery, Gynecology and Obstetrics*, **141**, 405–408.

Bargmann, J. M. (1990) Complications of peritoneal dialysis related to raised intra-abdominal pressure. *Dialysis and Transplantation*, **19**, 70–81.

Brezis, M., Rosen, S., and Epstein, F. H. (1991) Acute renal failure, in *The Kidney*, 4th edn, (eds B. M. Brenner and F. C. Rector), W. B. Saunders, Philadelphia, PA.

Cumming, A. D. and Winchester, J. F. (1994) Acute renal failure and poisoning, in *Renal Dialysis*, (eds J. D. Briggs, B. J. R. Junor, R. S. C. Rodger and J. F. Winchester), Chapman & Hall, London.

Davies, A., Reaveley, D. A., Brown, E. A. and Kox, W. J. (1991) Amino acid clearance and daily losses in patients with acute renal failure treated with continuous arteriovenous haemofiltration. *Critical Care Medicine*, **19**, 1510.

Dayton, K. D. and Lancaster, L. E. (1995) Effects of renal failure and its treatment on the immune system and assessment of immune system function. *American Nephrology Nurses Association Journal*, 22(6), 530–572.

Dolleris, P. M. (1992) Diuretic and vasopressor usage in acute renal failure: a synopsis. *Critical Care Nursing Quarterly*, **14**(4), 28–31.

Feinstein, E. I., Blumenkrantz, M., Healy, M. *et al.* (1981) Clinical and metabolic responses to parenteral nutrition in acute renal failure. *Medicine*, **60**, 124–137.

Hinds, C. J. and Watson, D. (1996) *Intensive Care: A Concise Textbook*, 2nd edn, W. B. Saunders, Philadelphia, PA.

Hutchinson, A. J. and Gokal, R. (1995) Peritoneal dialysis in the ICU: what is its role? *Care of the Critically Ill*, **11**(3), 111–113.

Kjellstrand, C. M., Jacobson, S. and Lins, L. (1992) Acute renal failure, in *Replacement of Renal Function by Dialysis*, 3rd edn, (ed. J. F. Maher), Kluwer Academic Publishers, Dordrecht.

Kjellstrand, C. M. and Solez, K. (1992) Treatment of acute renal failure, in *Diseases of the Kidney*, 5th edn, (eds R. W. Schrier and C. W. Gottshalk), Little, Brown & Co., Boston, MA.

Leblanc, M., Tapolyai, M. and Paganini, E. P. (1995) What dialysis dose should be provided in acute renal failure? A review. *Advances in Renal Replacement Therapy*, **2**(3), 255–264.

Meyrs, B. D., Millar, C. and Mehigan, J. T. (1984) Nature of the renal injury following total renal ischemia in man. *Journal of Clinical Investigation*, **73**, 329.

Reubi, F. C. (1974) The pathogenesis of anuria following shock. *Kidney International*, **5**, 106.

Rose, B. D. (1981) *Pathophysiology of Renal Disease*, McGraw-Hill, New York.

Schattner, A. (1994) Lymphokines in autoimmunity – a critical review. *Clinical Immunology and Immunopathology*, **70**(3), 177–189.

Smith, C. R., Lipski, J. J. and Laskin, O. L. (1980) Double blind comparison of the nephrotoxicity and auditory toxicity of gentamicin and tobramycin. *New England Journal of Medicine*, **302**, 1106.

Sponsel, H. and Conger, J. D. (1995) Is parenteral nutrition therapy of value in acute renal failure patients? *American Journal of Kidney Diseases*, **25**(1), 96–102.

Valeri, A., Radhakrishnan, J., Vernocchi, L. *et al.* (1993) The epidemiology of peritonitis in acute peritoneal dialysis: a comparison between open and closed drainage systems. *American Journal of Kidney Diseases*, **21**, 300–309.

Wardle, E. N. (1994) Acute renal failure and multiorgan failure. *Nephrology, Dialysis and Transplantation*, **9**(Suppl. 4), 104–107.

6 Principles of haemodialysis

Paul Challinor

LEARNING OBJECTIVES

At the end of this chapter the reader should be able to:

- Describe the principles of haemodialysis.
- Explain the effects of using different filters.
- Describe the effects of using different dialysis solutions.
- Describe the use of anticoagulants during haemodialysis.

INTRODUCTION

The principles of haemodialysis are dependent upon a number of simple phenomena, namely diffusion, osmosis and ultrafiltration. The term haemodialysis itself is derived from two roots: *haemo-*, meaning blood, and *dialysis*, meaning filtration or cleansing. The process of haemodialysis, then, is the filtration from the blood, *via* a semi-permeable membrane, of toxic substances that are then carried away by dialysis fluid. The process primarily employs diffusion for solute removal, and osmosis and ultrafiltration for fluid removal, although the role of osmosis is limited in haemodialysis.

DIFFUSION

All molecules in any substance, solid, liquid or gas, are in a continuous state of movement at body temperature because of the heat energy they contain. This random thermal motion of molecules in a liquid or gas will tend to redistribute them uniformly throughout the container – the process of diffusion. Some molecules are able to diffuse across cell membranes. The rate of spread of these molecules depends upon the concentration differences in solutions, size and electric charge of the particles. It is this diffusion of particles across a semi-permeable membrane that is the basis of dialysis.

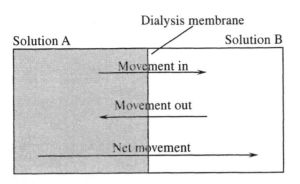

Figure 6.1 The two-way movement of solutes during the process of diffusion.

Diffusion is not purely a one-way movement of solutes from one compartment to another (Figure 6.1). Diffusion occurs in both directions between the two solutions involved; however, there is a net flux of the solute from the compartment containing the higher concentration to the lower. In haemodialysis, the removal of uraemic toxins from the blood into the dialysis fluid occurs because of the concentration gradient from blood to dialysate across the dialysis membrane, which acts as a semi-permeable membrane. If various solutes, such as acetate, bicarbonate and calcium, are added to the dialysate, these are transported from dialysate to blood because of the higher concentration of these solutes in the dialysate relative to the blood. This allows correction of plasma solute concentration abnormalities due to renal dysfunction. Uraemic toxins are removed, and hypocalcaemia and acid–base balance are corrected.

OSMOSIS

Water is a small, polar molecule about 0.3 nm in diameter that rapidly diffuses across cell membranes. Osmosis is the net diffusion of water from a region of high water concentration to a region of low water concentration when the movement of solute is inhibited. There are thus two components to osmosis: (1) the diffusion of water and (2) a barrier that limits solute movement but allows water movement.

The movement of water across a membrane that is permeable to water but not permeable to solute leads to an equilibrium state in which there is a change in the volumes of the two compartments caused by the net transfer of water from one to the other (Figure 6.2).

ULTRAFILTRATION

The majority of fluid removed during dialysis is achieved by the process of ultrafiltration (UF). Fluid removal occurs across the dialysis membrane *via* a transmembrane pressure gradient generated across the membrane. A

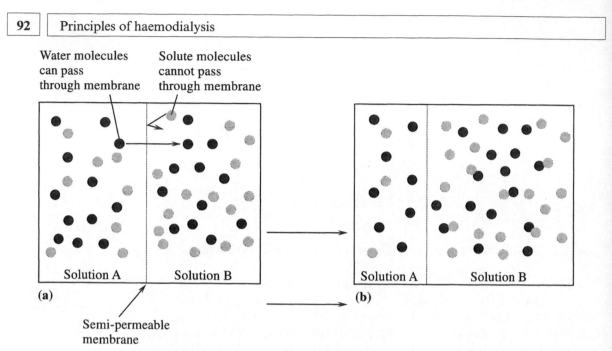

Figure 6.2 The movement of water by osmosis across a semi-permeable membrane. **(a)** Solutions A and B have the same volumes but different solute concentrations. **(b)** Through osmosis, the movement of water from solution A to solution B has resulted in equilibrium of the solution concentrations, but solution B has now increased in volume because of the influx of water from solution A.

hydrostatic pressure is created where the pressure of fluid is greater on one side of the dialysis membrane than on the other (Figure 6.3). These hydrostatic pressure gradients are created by either positive pressure on the blood compartment side of the dialyser or negative pressure on the dialysate side. These two forces conspire to create a loss of fluid from the blood into the dialysate, which is controllable by the adjustment of the pressure created across the dialyser membrane – otherwise known as the transmembrane pressure (TMP).

REMOVAL OF WASTE PRODUCTS BY HAEMODIALYSIS

Renal failure results in the accumulation of a great number of different toxins, which otherwise would have been excreted *via* the kidneys. These toxins are either the byproducts of normal cellular metabolism (e.g. creatinine, urea, uric acid, potassium, hydrogen and phosphate ions) or due to environmental poisons (e.g. antibiotics or other drugs). These toxins come in a variety of sizes, but the majority are relatively small molecules, with a molecular weight of less than 500 daltons. These smaller molecules diffuse across cellular membranes readily, according to their concentration gradients. This principle also holds true for diffusion across the dialyser (Figure 6.4). However, there are other metabolites, classed as middle molecules (mol. wt 300–2000 daltons), which diffuse poorly across most conventional membranes (Van Stone and Daugirdas, 1994). It is therefore molecules of

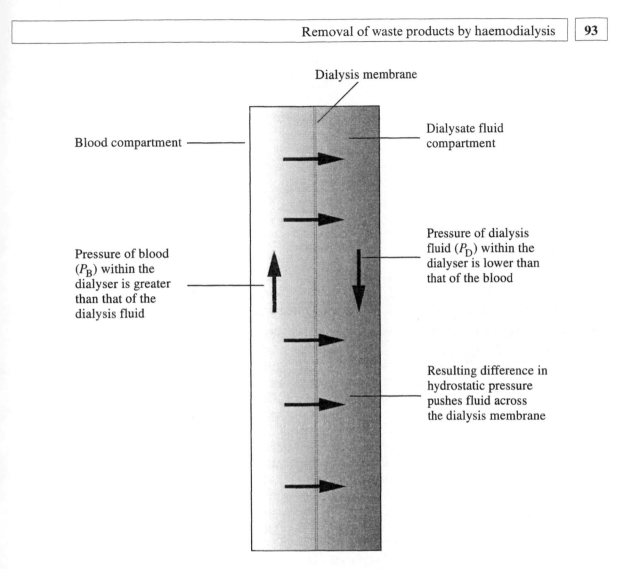

Dialysis membrane

Blood compartment

Dialysate fluid compartment

Pressure of blood (P_B) within the dialyser is greater than that of the dialysis fluid

Pressure of dialysis fluid (P_D) within the dialyser is lower than that of the blood

Resulting difference in hydrostatic pressure pushes fluid across the dialysis membrane

Figure 6.3 Ultrafiltration of fluid across the dialysis membrane due to higher fluid (hydrostatic) pressure in the blood compartment of the dialyser.

this size that are suspected of causing some of the uraemic symptoms still experienced by some individuals despite regular dialysis.

During dialysis, solutes move from the blood compartment of the dialyser down a concentration gradient into the dialysate. Dialysate contains specific concentrations of solutes to prevent 'overdialysing' of the patient, depleting the plasma sodium, calcium, etc. Various dialyses provide different concentrations of sodium, potassium, calcium, glucose, bicarbonate and acetate.

Clearance rates

The dialysis process occurs throughout the dialyser, so that by the time the blood reaches the end of the dialyser the uraemic toxin levels are lower than

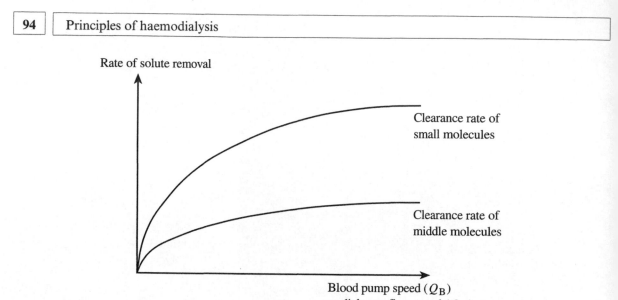

Rate of solute removal

Clearance rate of small molecules

Clearance rate of middle molecules

Blood pump speed (Q_B) or dialysate flow speed (Q_D)

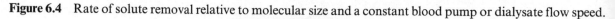

Figure 6.4 Rate of solute removal relative to molecular size and a constant blood pump or dialysate flow speed.

when it entered it. The rate of diffusion (clearance) depends upon the initial plasma concentration and the clearance rate of the dialyser. The higher the concentration, the faster the diffusional process will occur. Because of this, it is important that care is taken with patients who are suffering acute renal failure, or those with end-stage renal disease requiring dialysis for the first time. These individuals are at risk of disequilibrium syndrome because the body is not able to cope initially with the sudden drop in plasma levels of urea, creatinine and sodium.

The movement of solutes is not necessarily a one-way process. Excess salts such as sodium, potassium, chloride, urea and creatinine pass out from the blood into the dialysate solution. However, some of the therapeutic benefits of dialysis do not derive purely from removal of solutes. A buffer also passes across the dialyser membrane, but in this case it will be from the dialysate into the blood, helping to reverse the metabolic acidosis associated with end-stage renal failure. Throughout dialysis movement of waste products and excess salts occurs by diffusion into the dialysate, evening out the disparity in concentrations between dialysate and blood.

Initially during dialysis, it is only the concentrations of solutes and waste products that are affected. Intracellular concentrations alter only on a relatively long-term basis, over a matter of hours. Diffusion across the membrane causes a fall in the plasma concentration of solutes, which in turn creates a diffusional gradient difference between the intravascular and intercellular fluid compartments (Figure 6.5).

This in turn causes excess waste products and solutes to diffuse down their concentration gradients into the blood, creating another concentration gradient between the intercellular fluid and the intracellular fluid. It is for this reason that serum potassium levels appear to increase rapidly immediately after dialysis. Movement of potassium occurs over a number

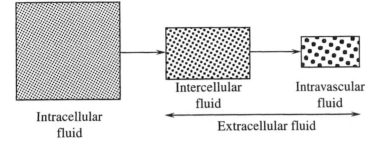

Intracellular
fluid

Intercellular
fluid

Intravascular
fluid

Extracellular fluid

Figure 6.5   Movements of fluid between body compartments during dialysis.

of semi-permeable membranes before final equilibrium after dialysis; hence the time lag.

To increase the removal of solutes, the trend has been to increase the blood flow rate through the filter. However, this has been found to be less effective than using high-flux dialysers, especially in the removal of larger molecules (Leypoldt and Cheung, 1996).

FLUID REMOVAL IN HAEMODIALYSIS

Fluid removal in haemodialysis is dependent upon a number of factors, all involving some form of pressure exerted across the dialyser membrane. It has already been mentioned that osmosis plays only a secondary role: the major driving force is the hydrostatic pressures created within the dialyser (Figures 6.3, 6.6). These forces work both ways across the membrane, although the main pressures to consider are the negative pressure created on the dialysate side and the positive pressure created on the blood side.

Blood-channel pressure (P_B) is defined for our purposes as venous pressure on the machine, and dialysate-channel negative pressure (P_D) can be defined as the dialysate pressure as indicated on the machine. It then follows that the greater the difference between blood-channel pressure and the dialysate-channel negative pressure the greater the amount of fluid removed during dialysis, although fluid removal is also influenced by the clearance rate of the filter.

Dialysate-channel negative pressure is created by the machine and can be altered to remove the amount of fluid required. Different filters have differing ultrafiltration rates and it is important that, if you are using a machine that does not have volumetric control, you understand how to calculate the correct TMP for that filter using simple maths and the data sheet that comes with each filter.

Allied with the principle of ultrafiltration is the concept of bulk flow. This is more important in haemofiltration but may also have a bearing in dialysis where large amounts of fluid are removed (Jaffrin, 1995). As fluid is removed it carries with it solutes. This loss of solutes is not by diffusion.

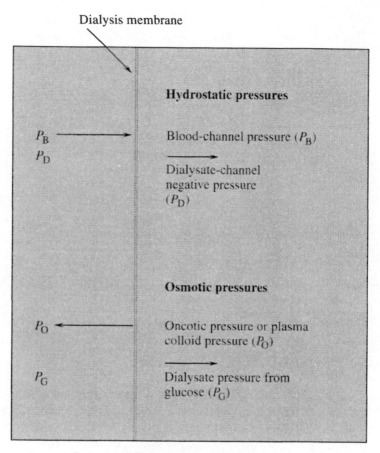

Dialysis membrane

Hydrostatic pressures

P_B — Blood-channel pressure (P_B)

P_D — Dialysate-channel negative pressure (P_D)

Osmotic pressures

P_O — Oncotic pressure or plasma colloid pressure (P_O)

P_G — Dialysate pressure from glucose (P_G)

Pressure difference over dialysis membrane
$$= (P_B + P_D) - (P_O + P_G)$$

Machine transmembrane pressure (TMP)
$$= (P_B + P_D)$$

Figure 6.6 Forces involved in the creation of transmembrane pressure.

So the larger the amount of fluid removed by UF, the larger the amount of solutes also carried across the membrane, although the amount lost is small in comparison to the effects of diffusion.

It is important that the correct pressures are applied across the dialyser membrane. Because of osmotic pressure created by the plasma proteins, the actual TMP is approximately 30 mmHg less than the pressure set on the dialysis machine (Kaplan, 1994). Too little fluid may be removed during dialysis, requiring either a longer session than usual or more fluid to be taken off in the following session. Too much fluid lost through UF leads to the all-too-common complications of hypovolaemia and hypotension. This is very uncomfortable for the patient and may result from a failure on the nurse's part to dialyse properly.

DIALYSATE FLOW

There are two directions in which dialysate can flow through the dialyser; either in the same direction as the blood (co-current flow), or in the opposite direction (counter-current flow). Co-current flow is very rarely used (unless the dialysate line has been connected incorrectly!) because it does not afford a very efficient dialysis (Figure 6.7). If the blood and dialysis fluid are travelling in the same direction through the filter, the diffusional gradients between the dialysate and the blood are reduced as the fluids travel through the dialyser, leading to less solute transfer towards the end of the dialyser than can be achieved by counter-current mechanisms.

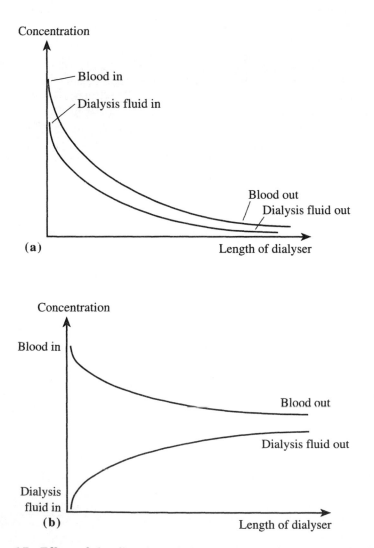

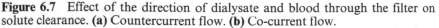

Figure 6.7 Effect of the direction of dialysate and blood through the filter on solute clearance. **(a)** Countercurrent flow. **(b)** Co-current flow.

Counter-current flow, on the other hand, provides an efficient dialysis for a given blood and dialysate flow. At any one point within the dialyser the blood is exposed to different dialysate fluid, creating a greater opportunity for diffusion to take place throughout the filter and increasing efficiency (Van Stone and Daugirdas, 1994).

HAEMODIALYSERS

All dialysers share the same four common basic components:

- the blood compartment, through which the blood passes;
- the dialysate compartment, through which the dialysate travels;
- the semi-permeable membrane, which separates the blood from the dialysate and is made of a variety of cellulose derivatives;
- the basic support structure of the dialyser.

The dialyser is constructed to create the greatest surface area against which dialysis can occur. Over the last 20 years changes in the supporting material and dialyser membranes have allowed dialysers to reduce in size but still maintain the equivalent surface area against which dialysis can occur. The efficiency of the filters has also increased markedly over this period. Cellulose-based membranes show a 47% improvement in clearances for small molecules (Woffindin and Hoenich, 1995). These have been reflected in the reduction of treatment times.

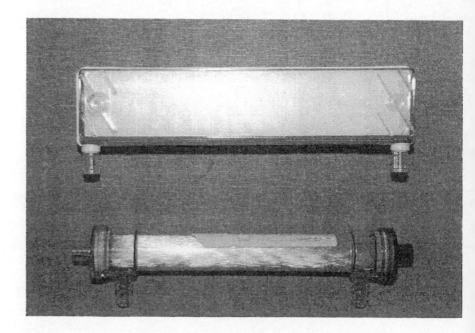

Figure 6.8 Two common forms of haemodialyser.

Key reference: Woffindin, C. and Hoenich, N.A. (1995) Hemodialyser performance: a review of the trends over the past two decades. *Artificial Organs* 19(11): 1113–1139.

Dialysers are produced in two main forms, flat plate and hollow fibre (Figure 6.8), the latter being the more common nowadays. Flat plate dialysers consist of parallel sheets of membrane arranged in layers, similar to a sandwich, with the blood and dialysate passing through alternate layers. Hollow fibre dialysers are made up of thousands of small capillary tubes through which the blood passes. These capillary tubes are surrounded by the dialysate fluid.

Membranes

The materials used for the dialyser membrane fall into two prime categories: cellulose and synthetic, although within each of these categories there are variations. Cellulosic membranes are produced from processed cotton and are the most common. More complex forms of the membrane include the addition of hydroxyl groups and synthetic material during the production in an attempt to make the membrane more biocompatible.

Synthetic membranes are not cellulose-based and are made from materials such as polysulphone, polycarbonate and polyacrylonitrile, among others. These tend to more expensive, but are considered to be more biocompatible.

Fluid–solute transfer and membranes

The transfer of solutes across the membrane is related to the design, chemical and physical structure of the material. The permeability of solutes in both forms of membrane can be affected by altering the pore size and thickness of the membrane. The larger the pores and thinner the membrane the greater the permeability. Because of these factors, clearance rates of solutes and fluid vary between dialysers.

Specification sheets accompanying dialysers give the clearance rates either within tables or in the form of a graph. These will assist the nurse in dialyser choice. The amount of fluid removal of which a particular dialyser is capable is called the ultrafiltration coefficient (k_{Uf}). This is the number of millilitres per hour of ultrafiltration for each millimetre of mercury of transmembrane pressure. The greater the k_{Uf} the greater the amount of fluid removed. Some synthetic membranes (high-flux dialysers) have the capability of removing large amounts of fluid at low TMP. Care needs to be taken in using these filters, as it is easy to dehydrate the patient very quickly unless a machine with volumetric controls is used.

Clearance rates for solutes such as urea, creatinine and vitamin B are also given in the data sheets provided with the dialysers. These are usually given at blood flow rates; the faster the blood flow the greater the efficiency of the dialyser and hence the greater the clearance of the solute. The efficiency of

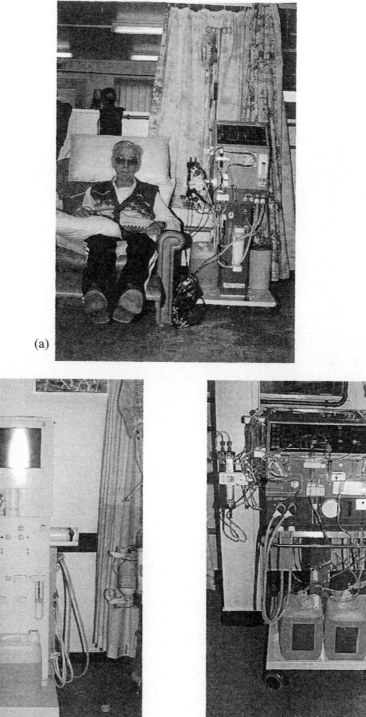

Figure 6.9 (a) A patient receiving haemodialysis; (b) two types of haemodialysis machine.

the dialyser is usually identified as the dialyser mass transfer area coefficient, k_{oA}. This is linked to the urea clearance rate at any blood and dialysate flow rate and is given as a nomogram within the data sheet. Care needs to be taken when interpreting these *in vitro* values, as they tend to be an overestimate of the efficiency of the dialyser in comparison to *in vivo* use during dialysis.

Biocompatibility

Much has been written about the effects of cellulose membranes on the patient during maintenance haemodialysis. In a recent comparative study, De Sanctis *et al.* (1996) found that, although all the membranes used increased the incidence of thrombogenesis and fibrinolysis, cellulosic membranes created a more marked increase. Parker *et al.* (1996) also suggested that bioincompatible membranes adversely affected the nutritional parameters of 'maintenance haemodialysis patients' in comparison to those dialysed with biocompatible membranes. However, despite such suggestions in the literature about the adverse effects of so-called 'bioincompatible' membranes, authors are now questioning the clinical relevance of these findings (Shaldon and Koch, 1995). Nevertheless, Locatelli (1996) argues that, despite the inconclusive effects of bioincompatible membranes on the morbidity and mortality of haemodialysis patients, only cost is in favour of the use of cuprophane membranes.

Key reference: Shaldon, S. and Koch, K.M. (1995) Biocompatibility in haemodialysis: clinical relevance in 1995. *Artificial Organs* 19(5); 395–7.

DIALYSIS FLUID COMPOSITION

The function of dialysis fluid is to correct the chemical composition of uraemic blood to normal physiological levels, removing excess uraemic wastes and electrolytes. In addition, it is also responsible for the movement of buffering agents from the dialysate into the blood to restore the acid–base balance of uraemic patients.

Acetate dialysis solution

The difficulty of preventing bicarbonate and calcium from precipitating into insoluble calcium carbonate in the early years of dialysis led to the search for an alternative buffering agent. The criteria for the substitution product for bicarbonate were, first, that it must be readily metabolized in the body, leading to the production of base equivalents. Secondly, it must be easily soluble and stable in a concentrated solution together with other electrolytes.

Acetate in the body

An activated form of acetate, acetyl-CoA, is one of the central metabolites in the body: it is involved in the metabolism of carbohydrates, lipids and proteins. For each conversion of acetate to acetyl-CoA, one equivalent molecule of bicarbonate is formed:

$$acetate + coenzyme\ A + carbonic\ acid \Rightarrow acetyl - CoA + bicarbonate + water$$
$$CO_2 + H_2O$$

This process takes place in mitochondria, which are especially abundant in liver cells. However, most of the acetate is metabolized in the muscle cells. Danielsson *et al.* (1987) found that there was an inverse relationship between body mass and plasma acetate levels during haemodialysis. Because of this, the malnourished and elderly appear to be more prone to the problems associated with acetate dialysis.

> **Key reference:** Danielsson, A. Gutierrez, A. Hultman, E. and Bergström, J. (1987) Patient-related factors influencing the plasma acetate concentration during hemodialysis. *Nephrol. Dial. Transplant* 2: 526–530.

The acetate concentration in blood is negligible, so, when present in the dialysis fluid, acetate diffuses into the blood in proportion to its concentration. After activation it is normally broken down to CO_2 and H_2O. If the acetate influx is larger than the normal metabolic pathway can accommodate, it will enter alternative biochemical routes and end up as carbohydrate or fat in the body (Ledebo, 1990).

Dialysis with acetate

During dialysis acetate is transported into the blood and bicarbonate out because of the difference in concentration gradients between the dialysis fluid and plasma. This is accompanied by a decrease in pH and P_{CO_2} (Leunissen and van Hooff, 1988). Many uraemic patients tend to be acidotic, and their situation is often exacerbated by dialysis with acetate. However, this is short-lived. The acetate is soon metabolized by the liver and bicarbonate released as a consequence, but it takes time to compensate for the outflow of bicarbonate from the plasma into the dialysate. During this time if the parameters are not changed the patient remains in a steady state until the end of dialysis. Following dialysis the remaining acetate is metabolized and the plasma bicarbonate level rises, increasing the pH.

During acetate dialysis a number of other factors need to be taken into consideration. Acetate has a vasodilatory effect, probably mediated by acetate itself (Keshaviah, 1982). Tissue hypoxaemia due to the metabolism of large amounts of acetate may also contribute to vasodilation. During dialysis the heart rate increases, and at low UF rates the cardiac output may be maintained. However, if the increased heart rate is not sufficient to accommodate for the reduction in stroke volume from UF, then the cardiac output will drop, in turn affecting the patient's blood pressure.

Bicarbonate dialysis solutions

During the 1980s the practical problems connected with the use of bicarbonate were solved one by one. Separate concentrates and proportioning

Table 6.1 Benefits from using bicarbonate in dialysis (Source: adapted from Ledebo, 1990)

Acute benefits	*Long-term benefits*
• No vasodilation	• Normalized acid–base balance
• Better fluid management	• Normalized protein metabolism
• Normal blood gases and breathing	• Optimized body weight
• No unphysiological accumulation of metabolites	• Fewer long-term complications
• Better phosphate removal	
• Less cytokine induction	
• Better correction of acidosis	

pumps were still needed, but highly automated and reliable equipment was developed that could cope with these problems. This increased the availability of bicarbonate dialysis and made it into the fastest-growing 'special treatment form' recorded by the EDTA Registry.

Unlike acetate, bicarbonate has no direct pharmacological effect on the cardiovascular system. A better preservation of plasma volume during bicarbonate dialysis has been shown, especially during the first part of dialysis. The better tissue oxygenation in combination with normal P_{CO_2} values during bicarbonate dialysis are thought to contribute to increased sympathetic tone and vasoconstriction. Bicarbonate dialysis has been shown to significantly reduce the incidence of hypotensive episodes, nausea and vomiting during dialysis (La Greca *et al.*, 1987; Oettinger and Oliver, 1989). Bicarbonate dialysate can reduce some of the morbidity factors associated with dialysis (Table 6.1).

Sodium concentration

Low sodium

In hypernatraemic patients low-sodium dialysate can be considered an option. Low-sodium dialysate leads to the transport of sodium from blood to the dialysis fluid. This creates an osmotic imbalance between the extra- and intracellular fluid compartments, leading to greater fluid shifts and intracellular swelling, resulting in a form of dialysis disequilibrium. The lower the sodium dialysate level the more efficient the dialysis and the more pronounced the effect. Care needs to be taken when using low-sodium dialysate because of the resultant extracellular volume depletion and hypotension.

High sodium

Patients who are overloaded may benefit from part of the dialysis being conducted using a high-sodium dialysate. Sodium diffuses into the blood from the dialysate, increasing the sodium concentration of the plasma. This osmotic imbalance helps to mobilize the intracellular fluid reserves, increasing the fluid shift from the intracellular fluid compartment to the intravascular compartment. Ultrafiltration is facilitated and the blood pressure remains stable. However, if dialysis is conducted throughout with a high-sodium dialysate then the risk of hypernatraemia is increased, resulting in increased thirst and a greater interdialytic weight gain (Robson *et al.*, 1978).

Physiological sodium

This is the most common sodium dialysate concentration (usually 135–140 mmol/l) and normally removes an adequate quantity of sodium and water during the dialysis procedure. The use of physiological sodium means that there is no large concentration gradient between plasma and dialysate so there is little or no net diffusion of sodium. Fluid movement is therefore not dependent upon variations in the sodium concentration but upon ultrafiltration. Sodium, if any, is removed by convection. Jenson *et al.* (1994) found that dialysing with a sodium concentration of 140 mmol/l resulted in a reduced incidence of dialysis-related hypotensive episodes.

> **Key reference:** Jenson, B.M., Dobbe, S.A., Squillace, D.P. and McCarthy, J.T. (1994) Clinical benefits of high and variable sodium concentration dialysate in hemodialysis patients. *ANNA Journal* 21(2): 115–120.

Potassium

Most dialysis concentrates use a hypotonic concentration of potassium of 2 mmol/l. This is usually enough to reduce the serum potassium levels of hyperkalaemic patients. However, no-potassium dialysate can be used for severely hyperkalaemic patients, although it should be used with care. Potassium-free concentrates should be used only at the start of dialysis, then changed to concentrate of 2 mmol/l. If this is not done the patient may become severely hypokalaemic, with attendant cardiac arrhythmias. Extra potassium can be added to concentrates if the patient is hypokalaemic. The patient scenario illustrates the difficulty of dialysing a hyperkalaemic patient, who may also be fluid-overloaded.

> **Patient scenario**
>
> Derrick was a 40-year-old man who had been on haemodialysis for 18 months but was never able to accept the dietary and fluid restrictions that his condition imposed on him. On Wednesday morning Derrick arrived for dialysis extremely short of breath and cyanosed. His interdialytic weight gain over 2 days was 4.3 litres and his blood pressure was 236/120 mmHg. Derrick was started on dialysis immediately and the system was placed in sequential ultrafiltration to remove 1.5 litres in the first hour of the treatment. Blood was sent off to the laboratory for an urgent urea and electrolyte analysis. Within half an hour the results came back showing a potassium of 6.3 mmol/l. Sequential ultrafiltration was stopped immediately and dialysis was commenced against a low-potassium dialysate for 1 hour. Transmembrane pressures were kept high to remove 1 l/h. Sequential UF was then recommenced and 2 litres was removed over the next 60 minutes. Derrick was then put back on dialysis against a normal dialysate for the remainder of the treatment session at a lower TMP. After a total treatment time of 5 hours, Derrick finished with a 4.8 litre fluid loss, a serum potassium of 4.3 mmol/l and a blood pressure of 160/90 mmHg.

Glucose

Glucose may or may not be used in dialysate solutions. When included it exerts an osmotic effect and aids ultrafiltration, although this effect is negligible if volumetric dialysis systems are used. Glucose-free dialysis leads to a larger osmotic drop in blood and loss of glucose to dialysate. To compensate, carbohydrate metabolism produces intermediates (e.g. aceto-acetate and β-hydroxybutyrate). These are lost in dialysis, especially in acetate dialysis (Ward and Walthen, 1982). These metabolic intermediates act as a buffer source, and their loss means an aggravation of acidosis. Fewer intermediates are produced during bicarbonate dialysis.

Ward *et al.* (1987) found that glucose-free dialysis aided removal of potassium ions. The reduced glucose gives rise to a reduction in plasma insulin, which leads to a favoured redistribution of potassium ions from the intracellular space, making them available for removal during dialysis.

Calcium concentration

Normal calcium dialysate levels are usually in the range of 1.5–1.75 mmol/l, slightly below physiological levels. The use of higher concentrations causes a positive calcium balance, with the long-term risk of developing metastatic calcifications. Lower concentrations induce release of parathyroid hormone, exacerbating the risk of secondary hyperparathyroidism. The increased use of calcium carbonate as a phosphate binder, instead of aluminium derivatives, may lead to the need to reduce calcium levels in dialysis fluid. Mactier *et al.* (1987) found that reducing the calcium dialysate level below 1.5 mmol/l was necessary to avoid hypercalcaemia in 11 out of 41 patients when using calcium carbonate. Slatopolsky *et al.* (1989) reduced the dialysate calcium to 1.23 mmol/l in a group of 21 patients and found no reduction in the quality of dialysis or appreciable plasma calcium levels. However, Fernandez *et al.* (1995) found that reducing dialysate calcium from 1.75–1.25 mmol/l increases the risk of hyperparathyroidism if used over prolonged periods.

WATER TREATMENT

Haemodialysis patients are exposed to large volumes of water during dialysis. It is, therefore, important that there are no contaminants in the water, chemical or biological, that can affect the patient's health. The adverse affects of poor water quality can be severe and potentially end in permanent injury or death (Chapter 8). Table 6.2 identifies some of the more important contaminants and their effects.

Water purification is usually carried out through a variety of means used in conjunction. Initially, suspended particles (mud, particulates, algae) are removed by filtration, removing particles as small as 5 μm. The water may then be further treated by passing through a water softener or a reverse osmosis (RO) unit. Water softeners remove calcium and magnesium, reducing patient exposure to high levels of calcium and magnesium but also

Table 6.2 Water contaminants and their effects

Contaminant	Effect
Aluminium	Dialysis dementia: neurological deterioration, personality changes, poor short-term memory, muscular spasms and weakness
Copper (from pipes)	Chills, nausea, headaches, liver damage, haemolysis
Nitrates (agricultural or bacterial contamination of water supply)	Methaemoglobinaemia, hypotension, cyanosis
High sodium levels (natural or from water softener)	Hypernatraemia, thirst, hypertension
High calcium levels	Hypertension, nausea, vomiting, muscle weakness, fits
Bacteria, endotoxins	Pyrogenic reactions

preventing the dialysis machine components from becoming clogged up with calcium from hard water. RO units use a semi-permeable membrane to create a pure ultrafiltrate. Many areas now use softeners in conjunction with RO units to increase the life of the semi-permeable membranes.

ANTICOAGULATION

Exposure of blood to the dialyser membrane induces fibrinolysis, resulting in a clotted dialyser if no anticoagulation is used. If clots form in the dialyser during the procedure then the effective surface area available for dialysis is reduced, affecting the efficiency of the treatment. The main aim of anticoagulation during dialysis is to anticoagulate the system, not the patient. This reduces the amount of anticoagulant needed, avoiding the risks of systemic *in vivo* anticoagulation.

Heparin

Heparin is the most common form of anticoagulant used, mainly because of its relative cost and short half-life. Heparin regimens are administered by either intermittent or continuous infusion. Both require a loading dose, usually between 25 and 50 units/kg body weight, with further bolus doses given during the dialysis (following an intermittent regimen) or an infusion administered continuously *via* a syringe pump. The amount given depends upon the needs of the patient and should be individually assessed using activated clotting times (ACT). Continuous infusion is the preferred regimen. Bolus heparinisation is associated with over- or under-anticoagulation (Ward, 1995). Once a patient has been established on the appropriate regimen, it should be checked monthly, or if there is a change in the patient's condition.

> **Key reference:** Ward, R.A. (1995) Heparinisation for routine haemodialysis. *Advances in Renal Replacement Therapy* 2(4): 362–70.

Regular anticoagulation (see marginal note) is given to maintenance haemodialysis patients who have no or little risk of bleeding. Acute renal failure patients, or end-stage renal disease patients having dialysis for the first time, should be dialysed against a moderate regimen. Individuals at risk of bleeding (postoperative, post-transplant, bleeding diathesis, pericarditis) should be carefully dialysed with minimal or no heparin if at all possible, to reduce the risk of bleeding complications.

In patients being dialysed *via* a fistula or graft the heparin infusion should be switched off 30 minutes before the end of the dialysis session to avoid the risk of bleeding from the access site post-dialysis. Prolonged pressure on the fistula post-dialysis, waiting for a clot to form after removal of the needles, could damage the fistula. Patients dialysed *via* a subclavian or femoral line should not have the heparin discontinued until the end of dialysis.

Protocol for ACTs and heparin requirements during dialysis

Regular
150–180 s
Medium
110–150 s
Tight
90–120 s

Regional heparinization

Patients at high risk of bleeding can be dialysed using regional heparinization. Here the heparin is given as usual in the arterial dialysis lines (those entering the dialyser), but before the blood re-enters the body, protamine sulphate is infused continuously to counteract the effects of heparin. This is a very tedious approach and has since been superseded by low-molecular-weight heparin.

Low-molecular-weight heparin

Low-molecular weight heparin (LMWH) is created by chemical degradation of crude heparin. It inhibits factors X and XII, but has little effect on thrombin and factors IX and XI, thus increasing clotting time *in vivo* but having a minimal *in-vitro* effect. There are no direct bedside tests that can ascertain clotting times, so LMWH is given on a body-weight basis. Because of the reduced systemic anticoagulant effect, LMWH is increasingly being used on ARF and patients with an increased risk of bleeding. Kerr *et al.* (1994) found that bolus doses of LMWH were as efficient in preventing clot formation within the filter as continuous infusion heparin.

Heparin-free dialysis

Prostacyclin is used as an anticoagulant in ARF for both intermittent dialysis and haemofiltration. Some reports have suggested that prostacyclin is inferior to heparin in its effectiveness, but Davenport *et al.* (1994) suggest that, in the case of patients with a high risk of haemorrhage, prostacyclin is more effective in maintaining the integrity of the haemofiltration system than heparin.

Assessing the effectiveness of anticoagulation

Ideally, following the dialysis session, when the dialyser has been flushed, there should be no clots visible and the patient should not be at risk of increased bleeding times. During dialysis, visual checks of the filter can indicate undercoagulation. If the colour of the blood within the filter becomes darker, or dark streaks appear, then clotting of the filter has occurred. Changes in arterial and venous pressure could also indicate the presence of clots forming in the filter or bubble trap. The easiest and most accurate form of assessment is through ACTs. In new patients a baseline should be established before dialysis to compare results during the procedure and heparin should be given accordingly.

INFECTION CONTROL

The control of infection in the haemodialysis unit is as important as elsewhere in the health-care setting, although, with the exposure to blood during dialysis, the risk of bloodborne infection presents a particular problem.

Hepatitis B and Hepatitis C

Following the outbreak of Hepatitis B (HBV) infections in dialysis units in the 1970s, strict control and procedures have been put into place to prevent and contain further outbreaks (Table 6.3). The mortality rates among both staff and patients were high. In 1972, 43% of European dialysis centres reported that 402 staff and 583 patients had contracted HBV, with a mortality rate of 2.4% among staff and 2% in patients (Crosnier *et al.*, 1989).

The concern over HBV has recently been transferred to include the risks concerning Hepatitis C (HCV), because the transmission process is very

Table 6.3 Guidelines for the prevention of HBV spread in dialysis units

- Routine screening of staff and patients for HBV
- Universal precautions
  - Protective gloves and clothing for use with all patients
  - Careful disposal of sharps
  - No recapping of sharps
- Blood spillages to be treated with hypochlorite solution and paper towels, to be disposed of by incineration
- In-service education for all staff
- Vaccination programme for staff and patients
- Careful screening of 'holiday patients'
- Isolation of HBsAg-positive patients
  - Dedicated dialysis machine
  - No reuse of dialyser from this group of patients
  - Clean machine externally with hypochlorite solution
  - Sterilize internally with formaldehyde solution

similar to HBV. It was originally thought that transmission among dialysis patients was through blood transfusion. However, a higher prevalence of HCV has been found in patients on dialysis for more than 2 years and in patients who have not had a blood transfusion, suggesting other routes of transmission (Hardy *et al.*, 1992; Crespo *et al.*, 1992). Although HCV-positive patients do not often exhibit signs of infection, the virus has been linked to chronic liver cirrhosis. Because of these factors, the prevention of HCV is as important an issue as the prevention of HBV.

CONCLUSION

There are many issues that need to be considered before a patient starts dialysis – dialyser, concentrate, anticoagulation are the most obvious. All these can and will impinge on the quality of the dialysis and the morbidity of the patient post-dialysis. Global assessment of the patient prior to commencing the procedure is important: nursing assessment and bio-chemical parameters all influence the choice of filter and dialysate. If these are mismanaged then the effects can be detrimental to the patient's health.

REVIEW QUESTIONS

- Describe the main principles of dialysis.
- Define the term 'transmembrane pressure'.
- What are the advantages to the dialysis patient of using bicarbonate dialysate instead of acetate solution?
- What system of water purification does your dialysis unit use?
- If a haemodialysis patient had undergone surgery 5 days ago, what anticoagulant regimen would you recommend and why?
- What are the advantages and disadvantages of using a hypertonic sodium dialysate solution?

REFERENCES

Crespo, R., Munoz, I., Tierno, C. *et al.* (1992) Hepatitis C virus infection in haemodialysis: further mechanisms of transmission. *Journal of the European Dialysis and Transplant Nurses Association–European Renal Care Association*, **18**(2), 37–38.

Crosnier, J., Degor, F. and Junger, P. (1989) Dialysis associated hepatitis, in *Replacement of Renal Function by Dialysis*, (ed. J. F. Maher), Kluwer Academic Publishers, Dordrecht.

Danielsson, A. Gutierrez, A. Hultman, E. and Bergström, J. (1987) Patient-related factors influencing the plasma acetate concentration during hemodialysis. *Nephrology, Dialysis and Transplantation*, **2**, 526–530.

Davenport, A. Will, E. J. and Davison, A. M. (1994) Comparison of the use of standard heparin and Prostacyclin anticoagulation in spontaneous and pump-driven extracorporeal circuits in patients with combined acute renal failure. *Nephron*, **66**, 431–437.

De Sanctis, L. B., Stefoni, S., Cianciolo, G. *et al.* (1996) Effect of different dialysis membranes on platelet function. A tool for biocompatibility evaluation. *International Journal of Artificial Organs*, **19**(7), 404–410.

Fernandez, E., Borras, M., Pais, B. and Montoliu, J. (1995) Low-calcium dialysate stimulates parathormone secretion and its long-term use worsens secondary hyperparathyroidism. *Journal of the American Society of Nephrology*, **6**(1), 132–135.

Hardy, N. M., Sandroni, S., Danielson, S. and Wilson, W. J. (1992) Antibody to hepatitis C virus increases with time on haemodialysis. *Clinical Nephrology*, **38**, 44.

Jaffrin, M. Y. (1995) Convective mass transfer in hemodialysis. *Artificial Organs*, **19**(11), 1162–1171.

Jenson, B. M., Dobbe, S. A., Squillace, D. P. and McCarthy, J. T. (1994) Clinical benefits of high and variable sodium concentration dialysate in hemodialysis patients. *American Nephrology Nurses Association Journal*, **21**(2), 115–120.

Kaplan, A. A. (1994) Maintenance haemodialysis: prescription and management, in *Renal Dialysis*, (eds J. D. Briggs, B. J. R. Junor, R. S. C. Rodger and J. F. Winchester), Chapman & Hall, London.

Kerr, P. G., Mattingly, S., Lo, A. and Atkins, R. C. (1994) The adequacy of fragmin as a single bolus dose with reused dialysers. *Artificial Organs*, **18**(6), 416–419.

Keshaviah, P. (1982) The role of acetate in the etiology of symptomatic hypotension. *Artificial Organs*, **6**, 378–387.

La Grecca, G., Feriani, M. Bragantini, L. *et al.* (1987) Effects of acetate and bicarbonate dialysate on vascular stability: a prospective multicentre study. *International Journal of Artificial Organs*, **10**, 157–162.

Ledebo, I. (1990) *Acetate Vs Bicarbonate*, Rahms, Lund.

Leunissen, K. M. L. and van Hooff, J. P. (1988) Acetate or bicarbonate for haemodialysis? *Nephrology, Dialysis and Transplantation*, **3**, 1–7.

Leypoldt, J. K. and Cheung, A. K. (1996) Removal of high molecular-weight solutes during high-efficiency and high-flux hemodialysis. *Nephrology, Dialysis and Transplantation*, **11**(2), 329–335.

Locatelli, F. (1996) Influence of membranes on morbidity. *Nephrology, Dialysis and Transplantation*, **11**(Suppl. 2), 116–120.

Mactier, R. A., Van Stone, J., Cox, A. *et al.* (1987) Calcium carbonate is an effective phosphate binder when dialysate calcium concentration is adjusted to control hypercalcaemia. *Clinical Nephrology*, **28**, 222–226.

Oettinger, C. W. and Oliver, J. C. (1989) An economical new process for incentre bicarbonate dialysate production: comparison with acetate in a large dialysis population. *Artificial Organs*, **13**, 432–437.

Parker, T. F., Wingard, R. L., Husni, L. *et al.* (1996) Effect of the membrane biocompatibility on nutritional parameters in chronic haemodialysis. *Kidney International*, **49**(2), 551–556.

Robson, M., Oren, H. and Ravid, M. (1978) Dialysate sodium concentration, hypertension and pulmonary oedema in haemodialysis patients. *Proceedings of the European Dialysis and Transplant Association*, **15**, 678–679.

Shaldon, S. and Koch, K. M. (1995) Biocompatibility in haemodialysis: clinical relevance in 1995. *Artificial Organs*, **19**(5), 395–397.

Slatopolsky, E., Weerts, C., Norwood, K. *et al.* (1989) Long term effects of calcium carbonate and 2.5 mEq/L calcium dialysate on mineral metabolism. *Kidney International*, **36**, 897–903.

Van Stone, J. C. and Daugirdas, J. T. (1994) Physiologic principles, in *Handbook of Dialysis*, 2nd edn, (eds J. T. Daugirdas and T. S. Ing), Little, Brown & Co., Boston, MA.

Ward, R. A. (1995) Heparinisation for routine haemodialysis. *Advances in Renal Replacement Therapy*, **2**(4), 362–370.

Ward, R. A. and Walthen, R. L. (1982) Utilisation of bicarbonate for base repletion in haemodialysis. *Artificial Organs*, **6**, 396–403.

Ward, R. A., Walthen, R. L., Williams, T. E. and Harding, G. B. (1987) Haemodialysate composition and interdialytic metabolic, acid-base and potassium changes. *Kidney International*, **32**, 129–135.

Woffindin, C. and Hoenich, N. A. (1995) Hemodialyser performance: a review of the trends over the past two decades. *Artificial Organs*, **19**(11), 1113–1119.

FURTHER READING

Gutch, C. F., Stoner, M. H. and Corea, A. L. (1993) *Review of Haemodialysis for Nurses and Dialysis Personnel*, 5th edn, C. V. Mosby, St Louis, MO.

Maher, J. F. (ed.) (1992) *Replacement of Renal Function by Dialysis*, 3rd edn, Kluwer Academic Publishers, Dordrecht.

Nissenson, A. R., Fine, R. N. and Gentile, D. E. (eds) (1990) *Clinical Dialysis*, 2nd edn, Prentice-Hall, Englewood Cliffs, NJ.

7 Vascular access in dialysis

John Sedgewick

LEARNING OBJECTIVES

At the end of this chapter the reader should be able to:

- Distinguish the different types of access used for acute and chronic dialysis therapy.
- Identify specific research factors influencing the optimal use of vascular access.
- Identify the associated anatomy and vascular physiology influencing blood flow within the access.
- Explain the complications associated with each form of access in dialysis.
- Understand the nursing care and associated management of varying vascular accesses.

INTRODUCTION

Dialysis requires the passage of blood extracorporeally through an artificial kidney (dialyser) for purification. To provide an adequate and efficient dialysis, vascular access has to provide optimal blood flows to the dialyser. Many factors are known to influence the success and efficiency of dialysis therapy and a good vascular access is one of the important mainstays of treatment. Nurses and other health-care staff providing dialysis therapy must have an understanding of the central role that vascular access plays in dialysis therapy (Berkoben and Schwab, 1995). Their role encompasses the day-to-day management of the access as well as educating patient and family about the care of his/her 'life-line'. The idea of a 'life-line' for dialysis cannot be underestimated. Waeleghem and Ysebaert (1995a) suggest that the maintenance and subsequent management of vascular access in dialysis is the Achilles heel of the haemodialysis patient.

Primary arteriovenous fistulae (AVF) are the preferred form of vascular access because they are most likely to provide long-term complication-free access. However, many patients entering haemodialysis programmes have vascular anatomy unsuitable for primary arteriovenous fistula creation; as a result, synthetic fistulae are currently the more common form of vascular access. Creating and maintaining a functioning vascular access is a goal for renal patients and the health-care team. Nephrology nurses play an important role in managing vascular-access-related complications through assessment and detection of possible complications. Inadequate dialysis and its complications can be minimized through attention to and documentation of factors leading to vascular access stenosis (Berry, 1996; Sherman *et al.*, 1997). Poor vascular access causes inadequate dialysis, while fistula failure disrupts the patient's lifestyle, results in the need for further surgical intervention, frequently leading to hospitalization, and also has financial implications for both patients and health-care provider. The morbidity and mortality of maintenance haemodialysis patients is largely determined by the ability of the nephrologist, dialysis staff and vascular surgeon to establish and maintain adequate vascular access.

> **Key reference:** Sherman, R.A., Besarab, A., Schwab, S.J. and Beathard, G.A. (1997) Recognition of the falling vascular access: a current perspective. *Seminars in Dialysis* 10(1): 1–4.

Survival rates of AV fistulae vary: it has been estimated that rates of survival vary between 56% and 75% at 3 years (Raja and Rasib, 1994). Patients who present with a poor vascular system as a result of either diabetes or atherosclerosis often experience difficulties with AVF creation. Many elderly patients are entering the haemodialysis programmes with co-morbid diseases, which increases the possibility of access failure, particularly in diabetic patients (Brothers *et al.*, 1996). The elderly undergoing haemodialysis have higher rates of access morbidity, the most common haemodialysis-related complications being hypotension, arrhythmias and gastrointestinal bleeding. Providing dialysis care to elderly patients presents nephrologists with many ethical issues and dilemmas (Grapsa and Oreopoulos, 1996).

> **Key reference:** Raja, M., and Rasib, M. (1994) Vascular Access for Hemodialysis. In Daugirdas J.T. and Todd S.I. (eds.) *Handbook of Dialysis*. New York. Little, Brown & Co., New York.

Prischl *et al.* (1995) examined whether age, gender, underlying renal disease or the skill of the surgeon performing the AVF were of prognostic value in the overall patency of vascular access in 108 haemodialysis patients with first Cimino–Brescia fistulae. The operating surgeon seemed to be the major determinant for the continuous patency of the fistula.

ACUTE VASCULAR ACCESS

A patient requiring urgent dialysis is usually suffering from a severe disturbance of biochemical balances and pulmonary oedema of a life-threatening nature. The type of acute therapy will often dictate the type of access needed and dialysis facilities available. The type of vascular access required for acute dialysis is different for those patients requiring long-term maintenance dialysis. Patients in acute renal failure usually have a temporary vascular access, of which there are principally three types: femoral catheters, AV shunts and central vein catheters/internal jugular catheters, which may also be used as a form of chronic vascular access.

Femoral catheters

The development of wide-bore femoral catheters has played an important role in the management of patients requiring various blood purification therapies. Their wide bore enables high blood flow to be achieved for dialysis. Femoral catheters are inserted under strict asepsis with the patient in the Trendelenburg position. Under local anaesthesia the femoral vein is cannulated and the femoral catheter is inserted. Extreme care is required to prevent accidental cannulation of the femoral artery. Complications of femoral catheterization mainly relate to their susceptibility to infection. Rarely, retroperitoneal haemorrhage may occur as a result of the cannulation procedure. Usually, following two to three treatments, femoral catheters are withdrawn and they are therefore only used on a short-term basis where a limited number of therapies is indicated.

Where the insertion of a subclavian line is not possible femoral catheterization may be the only solution for acute dialysis. In circumstances where patients have had recent groin surgery femoral catheterization should not be undertaken because of the risk of bleeding. The use of femoral catheters for dialysis is not common practice unless specific problems exist that prevent a temporary central line from being inserted. Kirkpatrick *et al.* (1996) undertook an extensive analysis of 120 patients requiring dialysis *via* femoral catheterization for 2 days or more to establish the frequency of catheter-related complications. Results indicated that the rate of clinically significant infection in femoral catheters was less than 3.5%; this compared favourably with infections in central vein catheters. Prolonged femoral vein catheterization for haemodialysis was associated with an acceptably low rate of complications when appropriate techniques for placement and catheter care were followed. Patients requiring femoral catheters usually only need them for 2 days or so. The anatomical siting of the catheters predisposes to infection and despite attention to asepsis and catheter management infections are a risk. Patients requiring femoral catheterization are required to be on bed rest and therefore they are also seen as restrictive.

Arteriovenous shunts

The external arteriovenous (AV) shunt, often referred to as the Scribner shunt, involves the surgical cut-down and cannulation with a Teflon–Silastic loop of an adjacent artery and vein, typically either the radial artery and cephalic vein at the wrist or the posterior tibial artery and greater saphenous vein at the ankle. The distal vessels are ligated, the Teflon ends of the shunt are secured to the proximal vessels and the Silastic tubing forms a loop on the external skin surface. This form of access is complicated by poor patency rates, leading to thrombosis or thrombophlebitis, distal ischaemia due to ligation of distal vessels, infection, haemorrhage due to dislodgement or skin erosion, and eventual exhaustion of peripheral vessels.

AV shunts are now rarely used in the management of patients requiring blood purification therapy. More efficient modes of access for acute dialysis have emerged with the developments in subclavian line and femoral catheters. Prior to these developments (AV) shunts offered an important means of access to the patient's circulation.

Subclavian catheter and internal jugular catheters

When urgent dialysis is required temporary subclavian or internal jugular catheterization can be performed. This mode of access has proved to be vital for patients who require dialysis while waiting for their AVF to develop adequately to support haemodialysis, for patients transferred to haemodialysis from peritoneal dialysis with no functioning internal AV access (graft or AVF), and for patients requiring plasmaphaeresis and venovenous continuous renal replacement therapy.

Placement of subclavian catheters or internal jugular catheters is undertaken under strict aseptic technique with the patient in the Trendelenburg position. Under local anaesthesia the subclavian vein is cannulated and the catheter is inserted and sutured into place. Before it is used a check X-ray is taken and the doctor verifies that the catheter is in the correct place. Patients who find it difficult to lie supine or have respiratory problems are not suitable for central vein cannulation. Complications that can occur following cannulation of the subclavian vein or internal jugular vein are pneumothorax, haemothorax, air embolism and haemorrhage.

Preventing infection of a central line is a challenge for the renal health-care team. The use of catheters coated with antibiotics is of growing interest in the prevention of infection although their efficacy is still being established. Thornton *et al.*'s (1996) experimental study compared antibiotic-coated catheters with plain catheters in central venous lines. Patients were randomly selected to either a control group whose catheters were not pretreated or to an experimental group whose catheters were pretreated by the manufacturer with a cationic surfactant and bonded with vancomycin 1 g made up in 10 ml of water immediately prior to insertion. In the control group 80% of catheters became infected, compared with 62% in the study group. The commonest organism isolated was coagulase-negative *Staphylococcus*. In patients at risk of sepsis, the use of central venous catheters bonded with antibiotics offers an interesting challenge in patient management.

The efficacy of antiseptic solutions in skin preparation prior to insertion and removal of central venous catheters is an area for continued research. Mizumoto *et al.* (1996a) studied the effectiveness of a newly available antiseptic solution consisting of 0.25% chlorhexidine gluconate, 0.025% benzalkonium chloride and 4% benzyl alcohol, compared with povidone iodine 10%. Catheter colonization and catheter sepsis were significantly lower in the chlorhexidine group. The 0.25% chlorhexidine solution was superior to 10% povidone iodine in preventing catheter-related sepsis due to Gram-negative bacteria, although not significantly superior in the prevention of Gram-negative infections. The trial solution was generally more effective than 10% povidone iodine for insertion site care of short-term central venous and arterial catheters.

Nursing interventions related to caring for central vein catheters

A major focus for staff caring for subclavian catheters or jugular vein catheters is the prevention of infection. With thorough attention to strict asepsis infectious episodes can be minimized. The catheter must be able to provide adequate blood flows for dialysis, and nurses are therefore required to exercise vigilance in the care and management of a patient's catheter during dialysis. Local unit policies will dictate the general care and management of the patient's catheter throughout all phases of dialysis.

Nursing assessment of patients' access is an important aspect of dialysis care. During discussions with the patient questions can be asked concerning general care, problems associated with the catheter and whether any issues need to be addressed. Site assessment is important: staff must look for undue redness that might indicate infection. If infection is suspected a swab of the exit site should be taken, blood should be taken for culture and antibiotic therapy should be commenced according to local policy. In the presence of persistent infection a decision must be made about whether or not to remove the central line. Dialysing a patient *via* an infected line will promote the development of systemic sepsis. Removal and reinsertion of the line will be undertaken if catheter colonization is evident. Exit site swabs should be taken and dressings undertaken according to the unit protocol.

VASCULAR ACCESS IN CHRONIC HAEMODIALYSIS

The importance of vascular access in long-term haemodialysis cannot be overstated. The most common chronic vascular access used is the native arteriovenous fistula. An AVF involves the surgical anastomosis of the radial artery to the cephalic vein (Figure 7.1). Once created the vein distends over a period of weeks because of the high arterial blood flow within the fistula. Following fistula creation, blood flow rates may be as high as 400 ml/min, upper-arm fistulae showing flow rates of more than 1 l/min. The blood flow rate within the fistula is determined by the sum of the resistance of the arterial system between the left ventricle and the anastomosis and the resistance of the venous system between the anastomosis and the right atrium. Cardiac complications are known to occur where blood flows within the fistula are too high. The AVF is created in

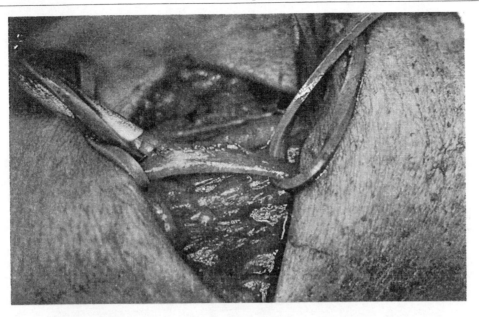

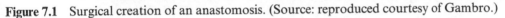

Figure 7.1 Surgical creation of an anastomosis. (Source: reproduced courtesy of Gambro.)

the patient's non-dominant arm. This makes it easier for the patient to undertake self-needling in the future and avoids unnecessary immobility of the dominant arm.

Different types of arteriovenous fistula exist: these include radio-cephalic, humerobasilic, brachiocephalic (upper arm), ulnobasilic and humerocephalic fistulae (Figure 7.2). The radiocephalic fistula is usually the first vascular access in a patient, the humerocephalic fistula being the least accessible vascular access and the one that presents the most problems for needling. Surgical anastomosis of the AVF may either join the side of the artery to the side of the vein or the side of the artery to the end of the vein. Both approaches ensure that blood flow through the artery distally is preserved. Venous hypertension may arise from a side-to-side anasto-mosis because the arterial pressure is transmitted to the veins distal to the anastomosis; this results in swelling of the hand known as steal syndrome.

PREPARATION OF THE PATIENT REQUIRING AN ARTERIOVENOUS FISTULA

Forward planning in the placement of access is important when a patient will require dialysis in the future. Preserving the quality of the proposed fistula arm is critically important and unnecessary venepuncture of the arm must be avoided. The creation of the AVF, usually on the patient's non-dominant arm, should be undertaken in sufficient time to enable the fistula to develop. Informing the patient preoperatively about how the fistula will be created and used for dialysis is important. Angiographic assessment of the patient's vascular system within the arm may be undertaken during the

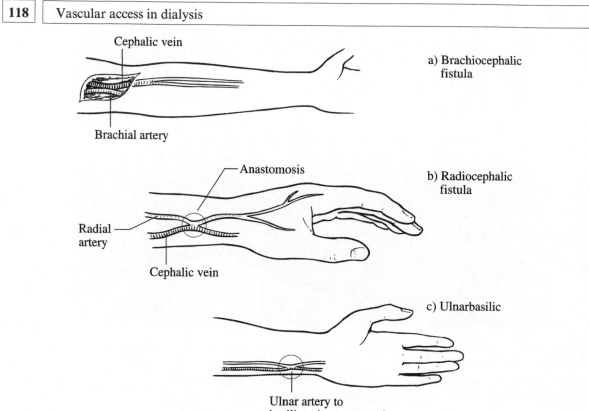

Figure 7.2 Various anastomoses that can be created for an AV fistula. **(a)** Brachiocephalic fistula. **(b)** Radiocephalic fistula. **(c)** Ulnarbasilic fistula.

preparation for an AVF; this may help to assess vascular damage due to previous insertions of subclavian catheters. Stenosis of the subclavian vein is a complication resulting from subclavian cannulation and can lead to blood flow problems within the fistula.

During the immediate period following the creation of the AVF the affected arm should be kept warm and elevated on a pillow to reduce oedema and dressing observed for unnecessary oozing. Tight restrictive dressings around the arm must be avoided since they may impede blood flow within the fistula, precipitating thrombosis of the access. Patency of the AVF can be assessed by auscultation for a bruit as well as manually feeling for the presence of a thrill over the anastomosis site. The colour and movement of the fingers is also an important observation in the detection of distal ischaemia. Early intervention in the presence of diminished bruit or thrill may save the AVF. In the postoperative period it is very important to ensure that the patient is kept sufficiently hydrated, which will minimize the likelihood of thrombosis occurring immediately following creation of the AVF. Thrombosis is often due to hypotensive episodes. The fistula should be allowed to mature before being cannulated: 6–8 weeks may elapse before it is sufficiently mature for cannulation. Patients should be taught to care for their AVF and learn to assess the bruit and thrill and report any changes promptly. Unit protocols will dictate the specific care and management of AVF.

CANNULATION OF AN ARTERIOVENOUS FISTULA

A thorough assessment must be made of the fistula prior to cannulation. This should consider the fistula anatomy, vein length, surgical formation of the fistula and whether any difficulties were encountered during its construction. Correct needle placement is an important factor in the longevity of a patient's AVF. The correct choice of needle for cannulation is also important as this plays a central role in the delivery of an efficient and adequate blood flow for dialysis. Various needles are available, each with their own advantages: 14, 15, 16 and 17 gauge needles are available for cannulation. Where a higher blood flow is required, as in high-flux dialysis, larger-bore, lower-gauge needles should be used (Figure 7.3). Blood flows of 400 ml/min can be obtained with 14 gauge needles. In the presence of small vessels, as in paediatric patients, smaller-bore, higher-gauge needles are used.

Newly created fistulae require a planned process of development whereby larger-gauge, smaller-bore needles, i.e. 17 gauge, are used when the fistula is relatively immature. The choice of needle is often dictated by unit policies. A standard 16 gauge needle is usually satisfactory for most adult fistulae, although in situations where blood flow rates need to increase to 350–500 ml/min the needle size will be 15 or 14 gauge. The bore of the needle tubing is also known to play an important role in the attainment of satisfactory blood flows for dialysis.

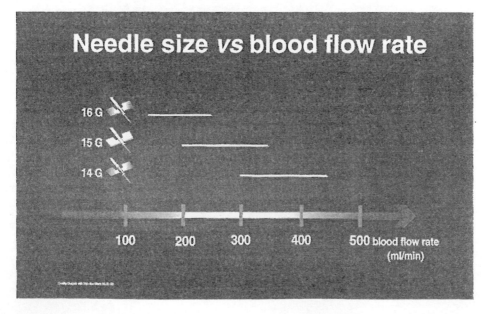

Figure 7.3 Needle size *versus* blood flow rate (Source: courtesy of Gambro).

Blood flow direction within the AVF is the main factor influencing needle placement. The venous needle is placed in the direction of the venous return (towards the heart) with the arterial needle pointing in either direction (preferably distally). Antegrade arterial needle placement means that the needle is pointing towards the direction of the blood flow, whereas retrograde needle placement is when the needle is pointing towards the arterial anastomosis; local unit policies will direct practices. In many situations there may be difficulty in the placement of two needles as is standard in dialysis therapy. The need to provide single-needle dialysis then becomes the focus of therapy although the efficiency of single-needle dialysis compared to double-needle dialysis is dependent upon establishment of good blood flows. Consideration must be given to the proximity of needles where they are placed in the same direction on the same limb. There is an increased chance of recirculation where needles are less than 3 inches apart from hub to hub (Figure 7.4).

With newly created or immature AV fistulae antegrade cannulation can be used. This provides a better and higher blood flow with less bloodline collapse or line sucking. Rotating needles should be considered when cannulating an AVF: this helps to prolong the lifespan of the AVF and reduce pseudoaneurysm formation. Cannulation along the whole length of the fistula promotes even development of the fistula, preventing soft areas developing and also preventing the formation of fibrous tissue, which can occur when the same site is cannulated continuously. Needle site rotation should be documented and recorded so as to ensure consistency

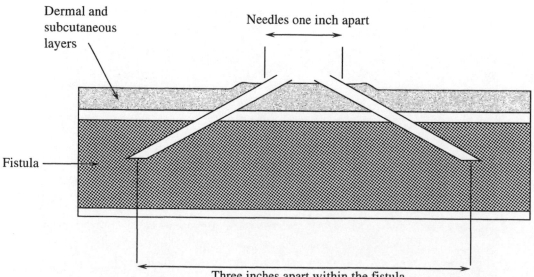

Figure 7.4 Correct minimum needle distance to prevent recirculation (Source: after Brouwer, 1995).

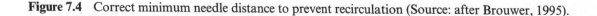

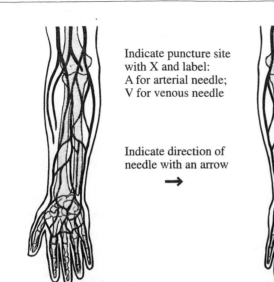

Indicate puncture site
with X and label:
A for arterial needle;
V for venous needle

Indicate direction of
needle with an arrow

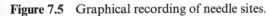

Figure 7.5 Graphical recording of needle sites.

among staff members dealing with the AVF. Graphical recording of fistula needle sites has been reported to be an important component in quality assurance in renal units (Serfaty *et al.*, 1994; Figure 7.5). The number of repeated punctures in vascular access can be used to develop an index to measure the quality of vascular access care within a renal unit. This was addressed by Alvarez *et al.* (1994), who identified the significance between the level of nurses' renal experience and the numbers of repeated AVF punctures undertaken. This led to the development of a clinical standard for measuring the quality of vascular access management.

Cannulation techniques

- **Area puncture**. This entails the development of a small number of cannulation sites for dialysis with the same sites being used repeatedly. The disadvantage of this technique is the potential for aneurysm formation as a result of repeated punctures over the same site.
- **The rope ladder technique**. This involves the equal distribution of needle sites along the length of the vessel, which results in uniform dilation of the vein with little or no stenotic deformation (Figure 7.6). During successive dialyses the vessel is punctured on alternate sides.
- **The buttonhole technique**. This involves the preselection of between one and three sites each for arterial and venous needles. The vessel is always punctured at the same site and at the same precise angle each time: this results in the creation of a conduit of scar tissue that is anaesthetic for the patient (Table 7.1).

Assessing the efficiency of AVF in providing optimum blood flows is an increasing part of fistula management. Techniques may include fistula flow studies (Aldridge *et al.*, 1984) and thermal dilution studies (Kramer and

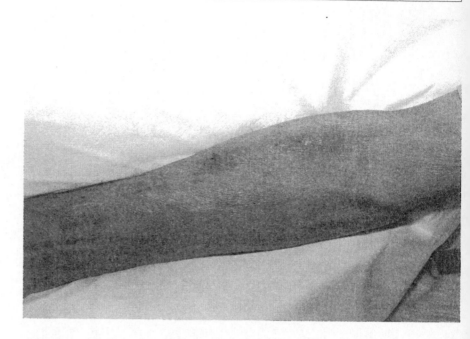

Figure 7.6 A mature fistula, showing distension of the venous system along the length of the forearm.

Polaschegg, 1993) to assess for recirculation. Martinez Barquinero *et al.* (1993) identified increasing complications with AVF associated with increasing age, particularly in patients over the age of 62 years. This study examined fistulae that presented needling difficulties and poor blood flows and whether a relationship existed between echo Doppler and anatomical changes found during surgical refashioning of AVF. Nursing staff in this study played a central role in the early diagnosis of non-functioning AVF, with nurses' clinical findings being confirmed by the results of the echo Doppler.

Limited research exists concerning the effectiveness and efficiency of the various strategies used to cannulate fistulae. An important development has been the formation of the Collaborative Research Programme

Table 7.1 Indications for various fistula cannulation techniques (Source: adapted from Byrne, 1994)

Vein characteristic	Cannulation technique
Vein long and wide	Rope ladder or buttonhole
Vein short and wide	Buttonhole
Vein long and narrow	Dilate with area puncture Rope ladder or buttonhole
Vein short and narrow	Dilate with area puncture Buttonhole

within the European Dialysis and Transplant Nurses European Care Association. Lindley (1996) highlights the results of a pilot project examining vascular access practices across Europe. In all centres studied, nurses were the health-care professionals who most frequently inspected and palpated vascular access. Variation in skin cleansing protocol was evident: in one unit patients simply washed the puncture sites with soap and water prior to needle placement. Many renal units used a combination of washing the site and use of disinfectant on the skin. Cannulation technique across those centres studied also varied, with 75% of centres using the rope ladder technique.

PREPARING PATIENTS FOR CANNULATION

Following the initial construction of the fistula staff will educate the patient, family and often carers on the general management of the newly created fistula until it matures. Patients should be advised of the importance of their role in the management of their access and all the information necessary should be given to allow them to make an informed decision regarding the use of the fistula.

Skin cleansing

Preventing infection in an AVF is one of the major goals in access management. Before cannulation patients should be encouraged to wash the AVF arm, usually with a bactericidal liquid soap, followed by cleansing of the forearm with an appropriate antiseptic agent. Iodine preparations are commonly used to clean the skin prior to the insertion of fistula needles. Patients should be encouraged to clean and care for their own access area. Universal precautions must be strictly adhered to during preparation of access sites, particularly the wearing of gloves. The use of protective eye shields/goggles and face visors during cannulation should also become standard practice so as to avoid accidental splash injuries with patients' blood during cannulation and the potential transmission of blood-borne viruses.

Use of anaesthesia

Cannulation is a painful and distressing procedure for many patients. Intradermal analgesia in the form of lignocaine can be administered immediately prior to cannulation, although care is needed to avoid inadvertent fistula infiltration. Along with intradermal lignocaine, chloroethane spray can be used or lignocaine 2% with prilocaine, in the form of Emla cream, where pain is experienced. Avoiding pain caused by needle placement is an important consideration since pain is known to influence patients' acceptance of haemodialysis (Gerrish *et al.*, 1996). Needle insertion is thought to damage the vessel wall due to the punch effect when needles are inserted. Placing the bevel of the needle face down or at an angle of 45° to the vein, particularly in the presence of a polytetrafluoroethene (PTFE) graft, is thought to reduce vessel wall damage, although conflicting views are evident concerning the placement of the needle bevel during cannulation.

Needle technique

Crespo (1994) undertook an examination of both upward and downward bevel position of fistula needles during cannulation. This single-blind, randomized study demonstrated an increase in puncture pain when the bevel of the needle was placed upwards. No significant differences occurred in blood flow rate or venous pressure between downward and upward bevel position. Cannulation with the bevel in the downward position resulted in a smaller puncture orifice with a reduction in bleeding time following needle removal. Manipulation of the needle by staff and twist manoeuvres to increase blood flow were also reduced.

During cannulation the needle should be held by the wings at an angle

---

Key reference: Crespo, R. (1994) Influence of bevel position of the needle on puncture pain in haemodialysis. *Journal of the European Dialysis and Transplant Nurses Association* 4:21–23.

---

of 20–35°, and at a 45° angle for grafts. On entry through the fistula or graft a flashback should be seen. Once in the fistula the needle should be inserted no further than 3 mm and then rotated through 180°. It has been suggested that the process of flipping the needle during the dialysis procedure may lead to further trauma of the intimal lining of the vessel, although further research needs to be undertaken on this topic. The act of rotation is designed to prevent back wall or posterior wall infiltration, which occurs if the needle tip punctures the bottom of the graft or fistula. The needle can be secured with a butterfly tape technique. Ensuring the security of needles throughout dialysis is important. This helps avoid needle displacement or movement, which might precipitate needle infiltration or impede adequate blood flow through the needle, reducing the effectiveness of the dialysis.

Vessel infiltration can occur with any needle cannulation. If this occurs prior to heparinization the needle should be removed and digital pressure applied with a sterile dressing. If infiltration occurs following heparinization a decision must be made as to whether to leave the needle in place until dialysis has been completed, providing the infiltration site remains stable. Where the haematoma increases in size the needle should be removed and digital pressure should be applied. When infiltration has occurred repeated cannulation should be performed as far away from the infiltration site as possible. In the case of venous infiltration the new needle can be placed above the previous needle infiltration site, although this is not always possible, in which case placing the new needle 4–5 cm away from the previous site will avoid accidental dislodgement of the haematoma. When dialysis is commenced the blood pump should be started slowly, allowing any increase in the size of the haematoma to be detected.

Table 7.2 Care and management of the arteriovenous fistula

Predialysis	Education of patients; information-giving concerning care of access and detection of problems
Skin preparation	Cleansing of area
Assessment of cannula sites	Skin characteristics (evidence of bruising, scars, general skin turgor, skin mobility)
Identification of sites	Previous evidence of scar tissue Vascular structure of access site Vascular filling of veins
Needle position	Length of vein Newness of fistula Anaesthetize (lignocaine creams) Needle placement (anterograde, retrograde) Single or double needle
Intradialytically	Observation of access sites (pain, bleeding, oozing) Presence of pain Safety of needles Secure and tape needles to skin Flow from fistula (arterial and venous)
Post-dialysis	Anticoagulation discontinuation prior to needle removal Needle removal Site care Maintenance of homoeostasis

Care must be exercised at the end of dialysis when dialysis needles are removed. Improper needle removal can further damage the vessel or graft (Table 7.2).

COMPLICATIONS ASSOCIATED WITH ARTERIOVENOUS FISTULAE

A summary of potential problems with arteriovenous fistulae is given in Table 7.3.

Thrombosis

Thrombosis is the most common cause of short-term access-related failure and hospitalization in long-term haemodialysis patients. Thrombosis of a native AVF usually occurs within 1 month of its construction and may be due to inadequate venous size or run-off. This problem is difficult to solve and requires a more proximal autogenous vein or prosthetic graft AVF. Thrombosis of AVF occurring later is uncommon and may be the result of anastomotic narrowing, discrete venous stasis due to multiple needle-sticks, aneurysm formation or post-dialysis hypotension; simple thrombectomy with or without anastomotic revision usually resolves the problem. Thrombosis occurring in a synthetic graft is usually the result of intimal hyperplasia at the venous anastomosis. While thrombectomy or graft curettage may be sufficient to deal with the

Table 7.3 Potential problems with arteriovenous fistulae

Size and location of veins	Takes time for veins to 'mature' to enable wide-bore cannula to be inserted.
Difficult blood flow through needle	May be due to vein size or diverted blood flow from branches feeding the fistula. Never place needle within 2 cm of the anastomosis. Side-to-side anastomosis may give rise to dilation of veins on back of hand more than in forearm.
Vessel spasm	Often occurs at the beginning of dialysis, possibly as a result of the needle 'sucking' against the vessel wall. Patients may feel a fluttering sensation in the fistula as well as pain.
Venous stenosis	Blood returning to the fistula may encounter resistance due to venous stenosis. Other factors accounting for resistance include needle position, position of extremity. The needles may need to be repositioned.
Accidental tearing of vessels during venepuncture	Formation of large haematomas.
Radial artery syndrome	Results in ischaemic changes in the fingers. Severe cases may result in cold, blue, painful and even gangrenous fingers. Caused by low arterial pressure at the fistula site due to diversion of radial artery blood to the vein. If detected early enough can be corrected by tying off radial artery distal to fistula.
Infection	Often due to poor aseptic technique during cannulation or general poor hygiene. Potential for thrombosis or sepsis.
Thrombosis	Most common complication, which may be precipitated by hypotension, stenosis of the fistula and infection. Direct pressure impeding blood flow within the AVF is another possibility. Patients should be encouraged not to sleep on their arm or to wear tight clothing around the fistula.
Aneurysm	Due to same-site cannulation over a period of time or to infection.

problem, the vein beginning at the venous anastomosis becomes progressively stenotic for as much as several centimetres. Intimal hyperplasia at the venous anastomosis usually progresses to complete thrombosis within 6-8 months of implantation.

Infection

Infection is the second most common cause of vascular access loss in the long-term haemodialysis patient. Churchill *et al.* (1992) indicated a 19.7% probability of PTFE graft infection at 1 year in comparison to 4.5% for native AVF. Although intraoperative graft contamination may occur it is generally believed that infections of prosthetic AV grafts occur through inoculation with skin flora due to poor needle insertion technique or contamination arising from distant sites such as intravascular catheters. Infection of native AVF can usually be managed with systemic antibiotics without loss of chronic vascular access. This is in contrast to prosthetic graft infections, which usually need surgical intervention that may include incision and drainage of graft infection and systemic antibiotics or the excision of a locally infected graft segment.

Arterial steal syndrome

A devastating complication of vascular access is distal ischaemia with an estimated occurrence of between 5% and 10% in patients with diabetes mellitus and more in individuals with peripheral vascular disease (Rivers *et al.*, 1992). Patients may present almost immediately following AVF creation with cool, pale, numb, painful fingers or they may present months or years later with ischaemic ulcerations or gangrene of the fingers. In the presence of a Brescia–Cimino AVF, ischaemia of the fingers is thought to be secondary to retrograde flow from the ulnar artery and palmar arch toward the low-pressure arteriovenous anastomosis. Treatment may include refashioning of the anastomosis or ligation of the distal artery. Distal ischaemia occurring in brachiocephalic or prosthetic graft AVF in the forearm or upper arm may be the result of global hypoperfusion and shunting of arterial blood through the graft.

Venous hypertension

Venous hypertension is increasingly being seen as a complication of haemodialysis access, especially with the increasing use of dual-lumen central venous catheters. Presenting symptoms include pain, oedema and hyperaemia and can progress to tissue necrosis if left untreated. Treatment consists of ligation of distal or collateral veins. Oedema of the entire arm is likely, because of subclavian vein stenosis or thrombosis due to previous ipsilateral subclavian vein cannulation. Percutaneous balloon angioplasty of the stenotic central vein with or without an intravascular stent or fistula ligation is an option in the management of this condition (Beathard, 1995).

Patient scenario

Debbie is a 34-year-old who has been receiving haemodialysis for 2 years. Following the creation of a native brachiocephalic fistula, access for dialysis was uneventful. Debbie is currently on home haemodialysis and has been self-caring with the support of her husband. She is reluctant to change her needling practices and has developed three sites that tend to be cannulated for dialysis. Her monthly blood figures indicate a reduction in her dialysis clearances and on questioning she states that she has been able to get 250–300 ml blood flow on dialysis. She says she has noticed that her venous pressure has been gradually increasing over a period of 6 weeks. Despite early home training Debbie has managed to care for herself very well. She is anxious about the need to transfer to centre haemodialysis for assessments to be undertaken of her access.

Review questions
- Identify the possible factors that may be responsible for Debbie's current access difficulties.
- Discuss the assessment and evaluation options that will need to be performed.
- Identify the nurse's role in supporting Debbie throughout the process of evaluation of her access.

Pseudoaneurysms

Aneurysms or pseudoaneurysms may develop in either native vein of prosthetic AV grafts as a result of repeated needle punctures in the same segment of the access. They can be avoided by careful rotation of needle sites. Infected pseudoaneurysms in prosthetic grafts may rupture, requiring emergency graft ligation or revision.

CENTRAL VENOUS CATHETERS FOR HAEMODIALYSIS ACCESS

Double-lumen central venous catheters are an important option for vascular access for haemodialysis. As well as providing access for acute dialysis they represent an important route of vascular access for chronic dialysis patients. Double-lumen catheters may be placed in the femoral, subclavian or internal jugular veins using the Seldinger technique (Figure 7.7). For longer-term temporary access (i.e. several weeks) either the subclavian or internal jugular route is used, although increasing recognition of the high incidence of ipsilateral subclavian vein stenosis following subclavian cannulation for haemodialysis has made the internal jugular vein the preferred route. The development of a double-lumen, Silastic, Dacron-cuffed central venous dialysis catheter inserted percutaneously or *via* surgical cut-down in the internal jugular vein and tunnelled on to the upper chest wall has greatly facilitated provision of prolonged temporary vascular access. Originally developed to provide temporary vascular access until an autogenous vein or prosthetic graft AVF was mature, recently they have been used successfully for long-term or permanent access in an

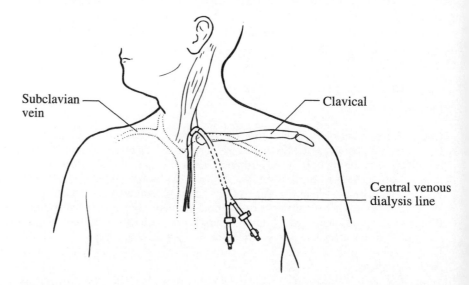

Subclavian vein

Clavical

Central venous dialysis line

Figure 7.7 Double-lumen tunnelled catheter. (Source: adapted from Uldall, 1993.)

increasing group of patients in whom an AVF cannot be created or maintained because of their age, co-morbid disease or multiple previous failed accesses.

COMPLICATIONS OF CENTRAL VENOUS DIALYSIS CATHETERS

Technical complications secondary to the insertion of catheters are known to occur with significant bleeding (1.4%), arterial puncture (0.8%), haemothorax (0.5%), pneumothorax (0.3%) and air embolism (0.1%) reported to occur (Vandholder, 1987). This study also identified that in a survey of 16 dialysis units five fatal complications occurred following 4000 catheterizations.

Thrombosis

The need for repeated access to the circulation, a feature of haemodialysis, and the requirement for a blood flow of 250–500 ml/ minute, along with the advent of high-flux dialysis requiring even higher flow rates, all increase the demands upon haemodialysis catheters. Poor flow rates may result from a kink in the tunnelled catheter or malposition. The tip of the catheter should be positioned in the right atrium to avoid flow-related problems. Correctly positioned, flow rates of 200–300 ml/min can be achieved. Poor flow rates and catheter thrombosis are the commonest complications of prolonged use of silicone dialysis catheters. Radiological studies often reveal a fibrin sheath around the catheter tip that acts like a ball-valve to restrict flow.

Subclavian vein stenosis

Concern about central vein stenosis, well described with the use of subclavian catheters in ESRD, has prompted the use of internal jugular vein permanent catheters to avoid this complication. Permanent catheter access is not without its own special problems (Rotellar et al., 1996). Suhocki et al. (1996) reviewed 163 consecutive episodes of catheter malfunctions that occurred in 121 catheters in 88 patients over a 3.5-year period. Instillation of urokinase successfully established flow rates of 300 ml/min in 74 of the episodes. In 38 of the remaining cases a fibrin sheath was detected encasing the catheter. The use of endoluminal thrombolytic therapy and percutaneous mechanical techniques extended the mean catheter survival to 12.7 months. Silastic-cuffed catheters are assuming a greater role in providing long-term vascular access for haemodialysis patients. However, catheter thrombosis, fibrin sheath formation and catheter malposition are recurrent problems that reduce extracorporeal flow rates and shorten catheter life.

Venous strictures or stenosis may occur in 42–50% of cases following subclavian vein catheterization with a stricture rate of 50% being reported in catheters in situ for an average of 11.5 days. Thrombosis may also occur in the brachiocephalic vein, superior vena cava and inferior vena cava following the long-term use of Silastic central venous catheters. Subclavian stenosis may lead to venous hypertension, elevated venous pressure or recirculation on dialysis, or thrombosis of an AVF placed distally to the ipsilateral extremity. Treatment of thrombosis may involve systemic thrombolytic therapy, percutaneous balloon angioplasty or intravascular stents. Thrombotic complications vary depending on the type of catheter material used: polyethylene catheters are more thrombogenic than Silastic and polyurethane catheters.

Infection

Infection represents the second major complication associated with central vein catheter use; maintaining asepsis and management of the catheter site are therefore critical. Minimizing the number of manipulations of the catheter plays a part in the reduction of infection (Corona *et al.*, 1990). Extensive research has focused on the use of various antiseptic solutions to prevent catheter-related infections. Chlorhexidine, an antiseptic that disrupts the microbial cell membrane, is particularly effective against Gram-positive bacteria, although less effective against Gram-negative bacteria and fungi. Iodine solutions are possibly the most widely used of the iodophor compounds, which produce their antiseptic actions by penetrating the cell wall of microorganisms (Gaudet and Beaufoy, 1996).

Key reference: Gaudet, D., and Beaufoy, A. (1996) Antiseptic solutions for haemodialysis catheters. *Canadian Association of Nephrology Nurses and Technicians* 6(4): 20–23.

Vandholder (1987) identified a significant increase in infections occurring in polyurethane catheters *in situ* for 10 days or more, in contrast to tunnelled, Dacron-cuffed silicone catheters, which show a reduced infection rate. The management of infection in the patient with a central venous catheter is still an area of continuing research, with standard practices including systemic antibiotics followed by a new catheter insertion once the infection has cleared. This represents a significant problem for the long-term dialysis patient where the focus is the preservation of vascular access site.

Differing views are evident on how to manage central venous catheter infections without losing a potential vascular access site. The use of parental antibiotics and guide-wire exchange have been advocated as successful approaches in managing catheter-related sepsis associated with tunnelled, Dacron-cuffed Silastic catheters. The organisms most commonly responsible for catheter-related sepsis include *Staphylococcus aureus* and *Staphylococcus epidermidis*. Exit-site infections can be treated with local care and systemic antibiotics, although grossly purulent tunnel infections require catheter removal. It has been identified that, within the haemodialysis patient, endogenous contamination due to the presence of *Staphylococcus* on the patient's skin is a potential source of infection even after skin cleansing with antiseptic (Kaplowitz *et al.*, 1988). The catheter hub and the infusate are major sources of exogenous catheter-relayed infections if health-care staff breach sterile technique.

SYNTHETIC GRAFTS

Subcutaneous autogenous saphenous vein graph is constructed from the patient's own saphenous vein, which is removed from the leg and tunnelled subcutaneously in the forearm, with the end attached to an artery and vein. These grafts are infrequently used today.

Specially treated bovine grafts, usually the carotid, have played an important role in vascular access for patients, although this form of access is more prone to thrombosis and infection. Venous stenosis, which accounts for the majority of thromboses, can be prospectively identified by performing routine measurements of venous dialysis pressure or urea recirculation. Prospective identification of venous stenosis followed by either angioplasty or surgical revision improves fistula patency and enhances the quality of life of the haemodialysis population.

Bhandari *et al.* (1995) compared the survival and complication rates of saphenous vein forearm grafts and Gore-tex® thigh grafts over a 12-year period. The survival of saphenous vein forearm grafts at 1 year was 89.4% and for Gore-tex® thigh graft 84.9%. Higher complication rates were evident in patients with Gore-tex® grafts (0.61 per patient year) in comparison to 0.22 for forearm grafts. Gore-tex® grafts had higher rates of infection (35%) with no infections evident in the saphenous forearm graft.

Complications associated with synthetic grafts

Synthetic grafts are at risk of development of infection. During the first 6 weeks post-insertion infection is usually attributable to contamination of the operative site during the procedure. *Staphylococcus aureus* is the organism most commonly responsible for graft sepsis, which often arises through infected needle puncture sites. Newly placed polytetrafluoroethene (PTFE) arteriovenous grafts require a period of wound healing and incorporation of fibrous tissue before use, a period typically lasting 6 weeks. An ideal PTFE graft would be one that could be used for vascular access immediately, obviating the need for temporary dialysis catheters. Despite the AVF being recommended as the best form of vascular access because of its limited complications the provision of vascular access through synthetic grafts is critical to successful therapy for many patients. Synthetic grafts provide excellent access to an individual's circulation but are prone to significant complications. Albers (1994) has compared the survival of synthetic grafts with native AVF and suggests that their 3-year survival rate is between 50% and 60%.

Vascular access complications are the most frequent cause of death among patients with end-stage renal disease on haemodialysis. The most common complication of prosthetic graft fistulae is thrombosis. Roberts *et al.* (1996) demonstrated the importance of directing unit policy towards effective graft surveillance, which involves measuring venous resistance, followed by fistulagram and percutaneous dilatation of identified stenosis, in the detection and management of potential access thrombosis. This retrospective review demonstrated the effectiveness of a policy of graft surveillance and percutaneous treatment of graft stenosis in prolonging primary surgical patency and graft survival. Waeleghem and Ysebaert (1995b) have identified a number of features that warrant a **colour Doppler ultrasound scan** or angiography.

Infection and thrombosis represent the two leading causes of loss in synthetic grafts (Windus, 1993). Anatomical stenosis is a leading cause of graft loss, venous stenosis being the most common anatomical lesion found. Hawkins (1995) suggests that more than 50% of these lesions occur at the venous anastomosis, stenosis at the arterial anastomosis being much rarer (fewer than 5% of cases). The development of intimal hyperplasia has been well documented as the cause of anastomotic lesions. Disruption of the graft's intimal lining has been associated with needle puncture and the subsequent development of thrombus formation. In cases of thrombosis occurring in the absence of anatomical lesions the probable predisposing factors are those resulting in low flow states through the access, including hypotensive episodes, excess pressure on needle sites post-dialysis, accidental graft compression during sleep and low cardiac output. Where there is evidence of hypercoagulability this is thought to predispose to thrombosis formation although conclusive evidence is lacking.

> **Key reference**: Hawkins, T.C. (1995) Nurses role in influencing positive vascular access outcomes. *American Nephrology Nurses Association* 22(2): 127–129.

When thrombus develops a variety of interventions have been suggested to ensure patency. Mizumoto *et al.* (1996b) demonstrated the benefit of directional atherectomy (DA) for vascular access failure with either poor blood flow or high venous pressure. This procedure, a therapeutic modality for coronary artery disease, demonstrated an 84% success rate. Despite re-stenotic events, the patency rate at 1 month post-intervention was 100%, at 3 months 93%, at 6 months 92% and at 12 months 75%. The short-term patency rate of DA was more satisfactory than the results of percutaneous transluminal angioplasty. The use of endovascular stents in the management of venous stenosis has been successful in a number of patients (Domingo *et al.*, 1996).

CONCLUSION

Complications associated with vascular access for haemodialysis represent one of the most important sources of morbidity among ESRD patients globally. The magnitude and growth of vascular-access-related hospitalization demonstrates that the costs of this morbidity are high in both personal

Indication for colour Doppler ultrasound scan or angiography

- Inadequate arterial inflow
- Increased venous pressure
- Changed urea recirculation
- Difficulty in returning blood into access
- Difficulty in cannulation
- Anatomical abnormalities in the access, including:
  - Enlarging aneurysm
  - Venous congestion or oedema of the access limb
- Repeated clotting of a graft post-thrombectomy
- Ischaemia of the access limb
- Sepsis of undetermined aetiology
- Planning for vascular access (Waeleghem and Ysebaert, 1995b)

and financial terms. Frequent hospitalization because of vascular problems is commonplace, the added cost to health-care resources being substantial (Civetta *et al.*, 1996). Although radial arteriovenous fistula continues to represent the optimal access modality, the appropriate roles for brachial arteriovenous fistulae, synthetic bridge grafts and central venous catheters are less certain because of inadequate data on the long-term function of the first and the high rates of complications associated with the latter two. To reduce vascular-access-related morbidity, strategies must be developed not only to prevent and detect appropriately early synthetic vascular access dysfunction but to better identify the patients in whom radial arteriovenous fistula is a viable clinical option (Feldman *et al.*, 1996; Hartigan, 1994)

Key reference: Hartigan, M.F. (1994) Vascular access and Nephrology nursing practice: existing views and rationales for change. *Advances in Renal Replacement Therapies* 1(2): 155–62.

REVIEW QUESTIONS

- Name the different types of vascular access available for dialysis.
- Identify the main complications associated with vascular access.
- What are the main considerations concerning the needling of AVF?
- Identify the role of the health-care team in the education of patients and families concerning chronic vascular access.
- Discuss the specific preoperative and postoperative management of a patient undergoing formation of a native AVF.
- How can the health-care team provide quality in terms of its management of vascular access?
- Discuss how infection can be prevented in (a) central venous catheters (b) native AVF (c) prosthetic AV grafts.
- Discuss the nursing assessment of a patient's access prior to commencing dialysis.

REFERENCES

Albers, F. J. (1994) Causes of hemodialysis access failure. *Advances in Renal Replacement Therapy*, **1**(2), 107–118.

Aldridge, C., Greenwood, R. N., Cattell, W. R. and Barrett, R. V. (1984) Assessment of arteriovenous fistulae from pressure and recirculation. *Proceedings of the European Dialysis and Transplant Nurses Association–European Renal Care Association*, **14**, 207–215.

Alvarez, R., Paris, C., Alvaro, A. *et al.* (1994) Repeated punctures as indicator of quality of vascular access care. *Journal of the European Dialysis and Transplant Nurses Association–European Renal Care Association*, **4**, 18–20.

Beathard, G. A. (1995) Thrombolysis versus surgery for the treatment of thrombosed dialysis access grafts. *Journal of the American Society of Nephrology*, **6**(6), 1619–1624.

Berkoben, M. and Schwab, S. J. (1995) Maintenance of permanent hemodialysis vascular access patency. *American Nephrology Nurses Association Journal*, **22**(1), 17–24.

Berry, C. (1996) Detecting hemodialysis vascular access stenosis: a tracking tool. *American Nephrology Nurses Association Journal*, **23**(4), 397–415.

Bhandari, S., Wilkinson, A. and Sellars, L. (1995) Saphenous vein forearm grafts and gortex thigh grafts as alternative forms of vascular access. *Clinical Nephrology*, **44**(5), 325–328.

Brothers, T. E., Morgan, M., Robinson, J. G. *et al.* (1996) Failure of dialysis access: revise or replace? *Journal of Surgical Research*, **60**(2), 312–316.

Brouwer, D. J. (1995) Cannulation: basic needle cannulation training for dialysis staff. *Dialysis and Transplantation*, **24**(11), 606–612.

Byrne, S. (1994) A new proactive approach to the management of arteriovenous fistulae. *Journal of the European Dialysis and Transplant Nurses Association – European Renal Care Association*, **4**, 10–15.

Churchill, D. N., Taylor, D. W. and Cook, R. J. (1992) Canadian hemodialysis morbidity study. *American Journal of Kidney Diseases*, **19**, 261.

Civetta, J. M., Hudson-Civetta, J. and Ball, S. (1996) Decreasing catheter-related infection and hospital costs by continuous quality improvement. *Critical Care Medicine*, **24**(10), 1660–1665.

Corona, M. L., Peters, S. G., Narr, B. J. and Thompson R. L. (1990) Infections related to central venous catheters. *Mayo Clinic Proceedings*, **65**(9), 979–986.

Crespo, R. (1994) Influence of bevel position of the needle on puncture pain in haemodialysis. *Journal of the European Dialysis and Transplant Nurses Association*, **4**, 21–23.

Domingo, E., Martinez, J., Ortells, R. *et al.* (1996) Self expandable endovascular stent for treatment of venous stenosis. *Journal of the European Dialysis and Transplant Nurses Association*, **22**(4), 29–30.

Feldman, H. I., Kobrin, S. and Wasserstein, A. (1996) Hemodialysis vascular access morbidity (editorial). *Journal of the American Society of Nephrology*, **7**(4), 523–535.

Gaudet, D. and Beaufoy, A. (1996) Antiseptic solutions for haemodialysis catheters. *Canadian Association of Nephrology Nurses and Technicians*, **6**(4), 20–23.

Gerrish, M. C., Chamberlain, H., Pammenter, K. *et al.* (1996) Quality in practice: setting a standard for the insertion of fistula needles. *Journal of the European Dialysis and Transplant Nurses Association–European Renal Care Association*, **22**(4), 34–35.

Grapsa, I. and Oreopoulos, D. G., (1996) Practical ethical issues of dialysis in the elderly. *Seminars in Nephrology*, **16**(4), 339–352.

Hartigan, M. F. (1994) Vascular access and nephrology nursing practice: existing views and rationales for change. *Advances in Renal Replacement Therapies*, **1**(2), 155–162.

Hawkins, T. C. (1995) Nurses role in influencing positive vascular access outcomes. *American Nephrology Nurses Association Journal*, **22**(2), 127–129.

Kaplowitz, L. G., Cornstock, J. A., Landwehr, D. M. *et al.* (1988) A prospective study of infections in haemodialysis patients: patient hygiene and other risk factors for infection. *Infection Control and Hospital Epidemiology*, **9**(12), 534–541.

Kirkpatrick, W. G., Culpepper, R. M. and Sirmon, M. D. (1996) Frequency of complications with prolonged femoral vein catheterisation for hemodialysis access. *Nephron*, **73**(1), 58–62.

Kramer, M. and Polaschegg, H. D. (1993) Automated measurement of recirculation. *Journal of the European Dialysis and Transplant Nurses Association–European Renal Care Association*, **19**, 6–9.

Lindley, E. (1996) Introduction to the research forum. *Journal of the European Dialysis and Transplant Nurses Association–European Renal Care Association*, **3**, 46–47.

Martinez Barquinero, M., Romero, L. and Perez, R. (1993) Evaluation of arterio-venous fistulae in haemodialysis with an echo–Doppler technique. *Journal of the European Dialysis and Transplant Nurses Association–European Renal Care Association*, **19**(2), 10–11.

Mizumoto, D., Watanabe, Y., Kumon, S. *et al.* (1996a) The treatment of chronic hemodialysis vascular access by Directional Atherectomy. *Nephron*, **74**(1), 45–52.

Mizumoto, O., Pieroni, L., Lawrence, C. *et al.* (1996b) Prospective, randomised trial of two antiseptic solutions for prevention of central venous or arterial catheter colonisation and infection in intensive care unit patients. *Critical Care Medicine*, **24**(11), 1818–1823.

Prischl, F. C., Kirchgatterer, A., Brandstatter, E. *et al.* (1995) Parameters of prognostic relevance to the patency of vascular access in hemodialysis patients. *Journal of the American Society of Nephrology*, **6**(6), 1613–1618.

Raja, M. and Rasib, M. (1994) Vascular access for hemodialysis, in *Handbook of Dialysis*, (eds J. T. Daugirdas and S. I. Todd), Little, Brown & Co, New York.

Rivers, S. P., Scher, L. A. and Veith, F. J. (1992) Correction of steal syndrome secondary to hemodialysis fistulas: a simplified quantitative technique. *Surgery*, 112, 593.

Roberts, A. B., Kahn, M. B., Bradford, S. *et al.* (1995) Graft surveillance and angioplasty prolongs dialysis graft patency. *Journal of the American College of Surgeons*, **183**(5), 486–492.

Rotellar, C., Sims, S. C. and Freeland, J. (1996) Right atrium thrombosis in patients on hemodialysis. *American Journal of Kidney Diseases*, **27**(5), 726–728.

Serfaty, M., Lopez, J., Granolleras, C. and Shaldon, S. (1994) The nursing use of a graphical record of arteriovenous fistulae. *Journal of the European Dialysis and Transplant Nurses Association–European Renal Care Association*, **20**, 12–14.

Sherman, R. A., Besarab, A., Schwab, S. J. and Beathard, G. A. (1997) Recognition of the falling vascular access: a current perspective. *Seminars in Dialysis*, **10**(1), 1–4.

Suhocki, P. V., Conlon, P. J., Knelson, M. H. *et al.* (1996) Silastic cuffed catheters for hemodialysis vascular access: thrombolytic and mechanical correction of malfunction. *American Journal of Kidney Diseases*, **28**(3), 379–386.

Thornton, J., Todd, N. J. and Webster, N. R. (1996) Central lines for haemodialysis access: central venous line sepsis in the intensive care unit. A study comparing antibiotic coated catheters with plain catheters. *Anaesthesia*, **51**(11), 1018–1020.

Uldall, P. R. (1993) Temporary vascular access for hemodialysis, in *Dialysis Therapy*, 2nd edn, (eds R. A. Nissenson and R. N. D. Fine), Hawey & Belfus, Philadelphia, PA.

Vandholder, R., Hoenich, N. and Ringoir, S. (1987) Morbidity and mortality of central venous catheter hemodialysis: a review of 10 years experience. *Nephron*, **47**, 274.

Waeleghem, J. P. and Ysebaert, D. (1995a) Vascular access in haemodialysis. *Journal of the European Dialysis and Transplant Nurses Association–European Renal Care Association*, **21**(1), 1–7 (Suppl.).

Waeleghem, J. P. and Ysebaert, D. (1995b) Vascular access in haemodialysis: part 2. *Journal of the European Dialysis and Transplant Nurses Association–European Renal Care Association*, **21**(12), 9–15 (Suppl.).

Windus, D. W. (1993) Permanent vascular access: a nephrologist's view. *American Journal of Kidney Diseases*, **21**(5), 457–471.

Complications of haemodialysis

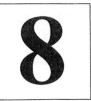

Paul Challinor

LEARNING OBJECTIVES

At the end of this chapter the reader should be able to:

- Identify the complications associated with haemodialysis.
- Describe the nursing care required to prevent the incidence of complications associated with haemodialysis.
- Discuss the importance of assessing the patient prior to commencing haemodialysis.
- Describe the care required to prevent the spread of infection in the haemodialysis unit.

INTRODUCTION

When one considers the haemodialysis process, it is sobering to reflect on the large number of complications that can occur during the procedure. If undetected, or through poor nursing care, many can be fatal. A large number of the complications associated with haemodialysis can be avoided through appropriate and careful patient assessment prior to commencing the treatment, and proper care during dialysis. However, because haemodialysis has a complex effect on individuals, the incidence of complications increases in association with the age of the patient and with medical conditions such as diabetes and cardiac disease (Lazarus and Hakim, 1991).

HYPOTENSION

Hypotension is a very common complication associated with haemodialysis, estimated to occur in around 25% of dialysis treatments (Henderson, 1980), and is probably a reflection of the large amount of fluid that is removed during the procedure as the patient nears his/her dry weight (de Vries *et al.*, 1991). Hypotensive episodes during dialysis occur in 25–30% of all bicarbonate treatments but this increases to 50% with the use of acetate dialysate (Orofino *et al.*, 1990; de Vries *et al.*, 1991).

Key reference: de Vries, P.M., Otholf, C.G., Solf, A., Sheunemann, B., Oe, P.L., Quellehost, E., Schneider, H. and Donker, A.J.M. (1991) Fluid balance during haemodialysis and haemofiltration: The effect of dialysate sodium and a variable ultrafiltration rate. *Nephrology, Dialysis and Transplantation* 6: 257–263.

Hypovolaemic hypotension

Symptomatic hypotension associated with relative hypovolaemia usually occurs towards the end of the dialysis session. Maintaining blood pressure is dependent upon the replacement of the fluid removed from the blood volume with fluid from the surrounding tissues. If fluid removal exceeds this intercompartmental shift then the venous return will be reduced, resulting in decreased cardiac output and hypotension (Hempl *et al.*, 1980).

To prevent hypotension fluid removal should be consistent throughout the session. To achieve this an ultrafiltration control should be used. Without this fluctuations in fluid removal can occur as a result of fluctuations in pressure across the dialyser membrane. If a large amount of fluid needs to be removed, because of excessive interdialytic weight gain or because the previous dialysis was short, consideration should be given to prolonging the treatment time to remove the fluid without resorting to an aggressive ultrafiltration rate. Large amounts of fluid can be removed by stopping dialysis and putting the machine into sequential ultrafiltration mode (Rouby *et al.*, 1980). Because relatively few electrolytes are removed in UF, only fluid, the patient is able to tolerate greater fluid removal. It is advisable to dialyse the patient for a short time (1 hour) to remove potassium before placing the machine into UF. This prevents haemoconcentration of potassium as fluid is removed, reducing the risk of cardiac arrhythmias. Once enough fluid has been removed, the session can then be returned to dialysis with a reduced TMP (Chapter 6).

If the patient is dialysed below his/her dry weight, hypotension results. The symptoms persist after dialysis and are associated with cramps and a 'washed-out feeling' (Lazarus and Hakim, 1991). Dry weights should be reviewed on a regular basis, especially if symptoms persist after dialysis (see patient scenario below).

Patient scenario

Mary Watkins had been on three-times-a-week dialysis for 6 months without any real problems of note. However, recently towards the end of dialysis Mary had begun to suffer severe symptomatic hypotensive episodes, occasionally accompanied by cramp in both legs. No change had been made to the dialysate solution and Mary's interdialytic weight gains had been on average only 1.5 kg. Mary's blood pressure had remained about 130/90 mmHg predialysis throughout. The recurrent hypotensive episodes were affecting Mary's mental tolerance of dialysis and she complained of feeling very thirsty the day after dialysis. It was decided to review Mary's dry weight and on assessment it was found that Mary had an increasing appetite and appeared to be gaining body weight. The dry weight was increased by 1 kg and the incidence of symptomatic hypotension and cramps diminished.

The use of a low-sodium dialysate concentrate inappropriately results in hypotension due to the excessive loss of sodium from the plasma. If a low-sodium concentrate must be used then the UF control should be utilized to reduce the amount of fluid removed.

Lack of vasoconstriction

Following plasma volume depletion the normal physiological response would be vasoconstriction and an increase in the heart rate as compensatory factors to prevent hypotension. However, dialysis interferes with this process and can lead to symptomatic **hypotension**.

Acetate dialysis concentrate has a known vasodilatory effect (Chapter 6), which is more evident in diabetics and women. Because the risk of symptomatic hypotension is reduced with the use of bicarbonate dialysis, the removal of larger amounts of fluid is possible. When high-flux dialysis is used, the use of a bicarbonate concentrate is mandatory (Collins and Keshaviah, 1988).

Many dialysis patients are hypothermic at the beginning of dialysis, and the body temperature often rises during dialysis, though the mechanism is poorly understood. It may, in part, be due to the exposure to the warming effect of the dialysate, which is normally kept at 37–38°C. Increases in core temperature have a vasodilatory effect, leading to an increased chance of symptomatic hypotension. Some writers have advocated using a lower dialysate temperature, but patients frequently complain of feeling cold and shivery when dialysed against a cool dialysate (Bregman *et al.*, 1994). However, Fine and Penner (1996) found that in patients with subnormal temperatures prior to dialysis, incidence of symptomatic hypotension was reduced when dialysed against a cool dialysate of 35°C.

Some patients experience hypotension following ingestion of food during dialysis, because of reduced constriction of some capillary beds, especially the splanchnic bed (Barakat, 1993), which makes the patient more prone to symptomatic hypotension. Large meals on dialysis should therefore be discouraged, and those at risk should be identified and the risks explained. The 'food effect' can last up to 2 hours (Bregman *et al.*, 1994), so eating just prior to dialysis should also be discouraged.

Symptomatic hypotension is also associated with antihypertensive drugs. A large proportion of dialysis patients receive such medication, and if taken before dialysis it may result in hypotension during it. Patients should be individually assessed to measure the risk and advice given appropriately.

Rare causes of dialysis-associated hypotension

- MI
- Occult haemorrhage
- Septicaemia
- Arrhythmias
- Anaphylaxis
- Haemolysis
- Air embolism

Treatment of dialysis-induced hypotension

Treatment is straightforward. The patient should be placed in the Trendelenburg position and the TMP should be reduced to as near zero as possible. If the hypotensive episode is severe, a bolus infusion of 100 ml (or more if necessary) of 0.9% saline should be administered. The amount of fluid given should be kept to the minimum. The equivalent amount of the infused saline needs to be removed during the remainder of the dialysis (unless the patient has been dialysed below his/her dry weight). Some centres use hypertonic saline, glucose or mannitol as alternatives to 0.9% saline.

Traditionally the use of hypertonic saline to relieve symptomatic hypotension during the last hour of dialysis has been discouraged because of the fear of hypernatraemia and interdialytic weight gain. However, Sanderson and Katz (1994) have demonstrated that giving hypertonic saline in the last hour of dialysis to treat hypotension does not significantly increase interdialytic weight gain.

> **Key reference:** Sanderson, N.A. and Katz, M.A. (1994) The fate of hypertonic saline administered during hemodialysis. *ANNA Journal* 21(4): 162–169.

Care and support may also be required if the patient is suffering from cramps, nausea or vomiting. These symptoms usually subside once the blood pressure is restored. Once the patient is stabilized, fluid removal can be resumed, but at a slower rate. If a large amount of fluid remains to be removed, then consideration should be given to extending the dialysis session, taking the fluid off slowly over a longer period of time.

Prevention

Preventative measures should include checking previous dialyses for hypotensive episodes and establishing the reason. Regular observations during dialysis should indicate and predict risk of hypotension. Patient education plays an important part, ensuring that antihypertensives are not taken on the morning of dialysis and encouraging patients not to exceed their fluid intake. Carefully setting the UF rate in relation to the amount of fluid to be removed should prevent large fluid losses in short time periods. Regular checks and reviews of dry weight are important, looking for loss of body mass or weight gain other than that attributable to fluid.

MUSCLE CRAMPS

Causes

The pathogenesis behind the incidence of cramps associated with dialysis is generally unknown, but it appears to be linked with a number of predisposing factors – hypotension, an incorrect dry weight, a dialysate too low in sodium and/or too large ultrafiltration volumes (Lazarus and Hakim, 1991). Cramps usually occur late on in dialysis, when the net amount of fluid removed is at its greatest.

Management

When cramp occurs on dialysis it can be a very painful and distressing condition for the patient, who is unable to move very much to alleviate the discomfort because s/he is still attached to the machine. A bolus infusion of normal saline or hypertonic saline may be beneficial, but care should be taken not to infuse too much fluid. Neal *et al.* (1981) found that a 50–100 ml bolus of 50% glucose brought relief within 5 minutes. The resulting period hyperglycaemia was short and no side-effects occurred as a result. Massaging the affected area helps to bring relief to the affected site, and the physical contact also helps to calm the patient.

If cramps persist, altering the dialysate sodium to a higher concentration may prevent any further incidences. The use of variable-sodium dialysis has been found to reduce the problem of dialysis-induced cramps (Flanigan *et al.*, 1997; Jenson *et al.*, 1994).

> **Key reference:** Jenson, B.M., Dobbe, S.A., Squillace, D.P. and McCarthy, J.T. (1994) Clinical benefits of high and variable sodium concentration dialysate in hemodialysis patients. *ANNA Journal* 21(2): 115–120.

Prevention

The link between the removal of large fluid volumes and cramp suggests that preventing too rapid fluid removal may result in a lower incidence of cramp. Educating the patient to prevent large interdialytic fluid gains should be a priority. Increasing the dialysate sodium concentration may be an option, but this may increase postdialysis thirst and consequent interdialytic weight gain. Administration of quinine sulphate before dialysis decreases the incidence of cramps on dialysis and has been found to be useful as a prophylactic measure (Blagg, 1992). However, Mandal *et al.* (1993) argue that, because cramp is a subjective symptom, the effectiveness of quinine may be open to question. But they do admit that most patients consider quinine to be beneficial.

NAUSEA AND VOMITING

Causes

Nausea and vomiting occur in approximately 10% of dialyses. The causes are multifactorial: although in the majority of cases the cause is probably hypotension. Nausea and vomiting may also be associated with disequilibrium and with acetate dialysate.

Management

The prime point of caring for patients suffering from nausea and vomiting during dialysis is to treat the cause. If the symptoms persist, antiemetics may be necessary.

Prevention

The most obvious preventative measure is to avoid hypotensive episodes. Reducing the blood flow rate at the beginning of dialysis occasionally helps, but may mean increasing the overall time of dialysis to ensure an adequate dialysis. If acetate dialysis is suspected then symptoms may disappear with a switch to bicarbonate dialysis.

ELECTROLYTE IMBALANCE

Haemodialysis is a relatively aggressive treatment. Plasma electrolyte balances are subject to large alterations during dialysis, and these changes now occur over shorter periods of time with the trend towards shorter dialysis times. Because of these factors, selection of the appropriate dialysate concentrate (Chapter 6) takes on greater importance. Inappropriate selection can at best lead to mild, but distressing complications and at worst to potentially life-threatening situations.

Hyponatraemia

This is associated with using a dialysate containing a hypotonic concentration of sodium (Blagg, 1992). Because of the osmotic imbalance between plasma and dialysate, sodium is removed from the plasma during dialysis, leading to hypotension, nausea, vomiting, cramps, headaches and in extreme cases symptoms associated with disequilibrium syndrome. If a patient complains of any of these symptoms the dialysate and conductivity should be checked, and dialysis should be reinitiated with an appropriate concentrate solution.

Hypernatraemia

This results from using a hypertonic sodium concentrate, purposely or accidentally (Lidner et al., 1972). It may also be due to inaccurate proportioning systems (Blagg, 1992) or inappropriate monitoring of the conductivity. Patients complain of headache, nausea and thirst. Dialysis should be discontinued and recommenced using the correct dialysate.

Hypercalcaemia

This complication is usually associated with water-treatment system failure, and primarily occurs in 'hard water areas' (hence the term hard water syndrome), although it can also occur if a hypocalcaemic patient is dialysed against a high-calcium dialysate (Kaplan, 1994). Symptoms include nausea and vomiting, agitation, muscle twitching and hypertension, which appear about an hour after starting dialysis. Again, dialysis should be stopped and recommenced with the correct dialysate or when the water softener is repaired. Because of the risk, in hard water areas the water should be checked daily before dialysis is started for the day.

Hypokalaemia

Hypokalaemia in patients undergoing maintenance haemodialysis is often associated with gastrointestinal loss through vomiting or diarrhoea

(Kaplan, 1994). The use of a concentrate with no potassium can also be the cause. Hypokalaemia is also common in normokalaemic patients in acute renal failure. Care should be taken to avoid hypokalaemia because of the risk of cardiac arrhythmias, especially in a patient on digoxin (Morrison *et al.*, 1980, cited by Kaplan, 1994). Dialysis against a dialysate with a higher potassium concentration should be considered, although this is not advisable for the whole dialysis; it is better to change to a lower concentration towards the end of the treatment. Potassium levels at the end of dialysis should be considered with care: there is a considerable potassium rebound 1–2 hours postdialysis (Ross and Nissenson, 1994).

Hyperkalaemia

Hyperkalaemia is usually associated with non-adherence to dietary advice but, although not associated with the dialysis treatment, it does affect decisions regarding time of dialysis, concentrate and filter to be used. Haemolysis during dialysis is the most likely cause of acute hyperkalaemia (Blagg, 1992), initiated by transfusion incompatibility or overheated dialysate (Kaplan, 1994).

DISEQUILIBRIUM SYNDROME

Disequilibrium syndrome is a combination of systemic and neurological symptoms that can occur either during or soon after dialysis. The syndrome is more prevalent in acute renal failure, during first dialysis for ESRD patients and in the elderly, but also occurs in any patient suffering from severe uraemia. In its more serious form it can lead to fits, coma and death from cerebral herniation.

The causative factors behind disequilibrium are open to dispute. Some believe that the symptoms are caused by a sudden reduction in plasma solute levels, leading to a variation in the osmotic balance between the plasma and the cerebrospinal fluid (Blagg, 1992). This results in a fluid shift into the cerebrospinal fluid, causing cerebral oedema. This is countered by Fraser and Arieff (1988), who argue that the increase in intracranial pressure is due to a disequilibrium between the pH of the plasma and the cerebrospinal fluid.

The incidence of severe forms of disequilibrium has fallen over the past 15 years. Acute and uraemic patients are no longer dialysed for prolonged periods. However, the incidence of mild forms of disequilibrium may be under-reported, because the symptoms can also be attributed to other causes.

Mild disequilibrium

In its mild form disequilibrium syndrome may present as a combination of, or any of nausea, vomiting, restlessness and headache. Although these symptoms are non-specific, they may constitute evidence of mild disequilibrium. If disequilibrium is suspected, reducing the blood flow and providing a gentler dialysis may induce equilibrium of solutes and fluid between the various compartments, thereby reducing the associated symptoms. However, early termination of dialysis if the symptoms continue or deteriorate should be considered.

Severe disequilibrium

In its more serious form symptoms associated with cerebral oedema – seizures, hypertension and coma – occur. They may appear in the last 1–2 hours of dialysis or not until dialysis has finished. The care given to a patient with disequilibrium is mainly supportive. If it occurs during dialysis, discontinue dialysis immediately. In the majority of cases symptoms decline within a few hours, but they may persist for 24–36 hours. Diazepam can be used to control fits, and i.v. mannitol may be administered to reduce cerebral oedema. In very severe cases ventilation may be necessary.

Prevention

Care must be taken when dialysing a patient with acute renal failure, or a patient with ESRD receiving his first dialysis. The session should be short, no longer than 2–3 hours, and with a slowish blood-pump speed, aiming to reduce the plasma urea level by no more than 30%. In hypernatraemic patients care should be taken in choosing an appropriate concentrate, to reduce the risk of dialysing too much sodium from the patient (Bregman *et al.*, 1994).

PYROGENIC REACTION

Causes

Alter *et al.* (1989) found that pyrogenic reactions occurred in 0.4–5% of all dialysis treatment. A patient who develops a fever or chill during dialysis or very soon afterwards can be defined as having suffered a pyrogenic reaction. There are many causes, and the time of onset gives an indication of the likely one (Table 8.1). Whenever a pyrogenic reaction is suspected the cause must be identified to reduce the incidence in the future.

The pyrogenic reaction is induced by production of interleukin-1 as a result of exposure to endotoxins. Exposure may be *via* direct infusion into the blood through contaminated lines, dialyser or an infected access site, or indirectly through exposure to contaminated dialysate. Endotoxins are too large to pass through the dialyser membrane, but smaller bacterial breakdown products are known to induce release of interleukin-1 from monocytes. Bicarbonate solution can support bacterial growth and is prone to contamination (Collins and Keshaviah, 1988). Once opened, bicarbonate solutions should therefore be discarded within 24 hours.

Table 8.1 Causes of pyrogenic reactions associated with haemodialysis

Cause	Likely time of onset	Symptoms
Dialyser	30 min into dialysis	Any of the following can occur:
Blood lines	30 min into dialysis	
Local infection	During or after dialysis	
Poor aseptic technique	During or after dialysis	Pyrexia
Contaminated dialysate fluid	30 min into dialysis	Rigor/shivers
Contaminated water	30 min into dialysis	General malaise
Reuse of equipment	Immediate – 30 min into dialysis	Convulsions
Poor sterilization		Inflammation at access site
Poor storage		Nausea
Inadequate rinsing		Loss of consciousness
Transfusion of contaminated blood	Immediate or soon after commencing transfusion	Confusion if hyperpyrexial

Key reference: Collins, A.J. and Keshaviah, P.R. (1988) Are these limitations to shortening dialysis treatment? *Transcripts of the American Society for Artificial Organs* 34: 1–5.

Nursing care

Serious consideration should be given to stopping dialysis, especially if the pyrexia develops at the start of dialysis. Antipyretics should be given and the patient should be kept comfortable and under observation for further symptoms. Cultures should be taken to identify the cause: blood (and take a white blood cell count), dialysate fluid, water supply, access/wound swabs, nasal swabs.

Care should be taken to remove the source of infection and commence antibiotics if necessary. Once the reaction is under control, if the equipment or dialysate was at fault then dialysis may be recommenced. Care should be taken to establish a new access for dialysis, especially if the present access site was the cause. The batch numbers of all equipment used should be recorded and dialysis should be restarted with new equipment.

Prevention

Prevention in this case is better than cure. Check all equipment before use, and if in doubt do not use. Bicarbonate concentrates should not be used if they have been open for more than 24 hours. The access site should be assessed before and after each dialysis, checking for inflammation. Clear protocols for cleaning fistulas and subclavian lines should be adhered to. Some units use access site check lists to ensure that this is followed. Maintain good aseptic technique during needling and connection procedures.

All staff need education in the use and setting up of equipment. It is especially important that careful monitoring of all reuse equipment is undertaken. The unit should have a policy of regular water sampling for colonization with bacteria.

Prior to dialysis the patient should have his/her predialysis temperature taken. This gives a baseline from which to work if s/he becomes symptomatic on dialysis. The patient may already have been pyrexial prior to dialysis. Patients should also be educated to check their own access for signs of infection, and to report any concerns to the unit staff.

AIR EMBOLISM

The invention and incorporation into dialysis machines of air detectors means that this potentially fatal complication is now rare. However, the risk still exists and the incidence may be under-reported.

Nursing care

Air embolism during dialysis is an emergency situation. The lines should be clamped immediately and the blood pump stopped. The patient should be laid flat on his/her left side, and the foot of the bed should be elevated. This should help trap blood in the apex of the right ventricle. 100% oxygen should be given. Heparin and plasma expanders should be given to support cardiac output. In extreme cases air may be aspirated from the left ventricle.

Prevention

All equipment should be checked regularly throughout dialysis, ensuring that all connections are secure. Care should be taken when priming the lines and the dialyser prior to dialysis to guarantee that all air has been expelled.

If the air detector sounds, it should never be bypassed without identifying the reason for the alarm. Ensure there are adequate clamps for immediate use by each machine in case of need. Intravenous fluids should be administered carefully; never allow the infusion to run unsupervised, especially if the fluid is in vented glass bottles. Ideally all i.v. fluids should be given *via* collapsable plastic bags.

All dialysis machines should be checked and maintained on a regular basis to ensure that all alarms are working adequately. If there is any concern over any machine it should be taken out of commission and checked.

FIRST USE SYNDROME

This is a collection of symptoms occurring during dialysis that have been noted when using new filters. There are two main classifications of first use syndrome, anaphylactic (type A) and non-specific (type B). Both are caused by an allergic reaction to either the filter membrane or the sterilizing

---

Air embolism

Causes
- Inadequate priming – lines, dialyser
- Faulty air detector
- Faulty de-aerator in the machine
- Access
  - Unclamped subclavian line
  - Disconnection of blood lines
- Faulty equipment
  - Holes in lines
  - Loose or cracked connector
- Careless i.v. fluid administration
- Unsupervised/careless air washback

Signs and symptoms
- Chest pain
- Cyanosis
- Cough
- Feeling of fullness – rushing sensation
- Loss of consciousness
- Convulsions
- Cardiac arrest
- Venous line – air in air/foam detector
- 'churning sound' on auscultation of heart

agent, usually ethylene oxide. The syndrome occurs as a result of acute activation of the complement system when the blood comes into contact with cuprophane or cellulose acetate membranes (Hakim *et al.*, 1984; Ing *et al.*, 1983).

Anaphylactic – type A

Signs and symptoms

- Dyspnoea
- Sense of impending doom
- Feeling of warmth at fistula site or over whole body
- Itching
- Coryza (watery eyes)
- Diarrhoea and abdominal pain
- Cardiac arrest.

Symptoms start in the first minutes of dialysis, but may be delayed by up to 30 minutes.

Management

Stop dialysis immediately, and clamp the blood lines and discard. Washing back the blood will only exacerbate the condition because the reactive agent will be returned to the patient. Antihistamines and steroids will alleviate the anaphylactic reaction associated with type A conditions. If the patient does arrest then cardiopulmonary resuscitation will obviously be necessary.

Prevention

The only effective treatment for this condition is prevention. It is important to ensure proper rinsing of the filter. If the filter is left for any length of time between priming and connection, then it must be rinsed again. The ethylene oxide will diffuse into the rinsing fluid from the potting compound. If filters are routinely primed in batches, labels should be attached identifying the time of initial priming. In patients with a history of first use syndrome the obvious preventative measure is to avoid using filters sterilized with ethylene oxide. The introduction of a reuse programme may be a valid consideration if there are a large number of patients who suffer first use syndrome on a frequent basis.

Non-specific – type B

Much more common than type A, but much less severe, this is still a distressing condition for the patient and makes him/her more prone to other complications such as hypotension and cramps. Symptoms include chest pain, which may or may not be accompanied by back pain. Symptoms usually occur in the first minutes of dialysis, but they may be delayed by up to 1 hour. Because the symptoms associated with the type B condition are much less severe and non-specific, they can often go unrecognized as being associated with first use syndrome.

Management is generally supportive with the provision of analgesia and oxygen. Dialysis can be continued, as the symptoms usually abate after 1 hour, but serious thought must be given to altering the filter or introducing a reuse programme.

BLEEDING COMPLICATIONS DUE TO HAEMODIALYSIS

Considering the constant use of anticoagulation during the haemodialysis procedure and the prolonged bleeding time associated with uraemia (Carvalho, 1983) it is no surprise that bleeding problems are commonly associated with haemodialysis (Table 8.2). Care should always be taken when considering the anticoagulant regimen to use (Chapter 6), especially in acute renal failure patients, those with bleeding disorders and those who have recently undergone surgery, invasive investigation or trauma. Episodes of unexplained hypotension should always be investigated, especially if associated with pain.

Prolonged bleeding of the access site after the removal of needles is an indication of overcoagulation. This appears to be a minor point but is an indication that, unless the overcoagulation is corrected in subsequent treatments, the risk of a more serious haemorrhage remains. Checks on the clotting times during dialysis should be conducted on a regular basis, monthly for established patients and more frequently for patients just starting dialysis, acutely unwell or following surgery.

Table 8.2   Site of haemorrhage associated with haemodialysis

Site	Risk factor
Subdural haematoma	Head injury, rapid ultrafiltration, hypertension, overcoagulation
Gastrointestinal haemorrhage	Uraemic gastritis, angiodysplasia, overcoagulation, nasogastric feeding
Retroperitoneal haemorrhage	Trauma, postrenal biopsy, displaced femoral line
Access site	Overcoagulation, displacement of line, trauma during insertion of needles or line, infection
Cardiac tamponade	Uraemic pericarditis, overcoagulation
Thoracic haemorrhage	Uraemic pleuritis, infection, pulmonary infarction, displaced subclavian catheter

Table 8.3   Common causes of cardiac arrest in haemodialysis patients

- Fits
- Severe hypotension
- Fluid overload
- Underlying cardiac problems
- Incompatible blood transfusion
- Excessive and over-rapid fluid removal
- Drug administration – either by patient before dialysis or during it
- Wrong concentrate – high potassium

CARDIAC ARREST

Cardiac arrests are relatively common, and it is no surprise considering the electrolyte and fluid changes that occur over such a short period of time during haemodialysis. The risk factors and causes are numerous, but the most likely are identified in Table 8.3. Space does not allow an in-depth discussion on the signs and symptoms of cardiac arrest, but there are a few important actions to undertake in the cardiac arrest situation if the patient is on dialysis at the time. Once cardiac arrest has been established, then cardiopulmonary resuscitation should be initiated. The blood lines should be clamped but access should be maintained for drugs. The blood can be recirculated for no more than 20 minutes; consideration should be given to a wash-back, but only if staffing levels allow. It is imperative to remember that the patient is all-important and the dialysis machine secondary – if enough staff are not available once the patient is disconnected the machine can be ignored.

Prevention

Before commencing dialysis, especially if the nurse is unfamiliar with the patient, it is important that a full check is made of the patient's history looking for potential trouble areas. Check choice of equipment – dialyser, concentrate – before dialysis, especially if the equipment is set up by other members of staff. Realistic weight gain and loss and accurate fluid removal during dialysis will reduce the chance of complications. Regular observations during the treatment can be a signpost to problems, but this is equally important for all potential complications. Preparation and careful dialysis can prevent a 'mundane hypotensive' episode from deteriorating into an emergency situation.

CONCLUSION

Considering the large number of possibly fatal complications associated with haemodialysis, it is worth considering how relatively seldom they occur. This is an indication of the high quality of care that staff deliver to their patients, and of the advances in technology that make haemodialysis safer. However, technology is no replacement for thorough predialysis nursing assessment.

REVIEW QUESTIONS

- If an elderly dialysis patient consistently suffers from symptomatic hypotension and cramps during dialysis what aspects of their care should be reviewed?
- If a patient suffers a pyrogenic reaction 25 minutes after commencing dialysis, what are the possible causes?
- Identify the preventative measures for the causes you have identified in question 2.
- What precautions should be taken to prevent an air embolism?
- List the symptoms of disequilibrium syndrome and describe the nursing care if you suspect a patient of suffering from this condition.

REFERENCES

Alter, M. J., Favero, M. S., Moyer, L. A. and Bland, L. A. (1989) High flux dialysis in the United States. *Transactions of the American Society for Artificial Organs*, **35**, 107–108.

Barakat, M. M (1993) Hemodynamic effects of interdialytic food ingestion and the effects of caffine. *Journal of the American Society of Nephrology*, **3**, 1813.

Blagg, C. (1992) Acute complications associated with hemodialysis, in *Replacement of Renal Function by Dialysis*, 3rd edn, (ed. J. F. Maher), Kluwer Academic Publishers, Dordrecht.

Bregman, H., Daugirdas, J. T. and Ing, T. S. (1994) Complications during haemodialysis, in *Handbook of Dialysis*, 2nd edn, (eds J. T. Daugirdas and T. S. Ing), Little, Brown & Co, Boston, MA.

Carvalho, A. C. A. (1983) Bleeding in uraemia – clinical challenge. *New England Journal of Medicine*, **305**, 521–522.

Collins, A. J. and Keshaviah, P. R. (1988) Are these limitations to shortening dialysis treatment? *Transactions of the American Society for Artificial Organs*, **34**, 1–5.

De Vries, P. M., Otholf, C. G., Solf, A. *et al.* (1991) Fluid balance during haemodialysis and haemofiltration: the effect of dialysate sodium and a variable ultrafiltration rate. *Nephrology, Dialysis and Transplantation*, **6**, 257–263.

Fine, A. and Penner, B. (1996) The protective effect of cool dialysate is dependent on patients' predialysis temperature. *American Journal of Kidney Diseases*, **28**(2), 262–265.

Flanigan, M. J., Khairuah, Q. T. and Lim, V. S. (1997) Dialysate sodium delivery can alter chronic blood pressure management. *American Journal of Kidney Diseases*, **29**(3), 383–391.

Fraser, C. L. and Arieff, A. I. (19988) Nervous system complications in uraemia. *Annals of Internal Medicine*, **109**, 143–153.

Hakim, R. M., Breillatt, J., Lazarus, J. M., and Port, F. K. (1984) Complement activation and hypersensitivity reactions to dialysis membranes. *New England Journal of Medicine*, **311**, 878–882.

Hempl, H., Paeprer, H., Unger, V. *et al.* (1980) Hemodynamic changes during hemodialysis, sequential ultrafiltration, and hemofiltration. *Kidney International*, **18**, (S83).

Henderson, L. W. (1980) Symptomatic hypotension during haemodialysis *Kidney International*, **17**, 571–576.

Ing, T. S., Daugirdas, J. T., Popli, S. and Gandhi, V. C. (1983) First-use syndrome with cuprammonium cellulose dialysers. *International Journal of Artificial Organs*, **6**, 235–239.

Jenson, B. M., Dobbe, S. A., Squillace, D. P. and McCarthy, J. T. (1994) Clinical benefits of high and variable sodium concentration dialysate in hemodialysis patients. *American Nephrology Nurses Association Journal*, **21**(2), 115–120.

Kaplan, A. A. (1994) Maintenance haemodialysis: prescription and management, in *Renal Dialysis*, (eds J. D. Briggs, B. J. R. Junor, R. S. C. Rodger and J. F. Winchester), Chapman & Hall, London.

Lazarus, J. M. and Hakim, R. M. (1991) Medical aspects of hemodialysis, in *The Kidney*, 4th edn, (eds B. M. Brenner and F. C. Rector), W. B. Saunders, Philadelphia, PA.

Lidner, A., Moskovtchenko, J. F. and Traeger, J. (1972) Accidental mass hypernatremia during hemodialysis. Simultaneous observation in six cases. *Nephron*, **9**, 99.

Mandal, A. K., Abernathy, T., Nelluri, S. N. and Stitzel, V. (1993) Is quinine effective and safe in leg cramps? *Journal of Clinical Pharmacology*, **35**(6), 588–593.

Neal, C. R., Resnikoff, E. and Unger, A. M. (1981) Treatment of dialysis-related muscle-cramps with hypertonic dextrose. *Archives of Internal Medicine*, **141**, 171–173.

Orofino, L., Marcen, R., Quereda, C. *et al.* (1990) Epidemiology of symptomatic hypotension in hemodialysis: is cool dialysate beneficial for all patients? *American Journal of Nephrology*, **10**, 177–180.

Ross, E. A. and Nissenson, A. R. (1994) Acid-base and electrolyte disturbances, in *Handbook of Dialysis*, 2nd edn, (eds J. T. Daugirdas and T. S. Ing), Little, Brown & Co, Boston, MA.

Rouby, J. J., Rottembourg, J., Durande, J. P. *et al.* (1980) Hemodynamic changes induced by regular hemodialysis and sequential ultrafiltration hemodialysis: a comparative study. *Kidney International*, **17**(6), 801–810.

Sanderson, N. A. and Katz, M. A. (1994) The fate of hypertonic saline administered during hemodialysis. *American Nephrology Nurses Association Journal*, **21**(4), 162–169.

9 Dietary and fluid considerations for the haemodialysis patient

Jane Torrington and Alison Shakeshaft

LEARNING OBJECTIVES

At the end of this chapter the reader should be able to:

- List the factors contributing to malnutrition in the haemodialysis patient.
- Describe the assessment methods which can be used to assess nutritional status in the haemodialysis patient.
- Understand the principles of calculating protein and energy requirements in the haemodialysis patient.
- Identify common foods that are high in potassium.
- Understand reasons for non-adherence to dietary and fluid regimens.
- Appreciate the role of the dietitian as a member of the multidisciplinary team.

MALNUTRITION IN THE HAEMODIALYSIS PATIENT

Patients approaching dialysis may show varying signs of malnutrition. The uraemia seen in end-stage renal failure causes nausea and often vomiting, leading to impaired appetite and poor food intake. Once haemodialysis has been established attention should be paid to both adequacy of dialysis and food intake.

In various studies signs of malnutrition have been observed in 10–70% of HD patients (Bergstrom, 1995a). Several studies have highlighted the relationship between malnutrition and morbidity/mortality in HD patients. Lowrie and Lew (1990) found an almost fivefold increase in the annual risk of death in HD patients with a serum albumin of 30–35 g/l compared with HD patients with a serum albumin > 40 g/l. Acchiardo *et al.* (1983) found that HD patients with low dietary protein intakes (DPI) had an increased number of hospitalizations per year and increased mortality rates when compared with patients with DPIs within the current recommended range (1.0–1.2 g/kg/d).

Key reference: Bergstrom, J. (1995a) Why are dialysis patients malnourished? *American Journal of Kidney Diseases* 26(1): 229–241.

FACTORS CONTRIBUTING TO MALNUTRITION

Table 9.1 highlights the many factors contributing to malnutrition in the HD patient.

Dialysis factors

Patients who are inadequately dialysed may remain uraemic. Uraemia leads to net protein catabolism, and nausea and vomiting that limits food intake. Some patients suffer with postdialysis fatigue and as a result eat less on dialysis days. This is often to the detriment of the patient's nutritional status. Protein requirements are raised in the HD patient, partly because of the loss of amino acids and peptides into the dialysate (10–13 g per dialysis session; Mitch and Klahr, 1988). Blood losses on dialysis may indirectly play a small role in increasing protein requirements. The dialysis procedure itself may well initiate an inflammatory reaction that leads to accelerated protein breakdown. This is more prominent with the use of

Table 9.1 Factors contributing to malnutrition in haemodialysis patients

Dialysis factors	Inadequate dialysis
	Postdialysis fatigue
	Amino-acid and peptide losses in dialysate
	Blood loss on dialysis
	Bioincompatible membranes
	Use of acetate and high-calcium dialysate
	Infection and sepsis
Biochemical factors	Acidosis
	Impaired insulin secretion and insulin resistance
	Increased glucagon levels
	High parathyroid hormone levels
	Anaemia
Factors affecting nutritional intake	Unpalatable diets
	Gastrointestinal disturbances, e.g. gastritis, gastroparesis
	Nausea and vomiting
	Altered taste acuity
	Poor dentition
	Weight loss
	Constipation
	Depression
	Inadequate social support
	Recurrent hospitalization
Factors affecting nutrient absorption	Malabsorption
	Medication

cellulose membranes. Acetate-containing dialysis fluid may increase acidosis and net protein degradation. High-calcium dialysate solutions have been associated with hypercalcaemia, which can cause nausea and vomiting (Mitch and Klahr, 1988). Nutritional requirements will be increased in the presence of dialysis-related infection and sepsis.

Biochemical factors

Patients with ESRF demonstrate disorders in endocrine and metabolic function. These include decreased biological activity of anabolic hormones such as insulin and increased circulating levels of catabolic hormones such as glucagon and parathyroid hormone (Mitch and Klahr, 1988). The combined effect of the above and uncorrected acidosis may lead to net protein catabolism. The symptoms of anaemia, e.g. tiredness, lethargy and shortness of breath, impair the ability to eat.

Factors affecting nutritional intake

Poor appetite is common among HD patients and as a result patients are unable to meet their increased protein requirements. Factors leading to reduced food intake include unpalatable diets, gastroparesis (in diabetic patients with autonomic neuropathy) and the nausea and vomiting associated with uraemia, anxiety and the haemodialysis procedure (Bergstrom, 1995b; Hakim and Levin, 1993). In practice altered taste acuity, poor dentition (especially in the elderly), weight loss and constipation are other important causes of poor dietary intake as are depression, inadequate social support and recurrent hospitalizations.

> **Key reference:** Hakim, R.M. and Levin, N. (1993) Malnutrition in hemodialysis patients. *American Journal of Kidney Disease* 21(2): 125–37.

Factors affecting nutrient absorption

Digestion and absorption of nutrients may be impaired in patients with coexisting malabsorption states, e.g. diabetic gastroparesis and Crohn's disease. Some drugs can affect the absorption and metabolism of nutrients: for example, phenytoin inhibits the absorption of some vitamins and minerals and ciprofloxacin binds with iron. All of the above are important factors that may lead to malnutrition in the HD patient and must be corrected in order to achieve optimal nutritional status.

ASSESSMENT OF NUTRITIONAL STATUS

Continuous monitoring and assessment of the patient's nutritional status is essential to diagnose, treat and prevent malnutrition. Table 9.2 lists practical ways of identifying malnutrition in the HD patient. Patients may exhibit any

Table 9.2 Practical ways of identifying malnutrition in the haemodialysis patient

Biochemical indices	Serum albumin < 35 g/l
	Serum cholesterol < 38 mmol/l
	Decreasing predialysis serum urea and creatinine
	Raised serum urea:creatinine ratio
	Decreasing predialysis serum potassium and phosphate
Dietary assessments	Dietary intake compared with recommendations
General appearance	Subjective assessment of patient
	Comparison of patient with a photograph of when s/he was well
Anthropometric measurements	Current weight compared to usual weight
	Current weight compared to ideal weight
	Body mass index (BMI)
	Recent weight loss
	Skinfold thickness
	Mid-arm circumference (MAC)
	Mid-arm muscle circumference (MAMC)
	Hand-grip dynamometry
	Bioelectrical impedance (BEI)
Urea kinetic modelling	Protein catabolic rate (PCR) < 0.8 g/kg/d

one or a combination of abnormal measurements and no one measurement should be used as a sole marker of nutritional status. The degree of malnutrition may be assessed by the number of abnormal parameters seen.

Anthropometric measurements

Determining the patient's weight status (**body mass index**) is one of the most practical tools in assessing the presence or risk of malnutrition. A comparison should be made between the patient's dry weight, their usual weight and their ideal body weight for height. Regular reassessment of dry weight is essential to identify those patients who are losing or regaining flesh weight. Patients often lose flesh weight prior to the commencement of dialysis. A **weight loss** of 10% or more over the past 3 months is a significant indicator of malnutrition (Thomas, 1994).

Skinfold thickness, mid-arm circumference and mid-arm muscle circumference can be used to measure muscle and fat stores. Although useful, these are impractical as they are time-consuming, inconvenient to the patient and need to be taken by the same clinician. Regular measurements are also required as single or infrequent measurements are of little value. Hand-grip dynamometry is an easier and quicker method of anthropometric assessment. Patients can relate to the hand-grip score and see positive results as their nutritional status improves.

Bioelectrical impedance (BEI) can be used to determine body composition. The HD procedure is known to alter the distribution of fluid within

Calculating body mass index (BMI)

This is a practical way of calculating ideal weight for height.

$$BMI = \frac{\text{weight in kg (dry flesh weight)}}{(\text{height in m})^2}$$

BMI	Interpretation
Under 20	= Underweight
20–24	= Healthy/ desirable weight
25–29	= Overweight
30–39	= Obese
Over 40	= Morbidly obese

N.B. Never take the patient's word for his/her height and weight

Calculation of % weight loss

$$\%W_L = \frac{W_u - W_c(kg)}{W_u(kg)} \times 100$$

where W_L is weight loss; W_U is usual weight and W_C is current weight extracellular and intracellular compartments (Madore *et al.*, 1994). The effect of hydration and acute volume changes during dialysis on the accuracy of BEI measurements needs further study (Madore *et al.*, 1994). More research is needed before BEI can be used as a regular assessment tool in the HD patient.

Biochemical results

Serum albumin is a commonly used marker of protein status. It provides an index of skin and muscle protein reserve and is usually reduced when protein stores are lost. Serum albumin levels should be monitored regularly and can be used equally to detect improving or declining nutritional status. However, serum albumin can be affected by other factors such as changes in fluid balance, proteinuria in the nephrotic patient and the presence of infection. As albumin has a mean half-life of 19 days and a large body pool it is unsuitable for use in short-term assessments (Taylor and Goodison-McLaren, 1992). These factors should be taken into consideration when using serum albumin as a marker of nutritional status.

A low serum cholesterol (< 3.8 mmol/l) is an indicator of inadequate energy intake and can be used to detect malnutrition (Hakim and Levin, 1993). Care should be taken not to interpret a low serum cholesterol as being healthy.

A low predialysis serum urea level (< 10 mmol/l) may indicate an inadequate DPI (Daugirdas and Ing, 1994). Decreasing predialysis levels of serum creatinine may indicate declining muscle mass (Hakim and Levin, 1993). Serum urea and creatinine levels should be examined together. A raised urea to creatinine ratio is due to either an excessive DPI or increased catabolic rate of body proteins (Daugirdas and Ing, 1994). In the catabolic patient provision of an adequate protein intake with additional non-protein calories will lead to normalization of the urea to creatinine ratio.

Predialysis serum potassium and phosphate levels may be low in patients consuming an inadequate protein (and therefore potassium and phosphate) intake (Daugirdas and Ing, 1994).

Urea kinetic modelling

Protein catabolic rate (PCR) can be used as an assessment of DPI. In a stable HD patient who is neither catabolic nor anabolic the PCR should be within the range 0.8–1.4 g/kg/d (Lopot, 1990). Patients with a PCR below 0.8 g/kg/d may have an inadequate DPI. Patients with a PCR above 1.4 g/kg/d may be eating an excessive quantity of protein. In both these cases the patient's dietary protein prescription should be amended.

Dietary assessment

A patient's dietary intake should be regularly reviewed by a dietitian, at least 6-monthly and more often if necessary. Attention should be paid to intakes of protein, energy, potassium, sodium, fluid, phosphate, fibre, vitamins and minerals. This should highlight any deviations from the dietary prescription for the individual patient and identify those at risk of malnutrition.

General appearance

Of equal value to the above objective measurements is the clinician's subjective assessment, based on the **general appearance** of the patient.

DIETARY REQUIREMENTS OF THE HAEMODIALYSIS PATIENT

Many patients presenting with ESRF are following the national healthy eating guidelines targeted at the general population. The guidelines are increased dietary fibre, less fat, sugar and salt and sensible alcohol consumption. A 'healthy diet' may conflict with the dietary restrictions needed by many HD patients. The message of increasing the intake of fruit and vegetables, jacket potatoes and high-fibre cereals may be inappropriate for those requiring potassium restrictions. Energy requirements will be difficult to achieve with diets too low in fat and sugar. With increased awareness of the healthy eating guidelines *via* schools, health and fitness clubs and the media patients may find HD dietary guidelines difficult to accept. Where possible the national guidelines should be incorporated into any dietary advice given. Table 9.3 summarizes the dietary requirements of the HD patient.

Assessment of general appearance

Asking the patient to provide a photograph taken when they were well, before the onset of dialysis, is an excellent way of comparing changes in nutritional status and overall wellbeing with time on dialysis.

Table 9.3 Dietary requirements of the haemodialysis patient (IBW = ideal body weight)

Protein	1–1.2 g/kg IBW/d (70–75% high biological value)
Energy	35 kcal/kg IBW/d
Potassium	1 mmol/kg IBW/d
Sodium	80–100 mmol/d
Fluid	500 ml plus previous day's urinary output
Phosphate	0.5 mmol/g protein
Calcium	700 mg/d
Fibre (Non-starch polysaccharides)	18 g/d
Water-soluble vitamins	Supplements usually required
Fat-soluble vitamins	Supplements not required
Iron	Supplements may be required
Zinc	Supplements may be required

Protein requirements

HD patients have increased protein requirements, as previously discussed. 1–1.2 g protein/kg ideal body weight/d is recommended, 70–75% of which should be high biological value (HBV; Bergstrom, 1993; Kluthe *et al.*, 1978). HBV protein contains all the essential amino acids.

How to calculate protein requirements

For example: a female patient

Height 1.65 m (5 ft 5 in)
Current dry weight 50 kg (7 st 12 lb)
BMI 18
Usual weight 59 kg (9 st 4 lb)
Usual weight of 59 kg gives a BMI of 22; therefore the patient's usual
    weight is her ideal weight.
1 g protein × 59 kg = 59 g protein/d
70–75% of total protein = 41.3–44.3 g HBV protein/d

Therefore, for this patient we would recommend a minimum total
protein intake of 59 g/d with 42 g being provided by HBV sources (6 × 7 g
HBV servings; Table 9.4). The remaining 17 g protein should be provided
by foods containing lower biological value protein, e.g. bread, cereals,
cakes, biscuits. In a patient whose actual body weight differs greatly from
the ideal weight it may be more appropriate to use a mid-point between the
two weights for the calculation.

Table 9.4   Protein and energy content of common foods; the average
protein and energy content represent a range of foods within the same
food group and a range of cooking methods

	Ave. protein content (g)	Ave. energy content (kcal)
HBV protein foods		
Meat (cooked weight) 28 g	7	60
Fish (cooked weight) 42 g	7	60
Egg 1 large	7	90
Hard cheese 28 g	7	120
Cottage cheese 56 g	7	50
Yoghurt 140 g	7	80
Milk 200 ml	7	98
LBV protein foods		
Bread 1 slice	2	70
Breakfast cereal 28 g	2	100
Biscuits 2–3	2	125
Cake 42 g	2	170
Potatoes, boiled or creamed 140 g	2	140
Potatoes, chips or roast 56 g	2	115
Rice, cooked 84 g	1	115
Pasta, cooked 56 g	2	53
Non-protein sources of energy		
Spreading fats 7 g (not low-fat spreads)		57
Vegetable oil 1 tablespoon		180
Cream 1 tablespoon		68
Sugar 1 teaspoon		20
Jam/marmalade/honey 2 teaspoons		28
Boiled sweets 112 g		327

Energy requirements

In the early years of HD treatment it was thought that HD patients had very high energy requirements. Studies by Monteon *et al.* (1986) and Slomowitz *et al.* (1989) demonstrated that patients on HD had energy expenditures similar to normal subjects. An adequate energy intake, i.e. 35 kcal/kg ideal body weight/d, is necessary to ensure that dietary protein is utilized efficiently. The above figure should be used as a guideline but energy requirements should be adapted for each patient depending upon any undesirable changes in body weight.

Meeting protein and energy requirements

Protein and energy requirements are calculated for each patient, as previously described. The dietitian will make an assessment of the patient's current dietary intake and will advise on how to make up any shortfalls identified. Wherever possible foods usually taken by the patient will be recommended to meet the requirements. Historically, high saturated fat intakes were used to meet energy requirements. This included the liberal use of cream and butter. In view of the link between hyperlipidaemia and coronary heart disease a higher polyunsaturated/monounsaturated to saturated fat ratio is recommended (Department of Health, 1991). Table 9.4 lists the protein and energy content of some common foods.

When requirements cannot be met by diet alone some form of nutritional support will be necessary. Where the patient is able to eat and drink, nutritional supplements will be prescribed in the first instance. Many supplements are available with varying nutritional composition. The dietitian will be able to advise on the most appropriate form of supplementation depending on the patient's requirements and individual preferences.

If requirements are not met by diet and oral supplementation, nasogastric or gastrostomy feeding should be initiated. Gastrostomy feeding may be more appropriate for patients requiring long-term nutritional support, e.g. patients with chronic dysphagia. The choice of feed will depend upon nutritional requirements, fluid balance and oral dietary intake.

Intradialytic parenteral nutrition (IDPN), i.e. an intravenous supply of amino acids, glucose and lipids during the HD sessions, has been used in several dialysis centres for the treatment of malnourished HD patients. Some studies have demonstrated favourable effects on nutritional status with IDPN (Bergstrom and Lindholm, 1993). Commercially prepared solutions can be used or individual regimens can be prepared by the pharmacist specializing in TPN.

The theory that malnutrition is unavoidable and untreatable in the HD patient is no longer tenable (Lowrie, 1994). A more aggressive approach to nutrition could prevent the costly and morbid effects of malnutrition.

Potassium requirements

Hyperkalaemia is a common occurrence in HD. Serum potassium levels are affected by several factors, including the frequency of dialysis, the

Table 9.5 Foods high in potassium

• Yoghurt	• Oranges	• Crisps
• Rhubarb	• Chocolate	• Parsnips
• Fruit cake	• Potatoes	• Dried fruit
• Fruit juices	• Nuts	• Bananas
• Muesli	• Spinach	• Coffee
• Mushrooms	• Baked beans	• Skimmed milk powder
• Salt substitutes	• Beetroot	• Pulses
• Evaporated and condensed milk		

presence or absence of residual renal function, medication and catabolism. One of the aims of HD treatment is to maintain serum potassium levels within the normal range. As a guideline, dietary potassium restrictions should be implemented when predialysis serum potassium levels exceed 5.3 mmol/l. The level of dietary restriction will depend upon predialysis serum potassium levels, the patient's usual dietary potassium intake, body size and frequency of HD.

When taking a dietary history attention should be paid to the type, quantity and frequency of dairy products, meat, fish, vegetables, fruit, cereals, cakes, biscuits, confectionery, convenience foods, take-aways, condiments and beverages. Attention should also be paid to the cooking methods used. Depending upon the assessment the patient will be advised on a potassium-restricted diet tailored to their individual needs. This may entail avoidance of a few high potassium foods only or a more prescriptive diet of approximately 1 mmol/kg body weight. Table 9.5 lists some of the common foods high in potassium. Patients will be advised to avoid or limit some of these foods.

Cooking methods may need to be adapted. Potassium from potatoes and vegetables will be leached into the cooking water during boiling. This water should be discarded and not used for making gravy. Steaming and microwaving are not recommended for cooking vegetables and potatoes. Patients should be advised to boil all vegetables, including those used in stir-fries, soups and casseroles, unless specialized low potassium recipes are followed, which may incorporate the use of limited quantities of raw vegetables. Patients may be advised to double-boil potatoes depending on the quantity usually consumed and the level of potassium restriction required.

Hypokalaemia should also be avoided. Patients on potassium-restricted diets who have low predialysis serum potassium levels should have their diets relaxed and if necessary should be encouraged to eat high potassium foods.

Sodium restriction

Patients are normally advised to control their sodium (salt) intake to help reduce thirst when fluid-restricted. The level of restriction is tailored to the individual but is often no stricter than no added salt (NAS), i.e. 80–100 mmol/d. A NAS diet limits the intake of salty foods, including:

- cured or preserved meats, e.g. bacon, ham, corned beef;
- processed meats, e.g. sausages, burgers;
- packet foods, e.g. dried soup, savoury rice;
- tinned foods, e.g. baked beans;
- salted snacks, e.g. crisps and nuts;
- cheese and milk.

Patients are advised to avoid adding salt to food at the table but are allowed to use a little salt in cooking. Advice on the use of herbs and spices should be given to ensure that the diet is not unpalatable. In practice, if patients can eat the above foods without exacerbation of thirst this should be permitted as meeting protein requirements can be difficult on a reduced sodium diet. Some patients may become salt-depleted on dialysis and require additional salt which may be taken either as salty foods or if necessary as sodium chloride capsules.

Fluid allowance

A common complaint among HD patients is the difficulties encountered when following a **fluid-restriction diet**. The fluid requirement of the body for normal physiological processes, e.g. temperature regulation and removal of waste products, is approximately 500 ml/d. The volume of urine excreted will influence the amount of fluid a patient can consume. In practice the daily allowance will be 500 ml plus a volume equivalent to the previous day's urine output. The fluid allowance must take into account all measurable fluids, e.g. drinks, milk on cereal, water with medication, soups, sauces and fluid-containing puddings.

Fruit, vegetables, potatoes, boiled rice and pasta contain a significant but difficult-to-measure amount of fluid. Whether on a potassium-restricted diet or not patients are advised to limit their fruit and vegetable intake to a total of four servings daily. Patients are encouraged to measure the fluid volume of their cups, glasses, etc. in order to control their fluid intake.

Phosphate and calcium considerations

The control of serum phosphate cannot be achieved by HD alone. Rather than restricting the dietary phosphate intake at the expense of DPI, attention should be given to the appropriate dosage and timing of phosphate binders, e.g. calcium carbonate preparations. Phosphate binders should be taken with all meals and snacks containing protein. Iron medication should not be taken with phosphate binders as the action of both will be diminished. If hyperphosphataemia persists despite the above, a prescription of 0.5 mmol/g dietary protein/d may be required. Calcium supplementation is not usually necessary as requirements are met by diet and the use of calcium carbonate preparations.

Coping with fluid restriction

An easy way to control the fluid intake is to use the jug method. Start with an empty measuring jug marked with the daily fluid allowance. Each time a drink or other source of fluid is taken, an identical amount of fluid is tipped into the jug until the allowed level is reached.

Useful hints to help with fluid restriction

- Use a small cup for all drinks
- Suck ice cubes to quench thirst
- Eat fruit chilled to quench thirst
- Reduce intake of salt
- Do not eat too many sweets
- Try sugar-free mints to freshen the mouth

Dietary fibre

Constipation is a common complaint in HD patients and can lead to severe complications if left untreated. The causes of constipation within this group include low fluid intake, inactivity and the use of phosphate binders and calcium resonium. Poor dietary fibre intake, often the consequence of potassium restriction, is also a major contributing factor. A balance must be achieved between the required potassium restriction and maintaining an adequate intake of dietary fibre. An increased intake of bread (preferably wholemeal) and suitable wholegrain cereals should be encouraged. Patients may be reluctant to eat breakfast cereals because the accompanying milk may take up a large proportion of their daily fluid allowance. Serum potassium levels permitting, an extra serving of fruit and vegetables can be recommended. The use of bran must be discouraged because of its mineral binding properties and the risk of faecal impaction with inadequate fluid intake.

Vitamin and mineral requirements

Vitamin requirements of HD patients differ from those of healthy individuals as a result of diet, uraemia, drugs and dialysis (Makoff, 1992). The vitamin intake of HD patients may be reduced for several reasons: dietary intake is often poor, the diet prescribed may limit foods high in B and C vitamins and the recommended cooking procedures reduce the vitamin content of potatoes and vegetables. It is possible that there is inhibited pyridoxine (vitamin B_6) metabolism with uraemia (Schmiker, 1995). Drugs given for concurrent disease can affect the absorption and activity of folic acid, pyridoxine and cobalamin (vitamin B_{12}). Such drugs include anticancer agents, anticonvulsants, alcohol and barbiturates (Makoff, 1992). Water-soluble vitamin losses on dialysis are well documented (Kopple and Swenseid, 1975; Descombes *et al.*, 1993). The recommended level of water-soluble vitamin supplementation is widely variable (Ramirez *et al.*, 1986; Westhuyzen *et al.*, 1993). As a consequence current practice varies widely from one renal unit to another. Supplements should be given to correct inadequate dietary intake to prevent subclinical/frank vitamin deficiencies. Megadoses are contraindicated.

> **Key reference:** Makoff, R. (1992) Vitamin supplementation in patients with renal disease. *Dialysis and Transplantation* 21(1): 18–24.

The requirements for vitamins A, E and K should be met by diet alone. Vitamin A supplements are contraindicated because of the risk of hypervitaminosis and potential toxicity, which have been reported in renal patients (Makoff, 1992).

Vitamin D plays a significant role in the interaction between calcium, PTH and bone metabolism. The kidney is the site where the inactive form of vitamin D is converted into the active form (1,25 dihydroxycholecalciferol). In renal failure this does not occur, leading to vitamin deficiency.

Supplementation with the active form of vitamin D can lead to hypercalcaemia and therefore should not be used without regular monitoring of serum calcium levels.

The intake and absorption of iron may be reduced in patients with diets poor in protein and vitamin C. Iron-containing medication may be prescribed if iron stores are low.

Dietary zinc intake may be low in patients with inadequate dietary protein intakes. Impaired taste acuity and loss of appetite are recognized signs of zinc deficiency. HD patients often complain of taste changes and, in practice, with zinc supplementation patients often report improvement in taste acuity and appetite. Whether this is a direct result of zinc supplementation or a placebo effect is not known.

COMPLIANCE WITH DIETARY AND FLUID REGIMENS

Non-adherence to dietary and fluid restrictions is common among HD patients. Compliance is influenced by several factors. Firstly, patients undergo many lifestyle changes with the onset of HD. These include potential loss of earnings, loss of personal freedom, self-fulfilment and self-esteem, loss of time, role changes within the family and adaptation to life on dialysis. These problems may be compounded by the patient feeling unwell. Patients may manifest signs of denial, anger and depression, leading to stress in the individual and within the family.

Changing social circumstances such as bereavement, loss of social support and family problems may cause further stress and create practical problems affecting diet; for instance, patients who previously did little cooking may find themselves in the position of preparing their own meals.

Poor understanding of dietary regimens, limited cooking skills and equipment, lack of interest in food and forgetfulness will also affect compliance. Patients do not necessarily feel any benefit from following the prescribed diet and non-compliance may not lead to unpleasant symptoms (De Motte, 1990).

How to encourage dietary compliance

- A good understanding of the patient's lifestyle, culture, food preferences and social support is essential.
- Advice should be individualized and kept as simple as possible. Too much information should not be given at any one time. The most important aspects of the diet should be explained first and further advice given at regular intervals, checking that the advice previously given has been understood.
- Written instructions should always accompany verbal advice. Audiotapes are useful for the blind patient. Written advice in languages other than English may be required.
- Practical information should be given where necessary. This may include help with meal planning, eating out and choosing appropriate

foods at festive occasions and when on holiday. Advice may also be needed for those relying on convenience foods and ready-made meals.

- Enlisting the support of family, friends and carers is of benefit to all concerned. Care should be taken that dietary restrictions are not imposed on the whole family.
- Where Meals on Wheels/attendance at day care facilities are required education of the food providers is essential.
- Regular review of the patient will provide the opportunity to offer continued support, answer questions and reinforce dietary advice. Positive feedback of blood results and acceptable interdialytic weight gains will give encouragement. A good rapport between the patient and dietitian is likely to lead to better understanding and compliance.
- Anticipating situations where non-compliance may occur and offering appropriate advice may prevent problems arising; for example as Christmas approaches practical advice on festive foods may help prevent hyperkalaemia.

Regular communication between members of the multidisciplinary team and the patient should highlight situations where dietary non-compliance may occur. Patients should be respected and involved in the problem-solving process.

CONCLUSION

Malnutrition is a common problem among HD patients and if left untreated has dire consequences. Malnutrition can be treated/prevented by identification of relevant risk factors, provision of optimal dialysis and aggressive nutritional support.

The dietitian can assess the nutritional status and dietary intake of the HD patient, calculate nutritional requirements and provide appropriate advice.

The responsibility of the patient's nutritional status lies not only with the dietitian and patient but with every member of the multidisciplinary team. A team approach will identify nutrition-related problems, including non-compliance, and work towards better patient care.

REVIEW QUESTIONS

- Devise a checklist that can be used to identify HD patients with signs of malnutrition or at risk of developing malnutrition.
- Obtain the body mass index for the following HD patient and calculate his daily protein and energy requirements: weight 73 kg: height 1.78 m.
- Discuss possible reasons for non-compliance with dietary and fluid regimens and suggest ways of overcoming them.

REFERENCES

Acchiardo, S. R., Moore, L. W. and Latour, P. A. (1983) Malnutrition as the main factor in morbidity and mortality of hemodialysis patients. *Kidney International*, **24**(Suppl. 16), S199–S203.

Bergstrom, J. (1993) Nutrition and adequacy of dialysis in hemodialysis patients. *Kidney International*, **43**(41), S261–S267.

Bergstrom, J. (1995a) Why are dialysis patients malnourished? *American Journal of Kidney Diseases*, **26**(1), 229–241.

Bergstrom, J. (1995b) Nutrition and mortality in hemodialysis. *Journal of the American Society of Nephrology*, **6**(5), 1329–1341.

Bergstrom, J. and Lindholm, B. (1993) Nutrition and adequacy of dialysis. How do hemodialysis and CAPD compare? *Kidney International*, **43**(40), S39–S50.

Daugirdas, J. T. and Ing, T. S. (1994) *Handbook of Dialysis*, 2nd edn, Little, Brown & Co., Boston, MA.

De Motte, C. (1990) Renal nutrition and the non-compliant patient: some guidelines. *Nephrology News and Issues*, **Nov. 14**, 54–56.

Department of Health (1991) *Report on Health and Social Subjects 41. Dietary Reference Values for Food, Energy and Nutrients for the United Kingdom*, HMSO, London.

Descombes, E., Hanck, A. B., and Fellay, G. (1993) Water soluble vitamins in chronic hemodialysis patients and need for supplementation. *Kidney International*, **43**, 1319–1328.

Hakim, R. M. and Levin, N. (1993) Malnutrition in hemodialysis patients. *American Journal of Kidney Diseases*, **21**(2), 125–137.

Kluthe, R., Luttgen, F. M., Capetianu, T. *et al.* (1978) Protein requirements in maintenance hemodialysis. *American Journal of Clinical Nutrition*, **31**, 1812–1820.

Kopple, J. D. and Swenseid, M. E. (1975) Vitamin nutrition in patients undergoing maintenance hemodialysis. *Kidney International*, **7**(Suppl.), S79–S84.

Lopot, F. (1990) *Urea Kinetic Modelling*, EDTNA–ERCA Series vol. 4, European Dialysis and Transplant Nurses Association–European Renal Care Association, Ghent.

Lowrie, E. G. (1994) The principle of dialysis care: the importance of nutrition with special reference to intradialytic parenteral nutrition. *Journal of Renal Nutrition*, **4**(1), 2–4.

Lowrie, E. G. and Lew, N. L. (1990) Death risk in hemodialysis patients: the predictive value of commonly measured variables and an evaluation of death rate differences between facilities. *American Journal of Kidney Diseases*, **15**, 458–482.

Madore, F., Wuest, M. and Ethier, J. H. (1994) Nutritional evaluation of hemodialysis patients using an impedance index. *Clinical Nephrology*, **41**(6), 377–382.

Makoff, R. (1992) Vitamin supplementation in patients with renal disease. *Dialysis and Transplantation*, **21**(1), 18–24.

Mitch, W. E. and Klahr, S. (1988) *Nutrition and the Kidney*, Little, Brown & Co., Boston, MA.

Monteon, F. J., Laidlaw, S. A., Shaib, J. K. and Kopple, J. D. (1986) Energy expenditure in patients with chronic renal failure. *Kidney International*, **30**, 741–747.

Ramirez, G., Chen, M., Boyce, H. W. *et al.* (1986) Longitudinal follow-up of chronic hemodialysis patients without vitamin supplementation. *Kidney International*, **30**, 99–106.

Schmiker, R. (1995) Nutritional treatment of hemodialysis and peritoneal dialysis patients. *Artificial Organs*, **19**(8), 837–841.

Slomowitz, L. A., Monteon, F. J., Grosvenor, M. *et al.* (1989) Effect of energy intake on nutritional status in maintenance hemodialysis patients. *Kidney International*, **35**, 704–711.

Taylor, S. and Goodison-McLaren, S. (1992) *Nutritional Support: A Team Approach*, Wolfe Publishing, London.

Thomas, B. (1994) *Manual of Dietetic Practice*, 2nd edn, Blackwell Scientific Publications, Oxford.

Westhuyzen, J., Matherson, K. and Fleming, S. J. (1993) Effect of withdrawal of folic acid supplementation in maintenance hemodialysis patients. *Clinical Nephrology*, **40**(2), 96–99.

Principles of peritoneal dialysis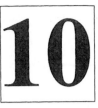

10

Coral Graham

LEARNING OBJECTIVES

At the end of this chapter the reader should be able to:

- Explain how to prepare the patient for insertion of a peritoneal dialysis catheter.
- Explain the specific care required following insertion of a peritoneal dialysis catheter.
- Explain the different forms of continuous and intermittent peritoneal dialysis treatments.
- State which patients are most suitable for peritoneal dialysis, and for what reasons patients are contraindicated for this form of treatment.
- State the advantages of automated peritoneal dialysis, and identify patients that are most suitable for this form of treatment.
- Describe the advantages and disadvantages of the various types of peritoneal dialysis fluids.

INTRODUCTION

Peritoneal dialysis (PD) has been accepted throughout the world as an established form of renal replacement therapy, and has many advantages over haemodialysis. Since continuous ambulatory peritoneal dialysis (CAPD) was introduced in 1975 there has been a steady increase in the number of patients, and at the end of 1996 there were 107 000 patients on PD worldwide. In the UK, PD is used to treat approximately half the total dialysis population.

Recent advancements in our understanding of the physiology of PD, and our increased knowledge of peritoneal dialysis kinetics have enabled nurses to be more proactive in the delivery of individualized therapy. Developments in systems, fluids and delivery machines have also progressed the science of PD, ensuring that it is a dynamic, challenging and rewarding area of nursing.

REVIEW OF THE ANATOMY AND PHYSIOLOGY OF THE PERITONEUM

The peritoneum is a membrane that holds certain properties, enabling it to be used for the purpose of dialysis. Until fairly recently, little was known about the peritoneum. Knowledge of the peritoneal ultrastructure is mainly due to the extensive peritoneal biopsy studies performed by James Dobbie during the 1980s.

The adult peritoneum is a continuous serous membrane of approx. 1–2 m². There are two distinctive layers: the parietal peritoneum lines the abdominal wall and the visceral peritoneum extends to the internal organs and lines the liver, stomach, intestines, etc. The peritoneal cavity is the potential space between the parietal and visceral layers. The normal peritoneal cavity contains approximately 10 ml of fluid to lubricate the membranous surfaces. However, the peritoneal cavity has the potential to accommodate large volumes of fluid, as seen in ascites (Figure 10.1). In peritoneal dialysis, patients of average-size, i.e. body surface area (BSA) of 1.73 m², can usually tolerate 2.5 litres in their peritoneum, and patients with a BSA greater than 2 m² can tolerate intraperitoneal volumes of 3–3.5 litres (Diaz-Buxo, 1996).

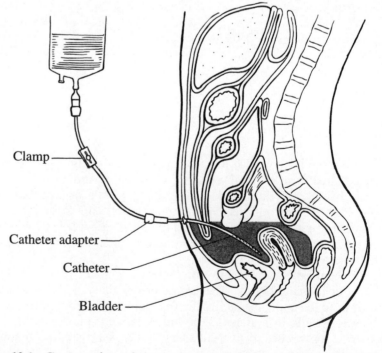

Clamp

Catheter adapter

Catheter

Bladder

Figure 10.1 Cross-section of the peritoneum, showing fluid in the abdomen. (Source: reproduced by courtesy of Fresenius from *Principles of CAPD*, Part 1 of a series of educational posters.)

Key reference: Diaz-Buxo, J.A. (1996) Enhancement of Peritoneal Dialysis: The P.D. Plus Concept. *American Journal of Kidney Diseases* 27(4): 92–98.

The normal peritoneum

The peritoneum consists of a serous membrane underlain by a simple monolayered, squamous mesothelial cell layer. The mesothelial cells have numerous microvilli, which are cytoplasmic finger-like processes believed to increase the peritoneal surface area up to 40 m^2. The interstitial tissue occupies the space between the mesothelial cells and the endothelial cells of the blood capillaries.

During the dialysis process, solutes are transported from the blood to the fluid in the peritoneal cavity. They pass through the peritoneal capillary walls, the interstitium (or connective tissue), the mesothelial cells and finally through the serous membrane.

The peritoneum after continuous exposure to dialysate

Mesothelium exposed to continuous dialysate has been observed to undergo certain changes. There is a proliferation of mesothelial cells, leading to an increased number of cells per unit area, and also a decrease in numbers and density of microvilli (Dobbie, 1994). The rough endoplasmic reticulum of the mesothelium undergoes hyperplasia, and there is a characteristic reduplication and thickening of the basement membrane of mesothelial cells and stromal blood vessels.

The effect of peritonitis

Most biopsies from patients with recent peritoneal inflammation show mesothelium that is either greatly damaged or the cells have been 'stripped' altogether. It takes approximately 4 weeks for the cells to recover and remesothelialize, but this process can be delayed for some months (Dobbie, 1994).

Sometimes, in extensive damage, the cells fail to remesothelialize, and fibrous tissue with abnormal bands of collagen develops instead of healthy tissue and mesothelial cells (Dobbie, 1994). It has been suggested that the continued use of glucose-based fluids during a peritonitis episode allows damage to occur to the stromal layer and exposed proteins (under the stripped mesothelium), which may inhibit remesothelialization and predispose to fibrosis (Hutchison and Gokal, 1992).

Key reference: Hutchison, A. and Gokal, R. (1992) Improved Solutions for Peritoneal Dialysis: Physiological calcium solutions, osmotic agents and buffers. *Kidney International* 42 Supp 38:153–159.

Blood supply and lymph drainage

The peritoneum receives a rich blood flow, which ensures that even during a hypotensive episode the blood flow remains fairly constant at 55–85 ml/min. The visceral peritoneum receives most of its blood supply from the superior mesenteric artery whereas the parietal peritoneum is supplied by the epigastric, lumbar and intercostal arteries.

The peritoneal lymphatics enable the continuous absorption of excess fluids, solutes, proteins and bacteria from the peritoneal cavity. Lymph drainage from the peritoneum is *via* lymph stoma situated under the diaphragm. There is an intricate supply of lymph vessels in both the parietal and visceral peritoneal tissues. Almost 80% of lymph is returned to the venous circulation *via* the right lymph duct.

On average 1 ml/min of fluid is drained from the peritoneal cavity *via* the lymphatics. It has been estimated that the daily lymphatic absorption rate during CAPD is 1 litre. Considerably higher lymph flow rates have been found in some patients with severe loss of ultrafiltration, in children and during peritonitis (Krediet, 1994).

THE PRINCIPLES OF PERITONEAL DIALYSIS

The principles of diffusion, osmosis and convection govern the exchange of solutes and water between the peritoneal capillaries and the peritoneal cavity. Solutes and water move through the peritoneum, which acts as an imperfect semi-permeable membrane, meaning that it is permeable to small molecules (e.g. urea) but less permeable to molecules of larger molecular weight (such as phosphates). It is impermeable to large particles such as blood cells.

Diffusion

Diffusion is the movement of solutes from an area of high solute concentration to an area of low concentration until equilibrium is reached (Figure 10.2). In the case of peritoneal dialysis, the area of high solute concentration

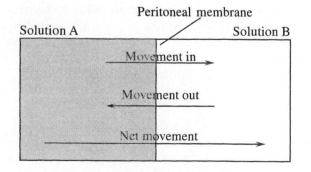

Figure 10.2 Diffusion.

is the blood capillaries of the peritoneum, in which excess uraemic toxins accumulate, and the area of low uraemic toxin concentration is the dialysate.

Diffusion occurs until equilibrium is achieved, when the dialysate is concentrated with toxins. At this point the concentration gradient has diminished and so diffusion ceases. Fresh dialysis solution must be introduced into the peritoneum to enable further diffusion to take place. All peritoneal membranes possess individual properties and characteristics, and thus solutes move at different rates.

Factors affecting the rate of diffusion

- **The molecular weight of the solute**. Solutes of lower molecular weight have greater diffusion coefficiency; for example, urea (mol. wt 60) diffuses more readily than creatinine (mol. wt 113; Winchester and Rotellar, 1994).
- **The solute concentration difference between the capillary and peritoneal cavity**. The greater the difference in concentration, the more diffusion will take place (Winchester and Rotellar, 1994).
- **The electrical charge of the solute**. The capillaries and mesothelium hold negative charges that repel certain solutes, e.g. proteins.
- **Membrane area**. This may be reduced by adhesions, sclerosis, etc.
- **Characteristics of the membrane** (Winchester and Rotellar, 1994).
- **Temperature of the dialysate**.

Osmotic ultrafiltration

Two main factors influence the rate of fluid removal across the peritoneum.

The hydrostatic capillary pressure gradient

The hydrostatic pressure in the capillaries is greater than in the interstitium, and therefore fluid is forced through the capillary pores into the interstitial spaces. The capillary colloidal pressure also aids this process. This outward pressure causes continuous leakage of ultrafiltrate into the interstitium, which is termed the 'interstitial free fluid'. Some of this fluid is reabsorbed in distal capillaries and venules, while some constantly enters the peritoneum to lubricate it. The remainder is absorbed by the lymphatics.

The capillary hydrostatic pressure remains fairly constant during peritoneal dialysis and does not influence ultrafiltration greatly. However, ultrafiltration has been shown to increase after the administration of intraperitoneal vasoactive drugs, e.g. dopamine (Leypoldt and Mistry, 1994).

The osmotic pressure gradient

During peritoneal dialysis, glucose is used as the osmotic agent as it generates a high osmotic pressure that induces ultrafiltration from the blood capillaries. There are three concentrations of anhydrous glucose –

1.5%, 2.3% and 4.25%. The most hypertonic solution (4.25%) will generate the most ultrafiltration, this being approximately 500–800 ml over a 4-hour dwell period. During this time lymphatic absorption would be approximately 350 ml, reducing the net ultrafiltration volume to 150–450 ml. Peak intraperitoneal volume would occur on average 2 hours into the dwell, when the lymph flow rate would equal the ultrafiltration rate. After this the intraperitoneal volume would begin to decrease. The lymph flow rate would exceed the ultrafiltration rate, because of the absorption of glucose, which causes the gradual dissipation of the glucose osmotic gradient.

The average ultrafiltration rate when using a weak glucose solution (1.5%) is 9 ml/min, whereas it is 21 ml/min for the strong solution (4.25%). Glucose equilibrium is achieved as late as 6–8 hours after the infusion (Khanna and Nolph, 1989).

Key reference: Khanna, R. and Nolph, K. (1989) The Physiology of Peritoneal Dialysis. *American Journal of Nephrology* 9:504–512.

Convective flow (or 'solvent drag')

Convection allows transport of water and solutes during peritoneal dialysis. During convective flow, large numbers of molecules are 'dragged' across the membrane, streaming through the pores as part of the total fluid loss, as opposed to diffusion, when there is random movement. A large ultrafiltrate will cause more solutes to be cleared by this 'solvent drag', independent of solute clearance by diffusion.

PERITONEAL ACCESS AND ITS NURSING CARE

Permanent, trouble-free access is one of the most important elements of a successful peritoneal dialysis programme. Up to 20% of patient transfers to haemodialysis are directly related to catheter problems (Gokal *et al.*, 1993).

Key reference: Gokal, R., Ash, S., Helfrich, G.B., Holmes, C.J., Joffe, P., Nichols, W., Oreopoulos, D., Riella, M., Slingeneyer, A., Twardowski, Z. and Vas, S. (1993) Peritoneal catheters and exit-site practices: Toward optimum peritoneal access. *Peritoneal Dialysis International* 13:29–39.

The peritoneal dialysis catheter

The peritoneal dialysis catheter allows the repeated instillation and drainage of dialysate. The catheters are normally 40 cm in length, are made of silicone rubber and are designed to be soft, flexible, biocompatible and atraumatic to the surrounding tissues. The catheter tubing is 2.6 mm in

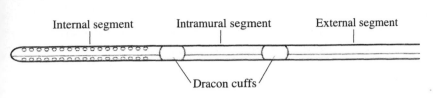

Figure 10.3 A straight Tenckhoff catheter.

diameter and usually has two (occasionally one or three) cuffs attached. Made of Dacron velour, the cuff facilitates fibrous tissue ingrowth and so anchors the catheter and minimizes the risk of infection tracking along the catheter length. When implanted a typical catheter has three segments:

1. **the intraperitoneal segment**, which has numerous perforations to allow flow of fluid;
2. **the intramural segment** with attached cuffs, which is situated in a subcutaneous 'tunnel' within the abdominal wall;
3. **the external segment**, which is situated outside the skin exit for connection to the delivery system.

Many catheters have been developed over the years, but the most prevalent type used in the world today is the Tenckhoff catheter (Figure 10.3). Developed in 1968, the two-cuff Tenckhoff catheter is favoured by the majority of surgeons in the UK. This catheter may be straight or coiled; the latter is potentially less prone to migration.

Preparation of patient prior to implantation

Prior to catheter implantation the nurse will explain the procedure, remove any abdominal hair and ensure that the patient is not constipated. This is vital as a full or impacted bowel can obstruct the flow of fluid and even cause catheter-tip migration. The exit site location will be identified by an experienced nephrology nurse or doctor with the patient upright. The exit should be at least 2 cm above or below the belt line and not on a scar. In obese patients it is necessary to place the exit above the skin fold to ensure the patient has good vision (Twardowski and Khanna, 1994).

Most centres favour the use of prophylactic antibiotics, but this has been associated with the emergence of resistant organisms and clinicians should therefore use prophylaxis with caution. Twardowski and Khanna (1994) recommend 1 g vancomycin intravenously.

Catheter implantation

The implantation must be performed by a dedicated, experienced surgeon/nephrologist under strict sterile conditions. Numerous implantation techniques have been described (which are too detailed to discuss here).

Local anaesthesia is preferred, as general anaesthesia predisposes to vomiting, coughing and constipation postoperatively, all of which would

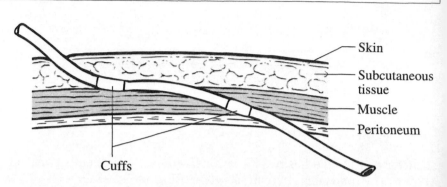

Skin

Subcutaneous tissue

Muscle

Peritoneum

Cuffs

Figure 10.4 Cross-section of the abdominal wall showing position of peritoneal dialysis catheter.

increase intra-abdominal pressure and predispose to leaks. The catheter is usually inserted through a paramedian incision *via* the rectus muscle, although some surgeons prefer a midline incision (Figure 10.4). The flow of fluid is checked during implantation. No sutures are placed at the exit site, as this promotes infection (Gokal *et al.*, 1993). The exit should be covered with gauze and secured with an air-permeable dressing or tape.

Post-implantation care and commencement of dialysis

Immediately following implantation, it is usual to flush the peritoneum with 1–2 litres of fluid (1000 units of heparin/l), using small volumes of 300–500 ml, to remove residual blood from the cavity. An X-ray to check the position is recommended.

To ensure good healing, it is important to avoid a pericatheter dialysate leak, as this interferes with fibrous tissue ingrowth into the cuff. Delaying dialysis for 1–3 days will permit good tissue healing. For those patients who require immediate dialysis, supine exchanges of 500–1000 ml will reduce the risk of leaks as the intra-abdominal pressure is lower in this position. The volume should be increased gradually by a maximum of 500 ml in 24 hours.

Ambulatory dialysis should be delayed for 10–14 days postimplantation. When dialysis is started early, the abdomen should be left dry for a part of the day to allow any leaked fluid to be absorbed.

The exit site dressing should be left undisturbed for 1 week, to minimize trauma and prevent infection. Thereafter, the site should be evaluated once or twice a week for signs of infection/quality of healing and the dressing should be changed weekly until the exit site has healed, which takes 4–8 weeks (Twardowski and Khanna, 1994). The catheter must be immobilized and secured at all times to prevent it from mechanical stress, as pulling and tugging can cause infection and cuff extrusion (Twardowski and Khanna, 1994).

If the catheter is not used, there seems to be no consensus on when to check it for patency. Most believe it should be flushed every 1–7 days, while others believe there is little danger of blockage and interference with the catheter would potentially introduce infection (Gokal *et al.*, 1993). Unless absorbable sutures have been used, the skin incision sutures should be removed after 7–10 days.

Care of the well-healed exit site

The peritoneal dialysis catheter is the patient's lifeline; correctly cared for it may survive for many years. Exit site and tunnel infections contribute to morbidity, catheter loss and technique failure (Prowant *et al.*, 1993). It is therefore essential to avoid these complications. Exit site and tunnel infections have become the primary infectious complications of peritoneal dialysis (Moncrief *et al.*, 1994). Many studies have examined exit site practices, but there is no consensus regarding optimal, long-term care. The following is based on a review of the current literature.

- **Frequency of dressing changes**. Daily examination and care is recommended. Scabs are not forcibly removed as this would break the epidermal layer and provide a haven for bacteria (Twardowski and Khanna, 1994).
- **Cleansing agent.** The results of a study by Prowant *et al.* (1988) indicate that cleaning with soap and water is inexpensive and prevents infections better than using povidone-iodine and/or hydrogen peroxide. An antibacterial liquid soap or bar soap used solely for the purpose of exit site care is recommended. Soap and water is also recommended by Twardowski and Khanna (1994) and Gokal *et al.* (1993). Povidone-iodine, although frequently used, is known to be disadvantageous. Twardowski (1992) stated that it is cytotoxic to mammalian cells and harmful to granulation tissue, and Gokal *et al.* (1993) have linked silicone degradation and cracking with the use of iodine as a cleansing agent. Furthermore, it is known to cause local irritation and alteration in skin flora, which has been associated with causing *Pseudomonas aeruginosa* exit site infections (Goetz, 1989).
- **Choice of dressing**. It is generally felt that sterile gauze should be applied over the exit site, then secured firmly with tape, although some centres do not cover the exit site once it has healed fully following Tenckhoff insertion, or if there is no evidence of infection or inflammation.
- **Immobilization**. The catheter should be secured at all times to prevent tension, which could lead to trauma around the exit site or along the catheter tunnel.
- **Showers/baths**. Showers are generally advocated, with avoidance of sitting in baths of stagnant water. Exit site care should be performed immediately after bathing.
- **Swimming/bathing**. Following healing, patients are advised to swim with watertight protection of their exit site.

Key reference: Twardowski, Z.J. (1992) Peritoneal Dialysis Catheter Exit Site Infections: Prevention, Diagnosis, Treatment and Future Directions. *Seminars in Dialysis* 5(4); 305–315.

DIFFERENT FORMS OF PERITONEAL DIALYSIS AND THEIR ROLE IN TREATMENT

When prescribing a peritoneal dialysis modality, one needs to consider the following:

- **Volume** – amount of solution used per exchange;
- **Dose** – amount of solution used over a period of time;
- **Method** – manual or *via* machine;
- **Regimen** – may be intermittent or continuous.

Peritoneal membrane transport characteristics

All peritoneal membranes have individual characteristics and transport properties. These have been categorized in the peritoneal function test (PFT; Keen and Gotch, 1994) and the peritoneal equilibration test (PET; Twardowski *et al.*, 1987). These tests provide us with information, such as the rate of urea and creatinine clearance from the peritoneum and the rate of glucose absorption from the dialysate, that influences ultrafiltration. These rates are defined as high, high average, low average and low transport rates (Table 10.1).

This information allows us to predict the patient's response to standard CAPD in terms of solute clearance and ultrafiltration, and to prescribe the most appropriate therapy to suit the patient's unique membrane transport characteristics.

When a patient has been on peritoneal dialysis for 2–4 weeks it is vital to perform an equilibration test, to ensure that the patient is receiving the correct therapy. During the first 2 weeks of peritoneal dialysis there may be a change in peritoneal transport characteristics (Rocco *et al.*, 1995). The variation in transport characteristics of individual peritoneums should lead to the individualization of dialysis regimen (see Patient scenario below).

Patient scenario

Gary Brown is a 35-year-old businessman who often returns home from work at 7–8 pm. He weights 74 kg. An equilibration test reveals high–average transport status and he currently has a urine output of 1.6 litres. He is commencing peritoneal dialysis.

- What type of treatment would you recommend for Gary? What are your reasons for this choice?

After 2.5 years on PD, Gary's weight has increased to 78 kg and his urine output has diminished to 100 ml. An equilibration test reveals that his membrane has changed to low–average transport status.

- How could the dialysis dose be increased to counteract the loss of residual renal function? What type of treatment would you now recommend for Gary, and how might the new treatment affect him in relation to his work?

Automated peritoneal dialysis (APD)

This refers to all forms of PD using a machine or 'cycler' to assist in the delivery and drainage of fluid, usually at night. The main advantages of

Table 10.1 Peritoneal membrane transport characteristics

Peritoneal transport	Drain volume	Ultrafiltration	Dialysis	Most suitable modality
High	Low	Poor	Adequate	NIPD, DAPD
High–average	Low–average	Adequate	Adequate	CAPD, NIPD
Low–average	High–average	Good	Adequate or inadequate	CAPD or high-dose CAPD
Low	High	Excellent	Adequate or inadequate	High-dose CAPD/CCPD

APD are that patients tolerate larger volumes of fluid when supine, which increases the efficiency of dialysis, and that because dialysis can be carried out overnight it obviates the need for manual exchanges during the day. It is therefore more acceptable for a helper to assist with this treatment. Another important factor in its favour is that the frequency of peritonitis is lower with APD (Woodrow *et al.*, 1994; Twardowski, 1990). The main disadvantages are the capital cost of the machine and the increased yearly therapy costs. However, it could be argued that the reduced incidence of peritonitis could go part of the way to negating this increase in cost.

Continuous regimens

- **Continuous ambulatory peritoneal dialysis (CAPD)**. Treatment is continuous over 24 hours: three or four manual exchanges are performed during the day and one before bedtime. The daily dose can be up to 15 litres. Patients with high transport status may absorb fluid in the long dwells.
- **Continuous cyclic peritoneal dialysis (CCPD)**. Three to five nightly exchanges of 1.5–3 litres are performed *via* a cycler at night. Fluid is in the peritoneum during the day, providing one long exchange of 14–16 hours.
- **High-dose CCPD**. The dialysis dose is increased by also performing one or two exchanges during the day, either manually or *via* a cycler. Compared to CCPD 'patients can accomplish a significantly higher clearance of small solutes with modest increases in dialysis solutions' (Diaz-Buxo, 1996). This is suitable for most patients, even large, anuric patients with low or low–average membrane status.

Intermittent regimens

These are most suitable for those patients who have high or high–average transport rates, maintain residual renal function and have a relatively low body surface area.

- **Daytime ambulatory peritoneal dialysis (DAPD)**. Manual exchanges of 1.5–3 litres are performed during the day when the patient is ambulatory. The peritoneum is empty overnight, so the treatment duration is 12–16 hours.
- **Intermittent peritoneal dialysis (IPD)**. Treatment of 10–20 hours' duration is given *via* a cycler two or three times a week. The dose per session

can be from 20–60 litres. In between dialysis sessions the peritoneum is empty. This form of therapy is increasingly being offered on an outpatient basis in hospitals in the UK, to accommodate those patients who are no longer able to dialyse independently.

- **Nightly intermittent peritoneal dialysis (NIPD)**. Treatment of 8–10 hours is delivered *via* a cycler at night while the patient sleeps. The dose is usually 12–20 litres. The peritoneum is empty during the day. This is appropriate for patients with hernias, leaks, etc., as intra-abdominal pressure is lower in the supine position.
- **Tidal peritoneal dialysis (TPD)**. This is delivered nightly *via* a cycler. There is an initial fill of 2–3 litres, followed by cycles in which approximately 50% of the dialysate is drained and replaced by fresh dialysate. These smaller cycles are the 'tidal' cycles and occur every 30–60 minutes. This leaves a large volume of dialysate in constant contact with the peritoneal membrane, which minimizes the dead exchange time and potentially increases clearances. Twardowski (1989) reported that TPD is approximately 20% more efficient than NIPD. However, Shah *et al.* (1992) showed no differences in clearance in the same patient during IPD and TPD using the same dialysate volume and flow rate. The disadvantage is that large volumes of dialysate are required – 30–36 litres per session (Khanna *et al.*, 1993).

INDICATIONS AND CONTRAINDICATIONS FOR PERITONEAL DIALYSIS

There are no categorical rules defining which patients should receive a particular form of treatment. All patients should be assessed individually by the team caring for them, and the decision should be based on their knowledge and experience. There are however, certain reasons why some patients will be strong candidates for peritoneal dialysis and it will be contraindicated for others. These are summarized in Table 10.2.

PERITONEAL DIALYSIS FLUID

Despite two decades of peritoneal dialysis the fluid remains largely unchanged, and cannot be considered as 'ideal'. However, given that the success of peritoneal dialysis lies in preserving the peritoneum as a dialysing membrane (de Fijter *et al.*, 1994), the fluids have been subject to continuous investigations in attempts to improve them, particularly in respect of the osmotic agent and buffer used.

Osmotic agents

Glucose has traditionally been used as the osmotic agent; it is cheap and reasonably effective in most patients. However, glucose absorption from

Table 10.2 Indications and contraindications for peritoneal dialysis (Source: adapted from Khanna *et al.*, 1993)

Medical / physical	Psychosocial

Strongly indicated for CAPD
 • Difficulty with vascular access
 • Diabetes mellitus
 • Heart failure or cardiovascular disease
 • Blood problems, i.e.
    – Transfusion problem
    – Bleeding disorder
	• Age 0–5 years and schoolchildren
	 • Strong patient preference; need for independence and flexibility
	 • Needle anxiety
	 • Living a long way from the centre
	 • University/college students

Questionably indicated for PD
 • Nutritional problems, e.g.
    – Chronic malnutrition
    – Eating disorders
 • Obesity
 • Chronic obstructive airways disease
 • Previous abdominal surgery causing multiple adhesions
 • Stomas
 • Recurrent hernias; hiatus hernias
 • Polycystic kidney disease, especially with large kidneys
 • Blindness
 • History of diverticulitis
 • Impaired dexterity skills
 • Chronic constipation
 • Low back pain
 • Chronic pancreatitis
	• Poor motivation/compliance
	 • Severe depression
	 • Drug abuse/alcoholism
	 • Unsatisfactory home environment, e.g.
	    – Cramped living conditions, lack of storage space
	    – Poor personal hygiene/cleanliness
	    – Nursing home
	 • Forgetfulness/dementia
	 • Absence of necessary home support
	 • Aversion to the PD catheter – poor body image

Contraindicated for PD • Severe inflammatory bowel disease, e.g. diverticulitis • Abdominal abscess • Severely impaired dexterity without a helper	• Strong patient resistance • Homelessness • Severe depression or psychosis • Severe intellectual impairment without a helper

Indications for APD (rather than CAPD)
 • Raised intra-abdominal pressure; pressure-related problems
    – Hernias
    – Large polycystic kidneys
    – Aortic aneurysms
    – Back pain
 • Frequent peritonitis during CAPD
 • Poor ultrafiltration due to high transport status
 • Inadequate small solute clearance
	• Children/college students
	 • Strong patient preference
	 • Poor compliance with CAPD
	 • Employed/active lifestyle
	 • Dirty work environment
	 • Helper preference/convenience

the dialysate can amount to one-third of the patient's daily calorific requirements and lead to obesity, hyperglycaemia and hyperinsulinaemia (Graham, 1995). Absorption of glucose causes dissipation of the osmotic gradient, which can result in net fluid reabsorption from the peritoneum. Also, the non-physiological nature of glucose is thought to be detrimental to the peritoneum and its host defences (Mistry and Gokal, 1994).

Glucose polymer at 7.5% and amino acids are alternative osmotic agents. Glucose polymers are larger molecules than glucose and do not permeate the peritoneum, ensuring a 50% reduction in carbohydrate load *via* the lymphatics (Gokal *et al.*, 1994). Ultrafiltration occurs slowly, achieving optimal fluid loss at around 10 hours. Therefore, glucose polymers are recommended for long overnight exchange only, and may benefit diabetics and patients who reabsorb fluid in this long dwell. Amino acids may also be used instead of glucose and can provide nutritional benefits for malnourished patients. However, the absorption of amino acids may exacerbate existing uraemia and acidosis. The increased cost of these fluids currently limits their use in the UK.

Buffers

Lactate is currently used as the buffer in peritoneal dialysis fluids, and the solutions have a pH of around 5.5, which is clearly bioincompatible. The disadvantages of this are:

- pain on instillation in some patients;
- mesothelial cell cytotoxicity;
- impairment of peritoneal host defence, which is thought to contribute to the development of peritonitis (Schambye *et al.*, 1992).

Also, lactate must be metabolized by the liver to generate bicarbonate, and this may be impaired in patients with liver disease. Bicarbonate as a buffer would avoid the acute toxic effects of lactate-based fluids and should not have any negative influence on physiological mechanisms of defence (Feriani *et al.*,1987). Furthermore, bicarbonate has not been shown to cause abdominal discomfort.

Calcium content

The traditional calcium concentration of peritoneal dialysis solutions has been 1.75 mmol/l, which was necessary to maintain calcium balance when patients used aluminium-based phosphate binders. However, accumulation of aluminium can lead to osteomalacia, anaemia and dialysis encephalopathy (Martis *et al.*, 1989; Pagliari *et al.*, 1991). Therefore, most patients now take calcium-based phosphate binders. Consequently, these patients dialyse against fluid with a low calcium concentration (1.25 and 1.00 mmol/l) to prevent excess absorption of calcium and subsequent hypercalcaemia.

CONCLUSION

It is essential that nurses working within the speciality of peritoneal dialysis understand the fundamentals, in order to give a standard of care that all patients deserve.

The aim of this chapter is to provide a basic, yet up-to-date view of all aspects of peritoneal dialysis, for use by both learners and experienced renal nurses. It is also the intention to encourage all health-care professionals to dispel the myth that PD is the 'second' dialysis option (to haemodialysis), as this is clearly untrue. PD is a dynamic therapy and deserves equal recognition with other forms of renal replacement therapy.

It is hoped that this information will meet the needs of learner nurses, and encourage experienced nurses to read further and develop a deeper knowledge and appreciation of the complexities of this subject.

REVIEW QUESTIONS

- What effect do (a) peritonitis and (b) continuous exposure to dialysate have on the peritoneum?
- Describe the preparation the patient requires prior to insertion of a peritoneal dialysis catheter. Why is it important that the patient is not constipated?
- What advice should be given to the peritoneal dialysis patient regarding showering and swimming?
- What patients are best suited to automated forms of peritoneal dialysis?
- In what way does high-dose CCPD differ from CCPD?
- What information can be obtained from performing a PFT/PET test? How does this information aid therapy prescription?

REFERENCES

De Fijter, C. W. H., Liem Oe, P., Donker, A. J. M. *et al.* (1994) Compatibility of peritoneal dialysis fluids containing alternative osmotic agents with cells present in the peritoneal cavity. *Peritoneal Dialysis International*, **14**(Suppl. 2), 33.

Diaz-Buxo, J. A. (1996) Enhancement of peritoneal dialysis: the PD plus concept. *American Journal of Kidney Diseases*, **27**(4), 92–98.

Dobbie, J. W. (1994) Ultrastructure and pathology of the peritoneum in peritoneal dialysis, in *Textbook of Peritoneal Dialysis*, (eds R. Gokal and K. Nolph), Kluwer Academic Publishers, Dordrecht.

Feriani, M., Biasioli, S., Chiaramonte, S. *et al.* (1987) Will bicarbonate CAPD strengthen the natural defence by having a physiological pH and a natural buffer? *Contributions in Nephrology*, **57**, 101–109.

Goetz, A. (1989) *Pseudomonas aeruginosa* infections associated with use of povidone-iodine in patients receiving CAPD. *Infection Control and Hospital Epidemiology*, **10**(10), 447–450.

Gokal, R., Ash, S., Helfrich, G. B. *et al.* (1993) Peritoneal catheters and exit-site practices: toward optimum peritoneal access. *Peritoneal Dialysis International*, **13**, 29–39.

Gokal, R., Mistry, C., Peers, E. and the Midas study group. (1994) A UK multicentre study of Icodextrin in CAPD. *Peritoneal Dialysis International*, **14**(Suppl. 2), 22–27.

Graham, C. (1995) The ideal peritoneal dialysis solution: fact or fiction? *RCN Dialysis and Transplant Nursing Forum Newsletter*, **2**, 8–10.

Hutchison, A. and Gokal, R. (1992) Improved solutions for peritoneal dialysis: physiological calcium solutions, osmotic agents and buffers. *Kidney International*, **42**(Suppl. 38), 153–159.

Keen, M. L. and Gotch, F. A. (1994) Peritoneal Function Test as a basis for assessment of adequate therapy and for urea kinetic modeling. *The Kidney and Blood Related Illnesses*, **23**(Suppl. 2), 141–143.

Khanna, R. and Nolph, K. (1989) The physiology of peritoneal dialysis. *American Journal of Nephrology*, **9**, 504–512.

Khanna, R., Nolph, K. D. and Oreopoulos, D. G. (1993) *The Essentials of Peritoneal Dialysis*, Kluwer Academic Publishers, Dordrecht.

Krediet, R. T. (1994) Fluid absorption in the peritoneum – it is less simple than you thought. *Nephrology, Dialysis and Transplantation*, **9**, 341–343.

Leypoldt, J. K. and Mistry, C. D. (1994) Ultrafiltration in peritoneal dialysis, in *Textbook of Peritoneal Dialysis*, (eds R. Gokal and K. Nolph), Kluwer Academic Publishers, Dordrecht.

Martis, L., Serkes, K. and Nolph, K. (1989) Calcium carbonate as a phosphate binder: is there a need to adjust peritoneal dialysis calcium concentrations for patients using $CaCO_3$? *Peritoneal Dialysis International*, **9**, 325–328.

Mistry, C. and Gokal, R. (1994). Icodextrin in peritoneal dialysis: early development and clinical use. *Peritoneal Dialysis International*, **14**(Suppl. 2), 13–21.

Moncrief, J. W., Popovich, R. P., Dombros, N. V. *et al.* (1994). Continuous ambulatory peritoneal dialysis, in *Textbook of Peritoneal Dialysis*, (eds R. Gokal and K. Nolph), Kluwer Academic Publishers, Dordrecht.

Pagliari, B., Baretta, A., De Cristafaro, V. *et al.* (1991) Short-term effects of low-calcium dialysis solutions on calcium mass transfer, ionized calcium and parathyroid hormone on CAPD patients. *Peritoneal Dialysis International*, **11**, 326–329.

Prowant, B. F., Schmidt, L. M., Twardowski, Z. J. *et al.* (1988) Peritoneal dialysis catheter exit site care. *American Nephrology Nurses Association Journal*, **15**, 219–222.

Prowant, B. F., Warady, B. A. and Nolph, K. D. (1993) Peritoneal dialysis catheter exit-site care: results of an International survey. *Peritoneal Dialysis International*, **13**, 149–154.

Rocco, M. V., Jordan, J. R. and Burkhart, J. M. (1995) Changes in peritoneal transport during the first month of Peritoneal Dialysis. *Peritoneal Dialysis International*, **15**, 12–17.

Schambye, H. T., Pederson, F. B., Christensen, H. K. *et al.* (1992) The cytotoxicity of CAPD solutions with different bicarbonate/lactate ratios. *Peritoneal Dialysis International*, **13**(Suppl. 2), 116–118.

Shah, J., Lane, D., Shrivastava, D. *et al.* (1992) Isovolemic tidal technique does not increase clearances in IPD (abstract). *Journal of the American Society of Nephrology*, **3**, 419.

Twardowski, Z. J. (1989) New approaches to intermittent peritoneal dialysis therapy, in *Peritoneal Dialysis*, (ed. K. D. Nolph), Kluwer Acadmic Publishers, Dordrecht.

Twardowski, Z. J. (1990) Nightly peritoneal dialysis. why, who, how and when? *Transactions of the American Society for Artificial Internal Organs*, **36**, 233–41.

Twardowski, Z. J. (1992) Peritoneal dialysis catheter exit site infections: prevention, diagnosis, treatment and future directions. *Seminars in Dialysis*, **5**(4), 305–315.

Twardowski, Z. J. and Khanna, R. (1994) Peritoneal dialysis access and exit site care, in *Textbook of Peritoneal Dialysis*, (eds R. Gokal and K. Nolph), Kluwer Academic Publishers, Dordrecht.

Twardowski, Z. J., Nolph, K. D., Khanna, R. *et al.* (1987) Peritoneal Equilibration Test. *Peritoneal Dialysis Bulletin*, **7**, 137–138.

Winchester, J. F. and Rotellar, C. (1994) Theory of dialysis, in *Renal Dialysis*, (eds J. D. Briggs, B. J. R. Junor, R. S. C. Rodger and J. F. Winchester), Chapman & Hall, London.

Woodrow, G., Turney, J. H., Cook, J. A. *et al.* (1994) Nocturnal intermittent peritoneal dialysis. *Nephrology, Dialysis and Transplantation*, **9**, 399–403.

11 Complications and nursing interventions associated with peritoneal dialysis

Krys Turner

LEARNING OBJECTIVES

At the end of this chapter the reader should be able to:

- Diagnose, treat and understand the implications of peritonitis.
- Understand the importance of maintaining the function of the peritoneum.
- Understand the effects of constipation on ultrafiltration and position of tube, and the use and side-effects of laxatives.
- Understand the principles of exit site care.
- Ensure patients are able to monitor and care for their exit site, reporting any signs of infection.

INTRODUCTION

Peritoneal dialysis is currently being used in all five continents and in at least 50 countries as a method of dialysis in end-stage renal failure. It is based on the use of the peritoneum as a dialysing membrane and of glucose solutions to remove the waste products of metabolism. However, this treatment involves direct access into the peritoneum and consequently an increased opportunity for infection.

More than 15 years after the introduction of PD, peritonitis is still considered an important complication of this treatment modality. Patients with a high incidence of peritonitis need to be transferred to haemodialysis, either short- or long-term. Modality transfer has far reaching implications for other hospital services – the chronic haemodialysis programme, theatre space for venous and peritoneal access formation, hospital beds – and most importantly for the patient's quality of life.

PERITONITIS AND ITS CONSEQUENCES

There are many opportunities for the introduction of infection into the peritoneum during PD. These include exogenous contamination from breaks in the technique, accidental disconnection, cracks in tubing and catheters, airborne skin scales, exit site infection or contaminated fluid. Endogenous infection may occur from inflamed or perforated abdominal viscera, through transmural migration of microorganisms across the gut and from other infected points in the body. The immune status of the patient, particularly cell-mediated immunity, is also affected by the uraemic state, making the PD patient highly vulnerable to peritonitis.

Peritonitis occurs readily among CAPD patients following apparently minor episodes of contamination. Because the peritoneum is permanently bathed with dialysis fluid, infection diffuses readily to the entire peritoneal cavity, even though the initial process might seem localized. However, the repeated drainage of the PD fluid offers a unique opportunity for the early detection of infection and direct access to the site of infection for immediate antibiotic treatment.

Peritonitis denotes inflammation of the peritoneum with a resultant increase in the number of white cells, leading to cloudiness of the peritoneal dialysis fluid when drained out of the peritoneum. This cloudiness, which is almost invariably present, should be seen as the earliest detector of infection; the majority of patients will also complain of abdominal pain or tenderness. Other accompanying symptoms may include nausea, vomiting, constipation, fever and chills. Treatment should begin at once and the consequences of not doing so will be discussed later. Patients who have recently started on CAPD may have cloudy fluid because of the presence of eosinophils. A differential cell count will establish this diagnosis and, if there is no growth, this condition will be self-limiting. It is thought to represent an allergic reaction to some constituents of the system.

Specimens of the dialysate fluid need to be sent to the laboratory for cell count, differential, Gram stain, culture and sensitivity. Antibiotic therapy should be initiated immediately using broad spectrum medication to include both Gram-positive and Gram-negative bacteria. Most patients can be successfully treated with intraperitoneal drug (i.p.) administration. However if the patient is seriously ill s/he may need parenteral antibiotics. Should there be a lot of pain and/or large amounts of fibrin, recent experience has found that a few half-hourly cycles using heparin should flush out some of the exudate and improve the patient's comfort. In addition, analgesic and antiemetic medication given intramuscularly will ensure the patient's comfort during the half-hourly flushes. Subsequently the patient can continue on CAPD using appropriate antibiotic therapy.

Recent studies (Dobbie *et al.*, 1994), show that the continued presence of irritating agents in the peritoneum, such as hypertonic glucose fluid, may retard the healing process. Glucose fluid causes a loss of macrophage activity just when that activity should be increased, and Dobbie suggests that a glucose-free physiological emollient dialysate should be provided for the acute and healing phase of severe peritonitis, or that all glucose should be drained from the peritoneum and the peritonitis should be treated with i.v. antibiotics.

Key reference: Dobbie, J.W., Anderson, J.D. and Hind C. (1994) Long term effects of PD on peritoneal morphology. *Peritoneal Dialysis International* 14(3):S16–20.

The peritoneal cavity is lined by mesothelium, which functions as a non-adhesive surface for internal organs. When damaged, the mesothelium produces fibrin, which, if not removed, may lead to adhesions between opposing serosal surfaces. It is therefore important to prevent the formation and deposits of fibrin and adhesions during peritonitis as they will reduce the chances of the patient remaining on this treatment. Although heparin, urokinase and streptokinase have been investigated (Vipond *et al.*, 1990) in the prevention of adhesions, and are commonly used in peritonitis, the results have been disappointing.

Gram-positive organisms usually respond to vancomycin. If a Gram-negative organism is present, aminoglycosides, cephalosporins or quinolones can be tried. If both Gram-positive and Gram-negative organisms are found or if there is no growth, then both antibiotics are given. Treatment of peritonitis has undergone many changes in terms of choice, route and duration of therapy. The use of i.p. aminoglycosides, either in every exchange or as a larger single dose, and once-weekly vancomycin delivered as a bolus dose and left to dwell for at least 6 hours with a repeat after 7 days has been recommended (Gokal *et al.*, 1993). Although such regimens involve considerably less work for both patients and staff, it is important to administer both Gram-positive and Gram-negative i.p. medication until the growth and sensitivity results are known. It is also vital to monitor the patient's progress regarding the clearing of the PD fluid and resolution of abdominal discomfort. If the infection is not seen to be resolving within a week, then the cannula is contributing to the persistence of infection; it should be removed and a new one not inserted for at least 3 weeks.

Fungal and yeast infections are best treated by removal of the cannula, using haemodialysis as an interim treatment. Using i.p. fungicidal drugs is usually ineffective as they can take 4 weeks or longer to have any effect, by which time severe adhesions have developed (Hoch *et al.*,1993).

Relapsing peritonitis is defined as the recurrence of peritonitis due to the same organism within 4 weeks of completion of an antibiotic course. After a second relapse, the catheter should be removed and the peritoneum rested for 3 weeks. Mixed infections and/or anaerobes strongly suggest that a bowel perforation has occurred and an urgent laparotomy is required (Tzamaloukas *et al.*, 1993).

The efficiency of some antibiotics may be affected by the length of time dialysate fluid has been warmed. Warming dialysate solution for longer than 4 hours may cause the pH of the solution to fall and become more acid. Insulin and heparin antagonize the effect of rifampicin when injected into dialysate fluid. This antagonism suggests that a significant degree of inhibition of antibiotic action may occur by the coadministration of agents in the treatment of peritonitis, particularly in diabetic patients using i.p. insulin (Richards *et al.*, 1993).

CONTAMINATION ACCIDENTS

If there is a break in the sterile technique (tubing dropped on to the floor, a leak from the bag, tubing or catheter), it should be regarded as a potential contamination. The system should be clamped between the site of contamination and the exit site, and the relevant contaminated part should be replaced. Prophylactic antibiotics are given when contaminated fluid has reached the peritoneum, although there is no literature to support their use. Furthermore, whether oral or i.p. treatment is necessary is also unknown (Lye and Lee, 1993).

If the Silastic catheter has a break there is grave risk of peritonitis. Sometimes small holes appear at the join of the titanium adapter to the catheter. This is due to wear on the catheter and needs careful examination at each clinic visit. The patient will notice that the dressing or skin is wet. It is necessary to trim the catheter beyond the holes, inserting a new adapter, and to give prophylactic antibiotics. If the extra-abdominal portion of the catheter becomes excessively short, it is possible to extend it using a commercially available kit.

EFFECTS OF PERITONITIS ON PERITONEAL MEMBRANE

Ultrafiltration failure is present in almost all episodes of peritonitis in PD patients (Boeschoten, 1996). Reports of the Peritoneal Biopsy Register (Dobbie *et al.*, 1994) indicate that patients who have experienced peritonitis show diabetiform changes in peritoneal capillary basement membrane. This suggests that during peritonitis there is a breakdown of the mesothelial barrier, which results in increased permeability to high glucose concentrations in the peritoneal interstitium, and glycosylation of the capillary basement membrane. Peritonitis also doubles the loss of protein from the body and this exacerbates an already malnourished patient further. Impaired ultrafiltration is due to the rapid influx of glucose into the bloodstream and a parallel fall in the osmotic gradient. Experimental data suggests that changes in permeability predominate as a consequence of histamine release and complement activation.

EFFECTS OF PERITONITIS ON MORBIDITY/MORTALITY

CAPD peritonitis appears to predispose patients with cardiovascular disease to cardiac death (Tzamaloukas *et al.*, 1993). Cardiac disease and malnutrition present before the onset of peritonitis and increase the risk of death, and mortality in peritonitis is also associated with *Staphylococcus aureus*, malnutrition, *Pseudomonas* infection and diabetes (Digenis *et al.*, 1990).

Peritoneal adhesions, sclerosis and loss of ultrafiltration

It was suggested as early as 1980 (Ghandi *et al.*, 1980) that recurrent peritonitis was a cause of sclerosing encapsulating peritonitis (SEP). This debilitating illness is characterized by a progressive formation of dense collagenous tissue and cocooning of the small bowel. Patients with this complication suffer with intermittent bowel obstruction, nausea, vomiting and malnutrition. These symptoms are usually preceded by a progressive loss of ultrafiltration (Krediet, 1993). The mortality rate of these patients is high – at least 50% – and in those patients who need surgical intervention the mortality rate is even higher. Evidence exists to suggest that the use of acetate dialysate buffer, cellular irritants such as plastic particles and hypertonic acidic use of dialysate fluid, together with the long-term use of intraperitoneally administered antibiotics such as vancomycin and amphotericin B, are all causative agents in SEP. Acetate is a known cellular toxin, and when used in the dialysate fluid its concentration is 350–450 times that normally found in the peritoneal cavity (Lo *et al.*, 1991; Bargman, 1994).

Prolonged and severe peritonitis will cause sclerosis of the membrane and PD will have to be abandoned. However, one study (Slingeneyer, 1987) suggests that cessation of PD is an important factor in the progress of SEP and that, although it seems sensible to stop PD as soon as SEP is diagnosed, it is possible that the dry peritoneum accelerates the encapsulating process (Boeschoten, 1996).

Occasionally, in the event of poor ultrafiltration, nocturnal cycling PD or intermittent overnight PD can be used. The effect of using the less affected upper parts of the peritoneum has sometimes made it possible to prolong the lifespan of PD.

MAINTAINING THE FUNCTION OF THE PERITONEUM

The peritoneum has an unknown lifespan, and it should be the renal nurse's role to ensure that peritoneal function is maintained as long as possible. The home PD patient's first contact during complications is usually the dialysis unit staff and it is their role to ensure that prompt action is taken to minimize the effects of peritonitis.

New catheter implantation techniques (Moncrief and Popovich, 1994; Twardowski *et al.*, 1993) have been tried recently to improve the bacteriological barrier between the outside contaminated skin and the internal sterile peritoneum. Numerous published anecdotal experiences and prospective randomized trials suggest a reduction in peritonitis rates with the use of disconnect, flush-before-fill and ultraviolet light devices (Li *et al.*, 1996). In spite of these published findings, some CAPD centres find it financially difficult to use these systems in bulk.

> **Key reference:** Moncrief, J.W. and Popovich, R.P. (1994) Moncrief-Popovich catheter: implantations technique and clinical results. *Peritoneal Dialysis International* 14(3): 56–8.

PATIENT INVOLVEMENT

One major aspect in ensuring a safe environment is maintained in the patient's community will be the quality of patient training and the specialist aftercare offered by the dialysis centre. Patient education during CAPD training using a varied format of input with constant reinforcement and assessment of information given will consolidate the importance of a scrupulously clean technique and the immediate reporting of infection symptoms. It is also important that the training nurse is aware of the influence of ethnic and cultural backgrounds upon the perception of illness and cleanliness, and is able to adapt the training and educational package to meet individual situations and patient needs. If there is any suspicion that the home circumstances may not be favourable to maintaining a safe environment, this should be clarified before discharge of the patient into the community. Once in the community, a gradual weaning from the training unit helps the patient deal with the transition from hospital to home and reinforces all that was taught during training. It is important that the patient has regular outpatient screening and community specialist support, as low patient motivation and minimal social support are significantly related to peritonitis rate (Stegman and Berger, 1984).

Another important feature is the training unit's access to new technological and innovative practices, and its ability to use this information in maintaining quality patient care. There is a plethora of international information available in specialist journals that are regularly available for members of the associations. Having access to such literature would both update the staff on the latest practices and motivate them to investigate and hopefully improve their practice.

OTHER PD COMPLICATIONS

Leakage

PD fluid leaking around the exit site or abdominal incision may be caused by mobilizing the patient too soon after placement of tube, or using too large a volume of fluid (Winchester and Kriger, 1994). It is important to reduce cycle volumes by half and avoid any dwell time and it may be necessary to stop PD for 12–24 hours. When restarting cycles, keep to low volumes, e.g. 500 ml cycles. The chances of leakage are much less if PD is avoided for 1 week after catheter insertion, and ensuring that the patient remains on bed rest for 24–48 hours after implantation of the catheter may lessen the likelihood of PD fluid leakage.

Inflow problems

A 2 litre bag of fluid normally takes about 15 minutes to drain in. More than 30 minutes is abnormal. Obstructions of inflow may be due to kinks in the tubing or an air lock. The tubing needs to be checked for obstructions and air locks can be dislodged by squeezing the bag. If simple measures fail, the cannula should be aseptically flushed using sterile water and heparin at a concentration of 500 u/l. Failure to obtain a good inflow despite flushing is an indication for a plain abdominal X-ray to show the catheter position. If it is in the pelvis, attempts to clear it with urokinase should be made. If the catheter is in the wrong position or cannot be cleared it will require replacement or manipulation.

Pain

Some patients experience inflow pain, which has been attributed to the low pH of the dextrose fluid. Warming the fluid for long periods reduces the pH even more. PD fluid should not be left in warmers for longer than 12 hours and ideally should be then discarded. Many patients have had inflow pain reduced/removed by the addition of bicarbonate solution just before infusion (10 ml of 8.4% bicarbonate injection). There are studies in progress at present to find the ideal biocompatible PD solution.

Outflow problems

Normally, 2 litres runs out in about 30 minutes. More than 60 minutes is abnormal. Should there be a problem with the outflow, make sure the roller clamp is undone and the tubing is free with no kinks in the catheter. Get the patient to strain for a few seconds to overcome any air locks, and changing body position sometimes helps. Very occasionally, running a further litre of fluid may clear the obstruction. Check that the patient is not constipated and check position of the catheter with an abdominal X-ray. If these measures fail, the catheter can be flushed aseptically and urokinase can be used. If all these measures fail it can be assumed the catheter is trapped by omentum, producing a one-way valve effect. A cannulogram may diagnose this problem (Moncrief and Popovich, 1994).

Constipation

Constipation can be a side-effect of CAPD, especially with the overuse of hypertonic dialysate fluid. Many patients receive stool softeners, but this may not be adequate to keep the bowel movements regular. Migration of the catheter has been known to occur with constipation, giving rise to drainage problems. It has also been suggested that acute treatment of constipation in PD may lead to inflamed or irritated intestinal serosa, facilitating the transmural migration of intestinal bacteria. In the presence of dialysate, exacerbated by an impaired immune defence system in a debilitated malnourished patient, peritonitis may result (Singharetnam and Holley, 1996).

Hydrothorax

Pulmonary complications are facilitated both by the upward displacement of the diaphragm due to bowel distension and by pulmonary oedema induced by inadequate fluid removal. Occasionally, CAPD patients may develop a pleural effusion not due to fluid overload, and this can be caused by a leak between the peritoneal and pleural cavities. The patient will have fluid overload symptoms, be breathless, and have had a history of poor outflow volumes. A chest X-ray will show fluid in the pleural cavity. Initial treatment is to stop PD and to aspirate the pleural effusion, leaving the abdomen empty for 2–3 weeks. Subsequently, PD may be recommenced using slowly increasing volumes.

Obesity, hernias, fluid leaks and backache

Many patients with ESRD are malnourished, and after starting PD will slowly gain dry weight. However, the absorption of dextrose from the dialysate, particularly if many 3.86% bags are used, will cause some CAPD patients to become obese. It is vital that patients are given correct dietary advice before they leave the training unit, in order that their protein intake is sufficient for them to regain and maintain their body weight.

One of the recognized complications of CAPD is the development of hernias. These occur at various sites, including through catheter insertion holes, past or present. As hernias may strangulate, it is wise to repair them prior to catheter insertion. Following repair it is important to avoid excessive abdominal distension until the wound is secure to minimize reoccurrence. The patient should have 500 ml, no-dwell cycles increasing to 2 litres over 2 weeks, when CAPD may be recommenced.

Back pain is also a frequent complication of CAPD, probably related to the change of body posture with the presence of fluid in the peritoneal cavity. Reducing cycle volumes from 2 litres to 1.5 litres can be considered if the uraemia is still adequately controlled. Sometimes the only solution is to transfer the patient to IPD or haemodialysis. Haemorrhoids, abdominal and pericatheter leaks are not uncommon in CAPD patients. These are related to the constant presence of fluid in the peritoneal cavity coupled with the high intra-abdominal pressure in the vertical position during natural activities. Intra-abdominal pressure in the supine position is negligible in relaxed patients, hence the rise in popularity of overnight cycling peritoneal dialysis.

Access site infection

Exit site infection has been difficult to both define and treat, as there is a spectrum of exit site appearances. This has led to an imprecise definition of infection and, in many instances, antibiotic treatment has been commenced prior to obtaining microbiological results. For a very precise description of a normal exit site and a detailed description and classification of exit site morphology, reference should be made to the latest documentation available (Twardowski and Prowant, 1996a).

> **Key reference:** Twardowski, Z.J. and Prowant B.F. (1996a) Peritoneal catheter exit site morphology and pathology. prevention, diagnosis, and treatment of exit site infections. *Peritoneal Dialysis International* 16(3): S6–31.

Exit site care should be taught to the patient or carer and any suspicion of infection should be reported to the renal unit. Antibiotic treatment needs

Prevention of exit site infection

- Keep exit site clean and dry
- Wash hands prior to exit site care
- Avoid submersion during healing or infection
- Avoid swimming in lakes, rivers, public pools, hot tubs, whirlpools
- Use waterproof dressings when swimming
- Perform exit site care immediately after swimming
(Prowant and Twardowski, 1996)

to be commenced as soon as possible after swabs have been sent. It is important to take a culture swab from the drainage coming from the sinus tract without touching the skin around the exit site as the skin could be colonized with Gram-positive organisms, the most common being *Staphylococcal aureus / epidermidis*). It is well documented that *S. aureus* nasal carriage is a risk factor in *S. aureus* exit site infection (Luzar *et al.*, 1992) and there have been measures suggested to reduce *S. aureus* nasal carriage with the use of mupirocin (Perez-Fontan *et al.*, 1992).

The commonly accepted signs of **infection at the exit site** are redness, crusting and visible pus, and sometimes there will be pain and tenderness. A swab should be taken for culture, and the commonest causative organism is *S. aureus* (Gokal *et al.*, 1993). Local measures can be tried, consisting of daily or more frequent cleansing of the site with povidone-iodine, and gentle removal of soft or loose crusts followed by a dressing. Antibiotics are also given, the regimen depending on the unit's protocol. A small amount of crusting may occur around the exit site and, if not accompanied by redness or pus formation, it is probably not serious. The crusts should be treated daily by soaking in povidone-iodine and gently removed with gauze swabs. A dry dressing should then be placed around the cannula. If crusting is excessive and/or there is obvious redness then suspect an infection and treat appropriately. Sometimes overgranulation of the tissues surrounding the exit site will cause bleeding and crusting, leaving the area open to infection. This can be cauterized with silver nitrate, usually once a week, but care must be taken to protect the surrounding skin and to only apply the silver nitrate to the granulating tissue.

If the outer cuff is visible or close to the surface, it is likely that the infection will not be eradicated but will flare up again. It is then best to exteriorize the cuff by slitting the tunnel to just beyond the cuff under local anaesthetic (Scalamonga *et al.*, 1991) and then shaving the cuff. The wound usually heals in 2–3 weeks. Often the infection will then disappear but if not, the only long-term solution may be catheter removal and replacement at a new outlet site under antibiotic cover. Great care is necessary to prevent the cannula from being perforated. If the outer cuff totally erodes so that it is no longer attached to the skin, the infection may clear up.

Subcutaneous tunnel infection is particularly likely to occur if the outer cuff has come out of the skin. The signs are tenderness and redness over the cannula track and sometimes pus appearing at the exit site. There is a serious risk of peritonitis if this infection is not treated urgently (Twardowski and Prowant, 1996b).

Principles of nursing care for infection at the exit site

- Culture exit exudate
- Cauterize overgranulated tissue
- Use sterile dressings
- Immobilize the catheter
- Increase frequency of dressings to at least once daily
- Avoid use of cytotoxic agents in the scabs
- Reassess exit site every 7–10 days
(Prowant and Twardowski, 1996)

Key reference: Twardowski, Z.J. and Prowant, B.F. (1996b) Exit site healing post catheter implantation. *Peritoneal Dialysis International* 16(3): 51–58.

Occasionally the cannula appears through the abdominal skin and is most likely to be seen through the midline incision if the catheter does not lie in a smooth curve but is kinked. The inherent torsion may then force it up before wound healing occurs. An alternative cause is an untreated tunnel infection that bursts through the skin exposing the cannula. Urgent catheter removal is required.

CONCLUSION

Peritonitis associated with PD is a significant cause of morbidity, reduces the patient's quality of life and adds to the cost of care. Reduction of peritonitis rates has been influenced by the use of flush-before-fill systems, sound teaching of patients and staff, and early reporting, treatment and follow-up of infection. The setting of ground rules in aseptic technique, with emphasis on how to avoid contamination of PD equipment, will enable patients to understand the implications of not following strict hygiene during exchanges and to report cloudy fluid to the unit immediately. It is imperative that a core of highly trained staff is available to ensure that diagnosis and antibiotic treatment is commenced without delay and that microbiological results are followed and acted upon. The aim is to avoid adhesions from prolonged peritonitis and to reduce the need for hospitalization and modality change for the patient. Effective peritoneal dialysis should not cause discomfort, inflow/outflow problems, tissue leaks or hernias. Prolonged dialysis exchange times reduce the effectiveness of the treatment as less time is left available for dialysate fluid contact with the peritoneum. The aim is to successfully maintain a well-dialysed, healthy patient in the community, avoiding modality treatment changes and hospitalization.

Exit site infection is difficult to diagnose and treat correctly. It can lead to peritonitis, loss of access, further surgery and change of modality, with the inherent loss of quality of life. These infections are mainly due to *S. aureus* and as yet the treatment is less than optimal. Therefore, the primary goal should be prevention with prophylactic treatment such as intranasal mupirocin or the use of silver-impregnated catheters. Sound patient education on preventative measures, correct diagnosis, quick and effective infection treatment and careful patient follow-up will improve the maintenance of a bacteriological barrier between the outside skin and the peritoneum.

REVIEW QUESTIONS

- What are both the short and long-term consequences of peritonitis?
- What is the nurse's role in reducing the occurrence of peritonitis in PD patients?
- What measures can be taken to prolong the lifespan of the peritoneal membrane?
- How important is it for patients to have correct and suitable training for home PD?
- What steps would you take in the event of PD fluid leaks, postoperation and long-term?
- What are the roles of the nurse regarding PD catheter care?
- How urgent is the need for exit site infection treatment?

REFERENCES

Bargman, J. M., Nong, Y. and Silverman, E. D. (1994) The effect of in vivo erythropoietin on cytokine mRNA in CAPD patients. *Advances in Peritoneal Dialysis*, **10**, 129–134.

Boeschoten, E. W. (1996) Long term consequences of peritonitis. *Peritoneal Dialysis International*, **16**(1), S349–S354.

Digenis, G., Abraham, G. and Savin, E. (1990) Peritonitis related deaths in CAPD patients. *Peritoneal Dialysis International*, **10**, 45–47.

Dobbie, J. W., Anderson, J. D. and Hind, C. (1994) Long term effects of PD on peritoneal morphology. *Peritoneal Dialysis International*, **14**(3) S16–S20.

Ghandi, V. C., Huamyun, H. M. and Ing, T. S. (1980) Sclerotic thickening of the peritoneal membrane in maintenance peritoneal dialysis patients. *American Journal of Kidney Diseases*, **140**, 1201–1203.

Gokal, R., Ash, S. R. and Helfrich, G. B. (1993) Peritoneal catheter and exit site practices: towards optimum peritoneal access. *Peritoneal Dialysis International*, **13**, 149–154.

Hoch, B. S., Namboodiri, N. K., Banayat, G. *et al.* (1993) The use of fluconazole in the management of *Candida* peritonitis in patients on PD. *Peritoneal Dialysis International*, **13**(Suppl. 2), 357–359.

Krediet, R. T., Inholz, A. L., Struijk, D. G *et al.* (1993) Ultrafiltration failure in continuous ambulatory peritoneal dialysis. *Peritoneal Dialysis International*, **13**(Suppl. 2), S59–S66.

Li, P., Chan, T., So, W. *et al.* (1996) Comparison of Y disconnect system (ultraset) versus conventional spike system in uremic patients on CAPD: outcome and cost analysis. *Peritoneal Dialysis International*, **16**(1), 368–370.

Lo, W. K., Chan, K. T. and Leung, C. (1991) Sclerosing peritonitis complication prolonged use of chlorhexidine in alcohol in the connection procedure for CAPD. *Peritoneal Dialysis International*, **11**, 166–172.

Luzar, M. A., Coles, G. A. and Faller, B. (1992) SA nasal carriage and infections in patients on CAPD. *New England Journal of Medicine*, **322**, 505–509.

Lye, W. C. and Lee, E. J. C. (1993) Intraperitoneal vancomycin/oral pefloxacin versus IP vancomycin/gentamicin in the treatment of CAPD peritonitis. *Peritoneal Dialysis International*, **13**(Suppl. 2), 348–350.

Moncrief, J. W. and Popovich, R. P. (1994) Moncrief–Popovich catheter: implantations technique and clinical results. *Peritoneal Dialysis International*, **14**(3), 56–58.

Perez-Fontan, N., Rosales, M., Rodrigues-Carmona, A. *et al.* (1992) Treatment of *Staphylococcus aureus* nasal carriers in CAPD with mupirocin. *Advances in Peritoneal Dialysis*, **8**, 243–245.

Prowant, B. F. and Twardowski, Z. J. (1996) Recommendations for exit site care. *Peritoneal Dialysis International*, **16**(3), S94–S99.

Richards, G., Gaynon, R. and Obst, G. (1993) The modulation of rifampicin action against *S. epidermidis* biofilms by drug additives to PD solutions. *Peritoneal Dialysis International*, **13**(2), 345–347.

Scalamonga, A., Castelnovo, C., Devecchi, A. and Ponticelli, C. (1991) Exit site and tunnel infections in CAPD. *American Journal of Kidney Diseases*, **28**, 674–677.

Slingeneyer, A. (1987) Preliminary report on a cooperative international study on sclerosing encapsulating peritonitis. *Contributions in Nephrology*, **57**, 239–247.

Singharetnam, W. and Holley, J. L. (1996) Acute treatment of constipation may lead to transmural migration of bacteria resulting in Gram-negative polymicrobial or fungal peritonitis. *Peritoneal Dialysis International*, **16**(4), 423–425.

Stegman, M. R. and Berger, A. M. (1984) Peritonitis among CAPD patients: host, agent and/or environment? *Peritoneal Dialysis Bulletin*, **4**, 206–208.

Twardowski, Z. J. and Prowant B. F. (1996a) Peritoneal catheter exit site morphology and pathology. Prevention, diagnosis, and treatment of exit site infections. *Peritoneal Dialysis International*, **16**(3), S6–S31.

Twardowski, Z. J. and Prowant B. F. (1996b) Exit site healing post catheter implantation. *Peritoneal Dialysis International*, **16**(3), 51–58.

Twardowski, Z., Ryan, L. P. and Kennedy, J. M. (1984) Catheter break-in for CAPD. University of Missouri experience. *Peritoneal Dialysis Bulletin*, **4**(Suppl. 3), 110–111.

Tzamaloukas, A., Obermiller, L., Gibel, L. *et al.* (1993) Peritonitis associated with intra-abdominal pathology in CAPD patients. *Peritoneal Dialysis International*, **13**(Suppl. 2), 335–337.

Vipond, M. N., Whawell, S. A., Thompson, J. N. and Dudley, H. A. (1990) Peritoneal fibrinolytic activity and intra-abdominal adhesions. *Lancet*, **335** (8698), 1120–1122.

Winchester, J. F. and Kriger, F. L. (1994). Fluid leaks, prevention and treatment. *Peritoneal Dialysis International*, **14**(3), 543–548.

FURTHER READING

Freiman, J. P., Graham, D. T. and Reed, T. G. (1992) Chemical peritonitis following the IP administration of vancomycin. *Peritoneal Dialysis International*, **12**, 57–60.

Gokal, R. (1996) CAPD overview. *Peritoneal Dialysis International*, **16**(1), S13–S18.

Keane, W. F., Everett, E. and Golper, T. (1993) Peritoneal dialysis-related peritonitis: treatment recommendations 1993 update. *Peritoneal Dialysis International*, **13**, 14–28.

12 Dietary and fluid considerations for the peritoneal dialysis patient

Lesley Russel

LEARNING OBJECTIVES

At the end of this chapter the reader should be able to:

- Discuss the problems that peritoneal dialysis patients have in relation to malnutrition.
- Discuss the need to individualize the peritoneal dialysis diet.
- Identify the main differences between the peritoneal dialysis diet and a normal diet.

INTRODUCTION

Before considering what is special about the peritoneal dialysis patient, first consider that nutrition is an important component of any patient's care. Hospital malnutrition is still common, with figures of around 40% of hospital patients being identified as malnourished and only about half of these being properly identified (McWhirter and Pennington, 1994); among patients who are identified, nutritional treatment is often successful. Dietary recommendations for the PD patient are set against the knowledge that malnutrition is also present. Estimates suggest that malnutrition is also present in about 40% of all patients receiving renal replacement therapy, with around 8% of renal patients having severe malnutrition (Young *et al.*, 1991). Indeed, figures can be higher in units and routine assessment shows that 54% of the PD population have decreasing mid-arm circumference data, indicating loss of body mass. One of the most important nutritional recommendations is therefore to monitor the nutritional wellbeing of the PD patient.

Key reference: Young, G.A., Kopple, J.D., Lindholm, B. *et al.* (1991) Nutritional Assessment of Continuous Ambulatory Peritoneal Dialysis Patients: An International Study. *American Journal of Kidney Diseases* XVII(4): 462–471.

MALNUTRITION AND THE PERITONEAL DIALYSIS PATIENT

Why do PD patients form such a vulnerable group in terms of nutrition? There are many reasons for this. Social considerations should never be underplayed; in the non-PD population social considerations have a huge impact on all aspects of health, including nutrition. In the PD population there are people no longer able to work who have in the past been the family's main breadwinner: poverty should not be underestimated. Psychological considerations also impact on nutrition in the PD population, depression and altered body image, directly as a result of Tenckhoff placement or PD dwells, being just two examples. The relationship that PD patients have with other co-morbidity is also very important. PD patients who have additional illness, such as ischaemic heart disease or peripheral vascular disease, may do less well in terms of nutrition, having a suppressed appetite that is independent of dialysis dose (Davies *et al.*, 1995). Some patients may also have difficulty taking an adequate diet, which will further confound their nutritional status. The effect of peritonitis must also be considered, as this is a vulnerable time when nutritional requirements may be higher but difficult to meet.

> **Key reference:** Davies, S.J., Russell, L.H., Bryan, J., Phillips, L., Russell, G.I. (1995) Comorbidity, Urea Kinetics, and Appetite in CAPD patients: their interrelationship and prediction of survival. *American Journal of Kidney Diseases* 26(2): 353–361.

PD patients sometimes report that the PD process itself has some implication in reducing appetite: often at the time of dwelling-in they feel full and are unable to eat their normal meals. The role of dialysis dose may also be important and therefore the role that residual renal function plays may also need consideration. Peritoneal function and renal acidosis are attracting interest as factors that may also impact on the nutritional status of the PD patient. It is suggested that the bicarbonate levels in dialysis patients should be maintained at normal levels to benefit nutritional status and that to be markedly acidotic has an undesired affect, leading to worsening protein metabolism, possibly because of changes in branch chain amino acid metabolism (Walls, 1995).

> **Key reference:** Walls, J. (1995) Metabolic acidosis and uraemia. *Peritoneal Dialysis International* 15(5S): S36–38.

The original renal diagnosis is important: a diagnosis of myeloma may have a different nutritional outcome from one of polycystic disease. Use of other drugs such as steroids will also have implications in terms of appetite and body composition. Renal anaemia may also be responsible for decreasing appetite; often patients will report increased food intake once this has been corrected with erythropoietin. The use of hypertonic solutions has also been implicated in the reduction of appetite of the PD patient, but this has not been substantiated by some workers (Davies *et al.*, 1996).

The catabolic factors involved in the PD process are well documented (Heimburger *et al.*, 1994). These include:

- abnormal protein and amino acid metabolism due to uraemia;
- decreased levels of the anabolic hormones such as insulin;
- increased levels of the catabolic hormones such as parathyroid hormone;
- blood sampling and other tests;
- losses of amino acids, protein and other nutrients in the PD effluent;
- decreased physical activity;
- impaired lipid metabolism;
- carbohydrate intolerance and altered cell energy metabolism.

ASSESSING DIETARY REQUIREMENTS

Malnutrition is the key area for consideration in the nutritional management of the PD patient: malnourished patients do not do well. Assessing the nutritional status of PD patients varies according to the local preference of renal team members. Some considerations are detailed below.

- determine the original renal diagnosis and any co-morbidity;
- establish the usual dialysis pattern and any problems with dialysis;
- establish the usual dietary intake and any deviations from this;
- know what the biochemical trends are;
- take a social history, including significant others;
- check for signs of psychological stress or depression;
- assess PD patients routinely, track anthropometric data;
- dry weight, deviations and any related symptoms;
- look at the patient, possibly using a nutritional assessment scoring system such as SGA;
- action concerns and alert team members to nutritional problems.

There is no one single test for the presence of malnutrition and therefore any approach has to involve many elements: a careful history, physical, psychological and social elements. The list above gives a few examples of some of the common elements in assessment. Assessing the needs of the PD patient must also be part of an ongoing assessment and not done only at the time of commencement on PD but regularly, as any changes can impact on nutritional status. Any decrease in nutritional status is easier to act upon if dealt with as it arises rather than waiting for it to become a major problem or letting it go undetected.

The use of anthropometrics may be useful in plotting changes for individual PD patients and using a series of results to monitor that patient's progress rather than comparing the results with the population norms. Mid-arm circumference (MAC) has also been used to give an estimate of dry weight (Bennet *et al.*, 1986). This system does, however, rely on the initial assessment being accurate and the PD patient being at dry weight when the first MACs are measured as the subsequent results are dependent on this initial ratio. For example a patient having an initial dry weight of 52 kg and MAC of 26 cm has a ratio of 2 (weight in kg/MAC in cm).

When the patient is reassessed at clinic the MAC is noted to be 27 cm, the dry weight is calculated as the initial ratio times the new MAC, i.e. 2×27, giving a new dry weight of 54 kg. If the actual weight of the patient is over this then there may be the possibility that some fluid weight is responsible and this can be investigated. Using anthropometrics in this way helps to provide trends and gives another dimension to the assessment. Using weight as the only anthropometric tool is obviously flawed and it is useful to have a more complete picture. The anthropometric data collected on PD patients has been shown not to be significantly different from the haemodialysis population (Nelson *et al.*, 1990).

During the time taken to perform anthropometric assessment, which may also include the use of skinfold measurements, there is an opportunity to look at the PD patient. Some PD units have formalized this as Subjective Global Assessment. Scoring sheets may be devised to formalize such assessments and may include details of medical history and physical assessment. Medical history can include weight change, dietary intake, gastrointestinal symptoms and nutrition-related functional impairment. Physical assessment may include loss of subcutaneous fat, evidence of muscle wasting and presence of oedema. Formalizing the assessment of the PD patient is useful. This may be done in the predialysis setting, before the patient has a Tenckhoff catheter placed, when training is commenced, and may be built into the time of the peritoneal equilibration test or form part of the dietetic service to the PD clinic, depending on the local situation. What is important is that there is time for the PD patient to have his/her nutritional concerns assessed and dealt with so that any deterioration in nutritional health is prevented if at all possible.

Patient scenario

Joan is a 65-year-old widow who underwent a bilateral nephrectomy for cancer 6 months ago. Initially she made good progress and her anthropometric data improved: at review in CAPD clinic she was noted to have a Cr of 780, Ur 17.8, albumin 32, phosphorus 1.3, potassium 4.7. When she is assessed it is noted that her weight and anthropometric data have decreased slightly since her last clinic visit. Initially she dismisses this, but after the nurse has been talking to her for a little longer, she admits to not eating as well as she has done. Joan's friend who takes her shopping has been in hospital for the past 2 months; she finds shopping difficult and misses the company of her friend. A community volunteer is contacted and arranges shopping visits. Discussions take place about the nutritional value of frozen and tinned foods so that food stores can be maximized, as shopping trips take place less often than before. The community PD nurse arranges to visit next week and liaises with the dietitian. This case illustrates that PD patients may have satisfactory biochemistry and not initially report any problems. However, with a series of anthropometric data and good questioning and empathy skills, potential nutritional problems can be spotted and acted upon before they become serious problems, in this case with relatively simple practical help.

Against this background it is worth considering some specific nutrient requirements for the PD patient.

Calories

Calorie requirements are set at 35 kcal/kg ('kilocalorie' is the scientific term for the 'calories' in common use; they are also called 'medical calories', or 'Calories') inclusive of PD calories, PD calories supplying around 5 kcal/kg (Davies *et al.*, 1996) from dextrose within the PD fluid absorbed *via* the peritoneum. The uptake of dextrose from the peritoneal dwells is in the order of 60–80% (Lindholm *et al.*, 1981). Each gram of dextrose (glucose) is equivalent to 4 kcal in terms of energy; we can therefore calculate rough estimates for the calorie contribution of the dialysis fluid.

For example, a PD patient receiving a dialysis regimen of four 2 litre exchanges of 1.36% dextrose will be administering 27.2 g dextrose in each of the 2 litre dwells, 20×1.36 (1.36 g glucose in 100 ml of PD fluid and 20×100 ml in 2 litres). Therefore in four exchanges 108.8 g will be administered; this is equivalent to 435 kcal (each gram of glucose gives 4 kcal, 4×108.8). If we assume that there is 70% absorption this will give a final calorie contribution of $435 \times 0.7 = 304.5$ kcal. This can be worked out for the patient's actual dialysis pattern and is assuming that all PD patients absorb 70% of their dialysate, but it is useful to get some estimate of the contribution of PD calories, which will need to be considered in all types of nutritional care plans for the PD patient, including the estimation of energy requirements during nasogastric and parenteral feeding. There is increasing interest in the alternatives to glucose as the osmotic agent in PD fluid; products that are high-molecular-weight polymers of glucose may lessen the glucose load in the dialysis solution and are promoted for the obese or diabetic patient (Chapter 10).

It is important that the calorie needs are met so that the protein is not used for gluconeogenesis, i.e. for energy, particularly in the PD patient, where protein intakes need to be a little higher. Assessment of PD patients gives wide-ranging results in terms of calories: in a sample of 207 dietary assessments for PD patients we found that the oral calories ranged from 463 kcal to over 4000 kcal. What is interesting is that the means for different age ranges and sexes show that the women under the age of 55 have lower calorie intakes when expressed as a percentage of the estimated average requirements for sex and age. It is important to bear this in mind when advising young women in terms of diet, as they may be self-selecting lower calorie intakes and this may be associated with concerns over body image.

Calories are provided from carbohydrate, fat and alcohol in most normal diets. While it is fundamental to ensure that calorie requirements are met in the first instance, it is also prudent to look at the contribution of each of the calorie sources in terms of general health. PD patients have lipid abnormalities and assessment of biochemistry should include consideration of the lipid profile: mortality from heart disease is high in the dialysis population (Wheeler, 1996). Advice may include the use of complex carbohydrates, such as bread, potatoes, pasta, rice and cereals, as long as appetite can meet the calorie requirements. There may be advice about altering the fat content of the diet and substituting polyunsaturated or monounsaturated fats for saturated fats, e.g. using sunflower or olive oil rather than lard. The use of refined carbohydrates will need careful consideration: if total calorie intake is met easily it may be prudent to limit the use of sugars in the diet; if total calorie intake is not met then the priority becomes ensuring that calories are taken and it may be necessary to use a wide range of calorie sources including snack items such as biscuits or sweets. Alcohol should be asked about when assessing the diet; although many PD patients do not take alcohol because of medication or for fluid restriction preferences there are those who may be acquiring calories *via* this route.

Obesity in the PD patient must be viewed in the context of the whole patient scenario. Good nutritional assessment can help to pick up trends in unwanted weight gain and start to address this issue. It is, however, fundamental that all overweight PD patients are not automatically told to reduce their food intake and lose weight. An obese person can still be malnourished and correction of malnutrition should be the primary aim.

There may be occasions where it is not possible to use normal food to meet total calorie requirements and the use of nutritional supplementation is necessary. In the PD patient, supplementation needs to take account of other restrictions, such as fluid, and the most appropriate supplement should be prescribed. This may be provided in calorie-dense forms giving 1.5–2.0 kcal/ml while most normal supplements give 1.0 kcal/ml. Supplements can be in the form of ready-to-drink preparations, powders to be made up or powders that can be added to food; a range of supplements is useful so that use can be individualized and variety helps to ensure that flavour fatigue is lessened. Where possible the preference is to use food familiar to the PD patient as this helps to normalize the situation.

Protein

Protein has a special place in the PD patient's diet; protein losses in PD fluid are well documented and tend to be in the order of 3–14 g protein per day in PD effluent. Protein recommendations based on the original nitrogen balance studies by Blumenkrantz *et al.* (1982) are 1.2 g/kg. However, it is interesting to note that some patients achieve stable or increasing anthropometric data on diets with as little as 0.8 g/kg.

There are patients who manage to achieve intakes of 1.2 g/kg who are not able to maintain their nutritional status. There may be many reasons for this: the reasons so far outlined in this chapter will all have a role to play in affecting the nutritional outcome of the PD patient. It would seem prudent, as although we know that some patients manage quite well on less than 1.2 g/kg we are not in a position to predict this, that we should therefore take 1.2 g/kg as a general recommendation. Protein intakes vary considerably: in our cohort the range was 0.4–2.3 g/kg. When this is broken down into actual protein figures and divided by sex and age again it appears that young women have lower intakes, possibly because of body image and vegetarian influences on the diets of the women in this cohort.

The prescription of 30 oral kcal/kg and 1.2 g protein/kg sounds fairly divorced from food. If a PD patient took in the following:

- **Breakfast**: Cereal and milk; 2 slices toast;
- **Mid-morning**: 3 biscuits;
- **Lunch**: 85 g chicken, potatoes, peas; Rice pudding;
- **Mid-afternoon**: Apple;
- **Evening meal**: 60 g corned beef sandwich; slice of cake;
- **Supper**: 2 slices toast with jam;

the result would be 84 g protein and 2270 kcal, which for a 70 kg man would give 1.2 g protein/kg and 32 kcal/kg.

The use of urea kinetics needs careful consideration before it is used to estimate the protein intake of the PD patient and is discussed in the next chapter. Care must be taken to account for the urea generation that occurs with catabolism; this urea is the result of muscle breakdown rather than dietary protein intake. Dietary assessment by an experienced dietitian will provide data on nutrient intakes for this population. There may also be a need to look at other appetite measures rather than normalized protein catabolic rate (Ginsberg *et al.*, 1996).

Protein is quite often the most expensive part of the diet and during the initial assessment of the PD patient, the normal sources of protein should be elucidated. There are many reasons why people choose not to eat certain of the protein foods, which can include cultural and religious beliefs as well as food scares. Some PD patients report that they no longer enjoy traditional meals based on meat, potatoes and vegetables; they may need to be encouraged to have smaller meals and snacks to meet protein targets. Ensure that the time taken to prepare them is not prohibitive and that sandwiches and toast meals designed to meet protein targets are assessed in the context of the whole diet so that any vitamin deficits can be met from elsewhere in the diet.

Occasionally it will be necessary to supplement the protein intake of the PD patient and the choice of supplement will depend on what else they are managing, their potassium and phosphorus status. Protein foods have associated with them potassium and phosphorus and therefore need to be considered along with these.

Supplementation may also be considered when there is intercurrent illness or peritonitis. Peritonitis is catabolic and can take some time to recover from. Peritonitis needs special consideration: it can lead to a decreased food intake at a time of increased requirement, increased losses of protein *via* the peritoneum, increased catabolism and decreased protein synthesis. The use of other methods of nutritional support such as nasogastric or peripheral intravenous feeding may be considered (Rubin, 1990). The use of intraperitoneal amino acids (IPAA) is gaining interest. Instead of the peritoneal dialysis fluid containing glucose, it contains 1.1% amino acids, a 2 litre bag giving 22 g amino acid. The amino acids act as an osmotic agent and are absorbed from the peritoneal cavity, available to the body for protein synthesis. The exchange containing the amino acids is usually given as the third exchange in a four-exchange pattern. There is a need to ensure that the patient is receiving adequate calories from the rest of the diet before the treatment is considered. IPAA can be included in the normal dialysis regimen and may be worth considering when it is not possible to meet protein requirements with other forms of nutritional support. Further clinical trial data is awaited on the use of IPAAs.

Fluid

Fluid requirements will vary for different PD patients depending on residual renal function. Many PD patients are following fluid restrictions and will report that this is the most difficult part of the PD dietary regimen. When assessing the PD patient, fluid restriction should be considered carefully and not given as part of a standard routine procedure. In order to help those people who need fluid restriction there must be careful explanation at the start of treatment and the fluid restriction must be translated into terms familiar to the patient, e.g. six small cups.

Ideas on how to keep track of fluid consumed during the day are also helpful, using measuring jugs filled with the appropriate amount and decanting these back as drinks are taken. To deal with thirst some patients prefer to limit the amount of salt that they take, using less salt in cooking, not adding it to food at the table and limiting very salty foods.

Strategies for coping with fluid restriction vary from patient to patient. Some patients find it helpful to use thin ice cubes, counted as part of their fluid restriction. Freezing various fluids may also help some patients, e.g. ice cubes made with lemon squash. The use of mouthwashes, lip balms, sweets and chewing gum may also help. Careful teaching of the importance of keeping to the correct dry weight is necessary for all team members. Units will vary in their approach to teaching and use of hypertonic bags.

Patients will need to be reminded that in very hot weather their dialysis regimen may require less hypertonics and possibly more fluid.

Fibre

Constipation is a reported problem in PD patients. This may be caused by reduced activity or fluid restrictions; dialysis itself may also be implicated. The dietary fibre intakes of patients vary tremendously, ranging from 2 g to 49 g in our group with a mean of 14.3 g; this is below the target of 20 g, based on 12 g fibre/1000 kcal. PD patients may need help in trying to aim for a mixture of fibre in the diet. The use of bran is not recommended.

Vitamins

Several workers have looked at vitamin requirements in the PD population (Lindholm *et al.*, 1981; Blumberg *et al.*, 1983; Kopple and Blumenkrantz, 1983; Digenis, 1987; Thomson *et al.*, 1988)

It is difficult to determine the exact requirements for vitamin supplementation and recommendations in renal patients as uraemia and anaemia may alter the clinician's perception of symptoms that could relate to subclinical deficiency. There are very few reliable and easily reproducible tests that can give definitive answers with regard to the vitamin status of PD patients. Assessment of the PD patient is necessary to ensure that s/he is not likely to become deficient and there may be a need to supplement some of the vitamins where dietary intake is not able to meet the recommended targets for the PD patient.

Fat-soluble vitamins

PD patients have increased circulating levels of vitamin A. It is not recommended that the PD patient takes any additional vitamin A. Dietary vitamin E appears to be sufficient for the PD patient's requirements, they may have elevated levels and supplementation is not recommended. Vitamin D has a special place in renal nutrition: the levels of 1,25-dihydroxy vitamin D_3 ($1,25(OH)_2D_3$) are low in PD patients, the 1-hydroxylation being carried out in the kidney and helping to explain this. However with time on PD there may also be a drop in the precursor, 25-hydroxy vitamin D_3 ($25(OH)D_3$), possibly because of less exposure to sunlight and dietary vitamin D. As the final hydroxylation is necessary to activate the vitamin D, requirements and supplementation with1 are worked out on an individual basis where there is clinical need.

Water-soluble vitamins

Vitamin C is reported to have high peritoneal clearance. Recommended supplements are in the range of 70–200 mg with a consensus of 100 mg. Intakes are variable; in our group, dietary vitamin C intakes are in the order of 41–230 mg (207 patients), normal requirements being for a reference nutrient intake of 40 mg. If the target for PD is 100 mg then clearly some patients will need additional supplementation while those who are eating well will meet their needs through their diet.

There is some indication that thiamine levels are low in long-term PD patients. Thiamine (vitamin B_1) has an important role in carbohydrate metabolism and therefore assumes more importance in the PD setting. Recommendations for this are 1–40 mg; dietary intakes are in the order of 0.5–5.7 mg in PD patients.

Vitamin B_6 (pyridoxine) levels have been reported to be low in patients with uraemia. Vitamin B_6 coenzymes have an important role to play in amino acid metabolism and therefore are important to consider in the PD patient. There are some similarities between the symptoms of uraemia and vitamin B_6 deficiency, including impaired immunological function. The active form of vitamin B_6, pyridoxal phosphate, is low in the plasma and circulating erythrocytes of people with uraemia. Recommendations vary between 5 mg and 15 mg; dietary intakes are variable, in the order of 0.7–2.7 mg, and therefore supplementation may be necessary.

Folate may be deficient in PD patients as a result of inadequate intake, there may be interference in its metabolism due to uraemia, and actions of various drugs may also interfere with its absorption and activity. Folate is essential for the synthesis of purines, pyrimidines, glycine and methionine (two amino acids). Folate has a role in the prevention of anaemia. Ensuring adequate levels is important in the PD population and needs to be considered together with vitamin B$_{12}$, iron, and erythropoietin status for red blood cell synthesis. Recommendations for folate supplementation vary from 0–1 mg. There have been problems with the accurate food analysis, estimates from actual PD patients intakes vary from 29–467 g. Careful assessment of folate intake is necessary. Good dietary sources are green vegetables, some pulses such as soya, black-eyed beans, chick peas, baked beans, potatoes, oranges, fortified breakfast cereals, bread, wholegrain pasta and brown rice.

Minerals

Phosphate

PD improves hyperphosphataemia, but may fail to normalize it completely. Phosphate is absorbed along the whole length of the gut; it is not dependant on vitamin D like calcium. Dietary intake is usually in the order of 800–1200 mg per day. If we absorb 50% of this and of this 250–350 mg is removed in the PD dialysate, this leaves a further 100–200 mg, which needs to be removed by the use of phosphate binders such as calcium carbonate. The need to control phosphate levels is crucial and central to the whole scenario of renal osteodystrophy, which involves the management of calcium phosphate, parathyroid hormone and vitamin D. In terms of diet the management of phosphate so that serum levels are maintained at 1–1.5 mmol/l is crucial (Gokal, 1988).

> **Key reference:** Gokal, R. (1988) Renal Osteodystrophy and Aluminium Bone Disease in CAPD patients. *Clinical Nephrology* 30(Suppl 1): S64–67.

In the PD patient this may need careful management as phosphorus is associated with protein in the diet and as already stated PD patients have higher protein requirements. Usual protein foods such as meat contain 7–8 mg phosphorus per gram of protein, dairy produce, such as cheddar cheese, contains 25 mg phosphorus per gram of protein. Eggs contain in the order of 16 mg phosphorus/g protein and some tinned fish, such as sardines, give 23 mg phosphorus/ g protein, while other fish such as cod are more akin to meat at 9 mg phosphorus/g protein. Care therefore needs to be taken when advising the PD patient about reducing phosphorus foods to ensure that their protein intake is not compromised and that they will substitute other protein foods, e.g. swapping a cheese sandwich for a chicken one. Advice will also be given about the use of phosphate binders, ensuring that these are spread evenly through the day, taken with food and perhaps weighted in order that the meals containing the highest levels of phosphorus have more binders; for instance, a patient who misses breakfast may be better to take binders with his/her cheese and crackers at supper time. It is usually advised that calcium carbonate is taken at the start of meals, but some workers have reported no difference if taken at other stages of the meal. It is probably better to take them at the beginning, as there may be less chance of forgetting, and if forgotten they can be taken as the meal progresses.

The use of dietary supplements may need to be considered against the background of phosphate restriction. Generally, supplements are used when the intake of all nutrients is low, including phosphorus, and in the short term the aim is to correct malnutrition and prevent further deterioration. However if supplementation forms part of a longer-term strategy, the phosphorus content of the supplement must be taken into consideration. There are now a number of supplements available that have modified phosphorus levels.

Potassium

Whether a PD patient needs a potassium restriction or not has to be based on the individual biochemistry. Indeed some PD patients have low potassium levels and need to eat more potassium, or have potassium supplements. PD patients who are on APD may need more careful monitoring from a potassium point of view. If a PD patient needs a potassium restriction, this should only be as strict as is necessary and not overzealous. Consideration should also be given to vitamin C supplementation. See Chapter 9 for more information about potassium.

Other nutrients

Calcium, iron and zinc are considered on an individual basis and may be supplemented as necessary. Calcium carbonate given as a phosphate binder may also supplement calcium intake. Zinc supplementation is discussed (Kopple and Blumenkrantz, 1983). There may be a case for supplementing with zinc if the clinical picture indicates that this is necessary or if the PD patient has a habitually low dietary intake. Zinc deficiency may alter taste perception. Good food sources of zinc are meat, fish, pulses and wheat products.

THE PD PATIENT ON OTHER DIETS

There is usually little problem in helping a new PD patient who is already on a special diet of some kind. Problems may arise where there is a swallowing problem and fluid volume is now restricted, so that a person who has previously been using lots of fluid will need help in the choice of nutrient dense supplements and care must be taken to ensure that the diet is adequate.

Diabetics will need to continue to aim for good glycaemic control and to maintain an ideal body weight using a diet that is nutritionally adequate. At the start of PD training there is a good opportunity to assess the diabetic diet and if the patient is able to manage a normal diet suggestions on the types of fats and use of complex carbohydrates can be made while ensuring that s/he takes in adequate protein. Diabetics may have been advised previously to limit their intake of protein foods and this will need to be reassessed in the PD situation.

Feeding *via* enteral and parenteral routes entails considering all the dietary aspects and taking into account the contribution of calories from the PD dwells as well as how much fluid space is available for feeding. PD patients can be managed successfully on both these types of nutritional therapy should the need arise.

The nutritional management of the PD patient is the responsibility of all the care team members. Nutritional targets for the PD patient are not easy to define and may change in the light of new evidence and the production of new products specific to PD. In summary, peritoneal dialysis needs careful nutritional management as indeed do all people with end-stage renal failure. The PD patient should be assessed as an individual. There should be a system in place to look for and prevent malnutrition, help being given to meet nutritional requirements. Reassessment of the PD patient must be a continual process and should not be viewed in isolation.

REVIEW QUESTIONS

- What is the protein requirement for diet in peritoneal dialysis?
- List five factors that contribute to malnutrition in peritoneal dialysis.
- Which protein foods contain the most phosphorus?
- Do peritoneal dialysis patients need routine potassium restriction?

REFERENCES

Bennett, S. E., Russell, G. I. and Walls, J. (1986) Serial anthropometry as an adjunct to the assessment of dry weight in patients receiving dialysis therapy. *Dialysis and Transplantation*, **15**(3), 148–151.

Blumberg, A., Hanck, A. and Sander, G. (1983) Vitamin nutrition in patients on continuous peritoneal dialysis (CAPD). *Clinical Nephrology*, **20**(5), 244–250.

Blumenkrantz, M. J., Kopple, J. D., Morgan, J. K. and Coburn, J. W. (1982) Metabolic balance studies and dietary protein requirements in patients undergoing continuous ambulatory peritoneal dialysis. *Kidney International*, **21**, 849–861.

Davies, S. J., Russell, L., Bryan, J. *et al.* (1996) Impact of peritoneal absorption of glucose on appetite, protein catabolism and survival in CAPD patients. *Clinical Nephrology*, **45**(3), 194–198.

Davies, S. J., Russell, L. H., Bryan, J. *et al.* (1995). Comorbidity, urea kinetics, and appetite in CAPD patients: their interelationship and prediction of survival. *American Journal of Kidney Diseases*, **26**(2), 353–361.

Digenis, G. E. (1987) Supplements for CAPD patients. *Dialysis Bulletin*, **7**(4), 219–223.

Ginsberg, N., Fishblane, S. and Lynn, R. I. (1996) The effect of improved efficiency on measures of appetite in peritoneal dialysis patients. *Journal of Renal Nutrition*, **6**(4), 217–221.

Gokal, R. (1988) Renal osteodystrophy and aluminium bone disease in CAPD patients. *Clinical Nephrology*, **30**(Suppl. 1), S64–S67.

Heimburger, O., Bergstrom, J. and Lindholm, B. (1994) Maintenance of optimum nutrition in CAPD. *Kidney International*, **46**(Suppl. 48), S39–S46.

Kopple, J. D. and Blumenkrantz, M. J. (1983) Nutritional requirements for patients undergoing continuous peritoneal dialysis. *Kidney International*, **24**(Suppl. 16), 5295–5302.

Lindholm, B., Karlander, S. G., Norbeck, H. E. *et al.* (1981) Carbohydrate and lipid metabolism in CAPD patients, in *Peritoneal Dialysis*, (eds R. Aitkins, N. Thomson and P. Farrell), Churchill Livingstone, Edinburgh.

McWhirter, J. and Pennington, C. R. (1994) Incidence and recognition of malnutrition in hospital. *British Medical Journal*, **308**, 945–948.

Nelson, E. E., Hong, C. D., Pesce. A. L. *et al.* (1990) Anthropometric norms for the dialysis population. *American Journal of Kidney Diseases*, **16**(1), 32–37.

Rubin, J. (1990) Nutritional support during peritoneal dialysis-related peritonitis. *American Journal of Kidney Diseases*, **15**(6), 551–555.

Thomson, C. R. V., Roger, R. S. C., Baker, B. L. D. and Hamilton, P. J. (1988) Multivitamin supplementation and CAPD. *Lancet*, **i**, 473.

Walls, J. (1995). Metabolic acidosis and uraemia. *Peritoneal Dialysis International*, **15**(5S), S36–S38.

Wheeler, D. C. (1996) Abnormalities of lipoprotein metabolism in CAPD patients. *Kidney International*, **50**(Suppl. 56), S44–S46.

Young, G. A., Kopple, J. D., Lindholm, B. *et al.* (1991). Nutritional assessment of continuous ambulatory peritoneal dialysis patients: an international study. *American Journal of Kidney Diseases*, **17**(4), 462–471.

Adequacy of dialysis

Liz Ford

LEARNING OBJECTIVES

At the end of this chapter the reader should be able to:

- Explain what urea kinetic modelling is.
- State the recommended doses of both haemodialysis and peritoneal dialysis in terms of Kt/V.
- Describe how urea kinetic modelling can contribute to the nutritional management of chronic renal failure.
- List the advantages of implementing urea kinetic modelling.
- Describe the circumstances in which urea kinetic modelling calculations should be interpreted with great care.

THE HISTORY AND DEVELOPMENT OF UREA KINETIC MODELLING

Since the earliest days of maintenance dialysis there has been a continual search for ways of determining the appropriate dose of dialysis for individual patients and for assessing the adequacy of the delivered treatment. Before urea kinetic modelling (UKM) these were rather haphazard and treatment prescriptions relied upon generalized standard procedures and the experience and expertise of the renal team (Aldridge and Greenwood, 1990).

Long before the introduction of renal replacement therapy the idea that uraemia resulted from the accumulation of different solutes because of poor kidney function was established and accepted. The measurement of such substances could therefore be regarded as the first criterion for the assessment of uraemia severity. After the introduction of dialysis these measurements were used to assess efficiency (Lopot, 1990).

Although the measurement of predialysis concentrations of certain solutes can reflect the clinical status of a patient, its value as a tool in deciding how to improve treatment efficiency is rather poor. Astute, experienced nephrology staff are usually capable of detecting when a patient on dialysis is malnourished or developing severe complications of uraemia but routine predialysis blood chemical measurements alone are of little predictive value in avoiding such problems (Johnson and Schniepp, 1981).

For this reason interest turned away from purely clinically oriented parameters (plasma concentrations of a marker solute) towards physical parameters that described the efficiency of solute removal by an artificial organ (Aldridge and Greenwood, 1990). The era of performance measurement using permeability coefficients, mass transfer coefficients and clearance began in the 1970s. Of these parameters, clearance remains the principal parameter in any mathematical method of assessing dialysis adequacy.

Urea was first kinetically modelled in haemodialysis patients in the 1960s but the use of this technique for the clinical control and individualization of treatment had its origin in the 1970s with work done by Gotch and Sargent. Their work took on greater practical relevance after the publication of the National Co-operative Dialysis Study in the United States in the early 1980s (Lowrie and Laird, 1983). Meticulous analysis of the results of this study by Gotch and Sargent led to the well known term Kt/V being introduced in 1985.

It is now widely accepted that UKM, although not perfect, is superior to previous methods of prescribing dialysis treatments owing to its built in facility for quality assurance and assessment of the patient's nutritional status. From its foundation in haemodialysis UKM can now be applied to haemofiltration, haemodiafiltration, peritoneal dialysis and the treatment of acute renal failure. It has also been suggested that UKM may have a role to play in the assessment of predialysis patients, and in the prediction of the optimum timing of commencement of dialysis (Tattersall *et al.*, 1995).

THE THEORY BEHIND Kt/V

Urea kinetic modelling uses urea, a waste product of protein catabolism, as a marker molecule for clinically important uraemic waste products in order to assess dialysis efficiency, calculate individual dialysis prescriptions and measure protein intake. As a marker of dialyser clearance and dialysis effect in the patient urea has several advantages. It is present in high concentrations and is easy to measure using standard laboratory tests. It is a stable, low-molecular-weight compound that is uncharged, soluble in water and easily removed by dialysis. It distributes throughout total body water and can easily diffuse between different body compartments. Taken together, these characteristics far outweigh those of any other compound as an indicator of dialysis adequacy (Depner, 1994).

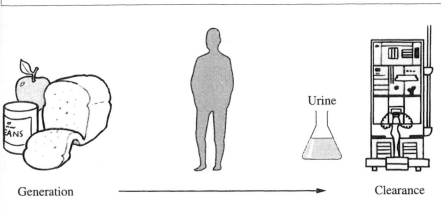

Generation   Clearance

Figure 13.1 Urea generation and removal.

Single-pool UKM

As previously mentioned urea is known to be evenly distributed in total body water. As a result of this single-pool UKM regards total body water as being in one compartment or 'pool' called the urea distribution volume (V). This volume can be estimated, taking total body water as 58% of lean body mass, or calculated more accurately using information about the patient's height, weight and gender (equations (13. 1) and (13.2); Watson *et al.*, 1980).

$$\text{Male } V = 2.447 - (0.0952 \times \text{Age (years)}) + (0.017 \times \text{Height (cm)}) + (0.336 \times \text{Weight (kg)}). \quad (13.1)$$

$$\text{Female } V = -2.097 + (0.107 \times \text{Height (cm)}) + (0.247 \times \text{Weight (kg)}). \quad (13.2)$$

The generation of urea into this pool is determined by the rate of protein catabolism. Removal of urea from the pool is equal to the sum of dialysis clearance and residual renal clearance (Figure 13.1).

The removal of urea during dialysis can be calculated using the equation Kt/V where:

K = clearance (both residual and that achieved on dialysis in ml/min);
 t = time (actual dialysis treatment time in minutes);
V = volume (the kinetically calculated urea distribution volume in litres).

Single-pool UKM takes a simplified view of the urea distribution within the body, which is more accurately described by a two-pool model.

Dual-pool UKM

Dual-pool UKM considers urea to be distributed in two pools in the body, the intracellular fluid (ICF) and the extracellular fluid (ECF). During dialysis, changes in the urea concentration of the intracellular fluid lag behind those of the extracellular fluid and following the end of dialysis a 'rebound' in the serum level of urea will occur (Smye *et al.*, 1994). This is due to the diffusion of urea from the ICF to the ECF, which continues until equilibrium is reached. During standard dialysis any rebound is usually minimal and a single-pool model suffices, but during rapid, high-efficiency haemodialysis the two-pool nature of urea distribution becomes more significant and higher Kt/V values are required for adequate dialysis (Haraldsson, 1995).

UREA KINETIC MODELLING AND HAEMODIALYSIS

Adequate dialysis dose

The estimation of an adequate dose of haemodialysis for patients with end-stage renal failure has been derived from studies such as the National Co-operative Dialysis Study (NCDS), which was completed in 1982. This study was intended 'to develop techniques by which haemodialysis could be prescribed on an individual and quantitated basis, and by which it would improve the minimum exposure that would keep dialysis patients free from dialysis related complications' (Wineman, 1983).

In that study, the participating patients were dialysed with less than the 'standard dose' of haemodialysis and their dialysis-related morbidity was monitored (Parker *et al.*, 1983). The original study used a time-averaged concentration of urea as the parameter of adequacy; however further analysis of the results indicated that a delivered dose of dialysis as defined by a Kt/V of approximately 0.9 three times per week was sufficient to maintain the morbidity of these patients at an acceptable level. A Kt/V of less than 0.9 was associated with a high probability (75%) of treatment failure, morbidity and mortality (Gotch and Sargent, 1985).

Key reference: Gotch, F. and Sargent, J. (1985) A mechanistic analysis of the National Cooperative Dialysis Study (NCDS). *Kidney International* 28:526–534.

Since its completion it has been suggested that the general applicability of the NCDS may be limited since the randomized participants of the study were approximately 10 years younger than the median age of the end-stage renal failure population, were free of major co-morbid conditions such as cardiovascular disease and were selected for their compliance. In addition, none of the patients in the study were diabetic (Hakim *et al.*, 1994). Despite these criticisms it is generally acknowledged that the NCDS established a useful, reproducible and valid technique for the quantification of prescribed and delivered dialysis (Parker *et al.*, 1994).

More recently it has been suggested that although Kt/V values can predict outcome, good outcome in terms of survival, severity of uraemic symptoms, hospitalization and intradialytic symptoms is based on much higher values of Kt/V than originally predicted. Several studies have shown that in large dialysis programmes the relative risk of mortality, adjusted for co-morbid conditions, age and diabetes, is significantly less for patients dialysed with a Kt/V greater than 1.2 than for patients who receive a Kt/V of 1.0 or less (Collins *et al.*, 1992; Hakim *et al.*, 1994; Parker *et al.*, 1994). These findings are further supported by Held *et al.* (1991), who reported a tendency to improvement in survival by 8% for each incremental increase in Kt/V of 0.1 up to a Kt/V of 1.4.

All Kt/V values mentioned above are for dialysis three times a week. This is because there is little clinically derived information relating to patients dialysing twice a week. An analysis based on UKM has suggested that a Kt/V of 1.8–2.0 should be aimed for when treating patients twice a week (Daugirdas, 1994). A twice-weekly dialysis schedule should only be used for smaller patients who have a substantial residual renal function and should be thought of primarily as a temporary treatment strategy (Renal Association, 1995).

Duration of dialysis

The duration of dialysis treatments has shown a tendency to decrease over the last decade. Weekly dialysis times of 25–40 hours in the 1960s were reduced dramatically to around 12–15 hours during the 1970s and 80s and in some units to as low as 7–8 hours in the 1990s (Valderrábano, 1996).

Studies completed in Europe and the USA have indicated that patients who dialyse for less than 12 hours per week have a significantly higher mortality rate than those who receive more than 12 hours of dialysis per week (Held *et al.*, 1991; Avram *et al.*, 1995; Kramer *et al.*, 1982). Various factors may be implicated to account for the increased mortality rate but the most important is thought to be insufficient dose of dialysis.

It is now widely recognized that following the NCDS the Kt/V modelling equation was frequently misapplied, often for commercial and logistical reasons. This led to the prescription of minimal dialysis and shortened dialysis times without proper assessment of the clinical and biochemical factors needed for optimum patient care (Mailloux, 1992). For this reason UKM should not be automatically linked with a reduction in treatment times but with the ability to manipulate treatments to suit the needs of the individual and to objectively assess the efficiency of the chosen regimen.

Prescribing dialysis dose

In order to develop a dialysis prescription it is first necessary to agree on a target Kt/V. As previously discussed this should be around 1.2–1.4 for patients dialysing three times per week. The next step is to calculate the patient's urea distribution volume (V) using either of the methods previously described. Once a specific dialyser has been chosen the predicted urea clearance can be calculated using a nomogram such as that developed by Daugirdas and Depner (1994), which requires data relating to dialyser urea clearance (KoA) and blood flow rate (Figure 13.2).

To use the graph, first find the dialyser KoA value which is available from the manufacturer. Identify the desired blood flow rate on the x-axis

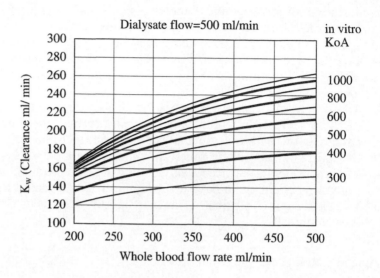

Figure 13.2 Predicted *in vivo* urea clearance. (Source: redrawn from Daugirdas and Depner, 1994, with permission.)

and follow it up to the appropriate *K*oA curve. Finally read the predicted urea clearance rate on the *y*-axis.

Once values for *Kt/V*, *V* and *K* are known the necessary dialysis duration can be calculated as shown in Figure 13.3.

This suggests that for a specific patient, using a dialyser with a *K*oA of 500 ml/h and a blood flow of 250 ml/h for 5 hours should result in a *Kt/V* of 1.2 being delivered. To ensure that this occurs regular monitoring of delivered dialysis dose should be performed.

Desired $Kt/V = 1.2$
Patient's urea distribution volume $(V) = 40$ l
Dialyser KoA $= 500$ ml/min
Blood flow $= 250$ ml/min
Predicted urea clearance $= 160$ ml/min

$$t = \frac{1.2 \times 40,000}{160}$$
$$t = 300 \text{ min or } 5 \text{ hrs}$$

Figure 13.3 Calculation of treatment duration.

Monitoring dialysis dose

The delivered dialysis dose is best monitored by regularly measuring pre- and postdialysis blood urea levels and calculating the delivered *Kt/V* using a computerized UKM package. Simplified methods of calculating Kt/V do exist but they are less accurate.

If the dialysis prescription is strictly followed, the amount of dialysis delivered should correspond to the prescribed dialysis dose. It has been shown, however, that as many as 50% of treatments deliver a dialysis dose that is less than that prescribed (Sargent, 1990). It is therefore very important that sufficient time is spent on training and education, so that all staff involved understand the need for precision and accuracy regarding blood flow rates, treatment duration, specimen collection and so on.

The most common reasons why a **delivered dialysis dose** may be less than that prescribed are summarized in the margin. Many of these causes can be eliminated by paying special attention to detail but others, such as access recirculation and residual renal function, need to be monitored in their own right.

Access recirculation may be measured using several methods and is usually expressed as a percentage. Once the amount of recirculation is known it must be incorporated into the UKM calculations to ensure that an adequate amount of dialysis is prescribed and delivered. The simplest way to do this is to reduce the blood flow used in the calculations by the recirculation factor. For example if the patient's blood flow is 300 ml/min but his/her recirculation factor is 15% the blood flow to be used in the UKM calculations is 255 ml/min.

Owing to its continuous action, even a small amount of residual renal function influences UKM significantly. Frequent and accurate measurement of residual renal function is essential because it declines to zero at varying rates in different individuals. The following procedure is recommended for calculating residual renal urea clearance (Daugirdas, 1994).

At the end of a dialysis session a blood sample for urea should be taken and the patient should be asked to void his/her bladder. After discarding this urine the patient should be advised to collect all the urine passed from this time until the start of the next dialysis session. An appropriate container should be provided that contains a small amount of dilute acetic acid to prevent the breakdown of urea during the collection period. At the beginning of the subsequent dialysis session a further blood urea sample should be obtained. Residual renal urea clearance can then be calculated as shown in Figure 13.4.

Common reasons for poor delivered dialysis dose

- Incorrect or inaccurate blood flow rate
- Incorrect dialysate/blood flow direction
- Incorrect or inaccurate dialysate flow
- Incorrect or inaccurate treatment time
- High negative arterial pressure
- Access recirculation
- Exaggerated residual renal function
- Incorrect dialyser
- Semi-clotted dialyser
- Blood sampling error
- Urea rebound
- Dialyser reuse
- Interrupted dialysis

COMPUTERIZED UKM PROGRAMS

Because of the amount of information that needs to be analysed and the number of calculations that need to be completed most units who implement UKM do so using computer software packages specially written for the purpose. Using rigorous mathematical techniques these programs allow the user to prescribe individual dialysis regimens and to periodically monitor the amount of dialysis received. Most computerized UKM packages contain several components, including:

$$KRU = \frac{\text{Urine Volume (ml)}}{\text{Collection Time (min)}} \times \frac{\text{Urine Urea (mmol / l)}}{\text{Mean Blood Urea}}$$

Example

Volume = 1220 ml
Time = 2420 mins
Urine urea = 94 mmol / l
Pre-collection serum urea = 10.1 mmol / l
Post-collection serum urea = 23.3 mmol / l

$$KRU = \frac{1220 \times 94}{2420 \times 16.7}$$

$$KRU = 2.8 \text{ ml / min}$$

Figure 13.4   Calculating residual renal function.

- patient information;
- clinic/doctor information;
- dialyser KoA information;
- residual renal function calculation;
- access recirculation calculation;
- urea distribution volume calculation;
- treatment prescription calculation;
- treatment assessment calculation.

Once information regarding the patients, their doctor, the clinic they attend and the dialysers used has been entered into the database, the computer can be used to provide individual dialysis prescriptions for any of the patients entered. Generally the program prompts the user to select a dialyser, dialysate buffer and flow rate and a desired Kt/V. The computer then calculates dialysis treatment times for a variety of blood flow rates. Any of the dialysis treatment parameters can be temporarily changed and the program will recalculate the dialysis prescription accordingly. This allows different dialysers to be compared or different blood flow rate scenarios to be viewed at the touch of a button, thus saving much time and effort.

After a dialysis prescription has been calculated and implemented computerized quality assurance programs can be used to assess how much actual treatment therapy was delivered during a dialysis session. The programs use actual treatment parameters together with pre- and postdialysis blood urea values. It is therefore important to be as accurate as possible when entering the data to reflect the actual treatment conditions.

The quality assurance programs calculate the delivered dialysis dose and are able to compare this to the prescribed dose, highlighting any discrepancies. Once data has been entered over a period of time various reports can be produced that show how patients are progressing.

UREA REDUCTION RATIO AND HAEMODIALYSIS

The urea reduction ratio (URR) is a simplified method of measuring dialysis adequacy and is calculated using equation (13.3) shown below.

$$URR\% = \frac{\text{Predialysis blood urea} - \text{Postdialysis blood urea}}{\text{Predialysis blood urea}} \times 100 \qquad (13.3)$$

It is less accurate than more complex methods, failing to consider volume changes, urea generation and residual renal function (Depner, 1994). It is however easy to perform and is better than no measurement at all.

The **URR correlation with Kt/V is curvilinear** and has been shown to correlate inversely with patient survival (Owen *et al.*, 1993). Dialysis is thought to be adequate if a URR of above 65% is achieved.

The primary goal of dialysis is to maintain a uraemic patient in the best possible condition and to prevent complications due to uraemic toxicity by providing as much dialysis as is practically possible and economically feasible (Khanna *et al.*, 1993). The clinical and laboratory indicators of **adequate peritoneal dialysis** are listed in the margin.

The amount of dialysis given to a peritoneal dialysis patient can be determined by either normalized creatinine clearance or normalized urea clearance.

Creatinine clearance

The mean peritoneal creatinine clearance can be calculated for a continual treatment such as CAPD by dividing the amount of creatinine removed during dialysis by the concentration of creatinine in the blood (equation (13.4)).

$$\text{Clearance } (C) = \frac{\text{Dialysate creatinine concentration} \times \text{Dialysate volume}}{\text{Blood creatinine concentration}} \qquad (13.4)$$

Creatinine clearance is affected by dialysis flow rate, ultrafiltration, membrane surface area and membrane permeability, and is independent of blood concentration (Khanna *et al.*, 1993). The mean creatinine clearance can be calculated per exchange, per day or per week.

As with haemodialysis residual renal clearance contributes to the overall clearance of low- and medium-molecular-weight molecules and fluid removal. It is suggested that peritoneal dialysis patients do well when they receive dialysis that , when added to their residual renal function, provides a creatinine clearance of at least 50–60 litres a week (Diaz-Buxo, 1994).

For patients on intermittent peritoneal dialysis therapy the average weekly creatinine clearance can be calculated using equation (13.5).

Adequacy and peritoneal dialysis

Kt/V	URR
1	58%
1.1	62%
1.2	65%
1.3	68%
1.4	70%
1.5	72%
1.6	75%
1.7	78%
1.8	80%

Indicators of adequate dialysis

Clinical indicators
- Patient feels well
- Blood pressure well controlled
- Stale lean body mass
- Good fluid balance
- Absence of uraemic symptoms

Laboratory indicators
- Serum creatinine
  < 16–20 mg/dl muscular
  < 12–15 mg/dl lean
- Normal electrolytes
- Stable nerve conduction velocities
- Normal serum albumin

$$\text{Clearance}(C) = \frac{\text{Intermittent therapy creatinine clearance (ml/min)} \times \text{Therapy time (h/week)}}{\text{No. of hours in a week}} \qquad (13.5)$$

The patient's intermittent therapy creatinine clearance should be calculated over a period of at least three exchanges using equation (13.4).

Urea clearance and Kt/V

Despite the fact that there has been no large cooperative study to investigate the minimum amount of peritoneal dialysis necessary it is widely agreed that the recommended minimum weekly urea clearance or Kt/V for continual therapies is 1.7. The minimum weekly Kt/V for intermittent treatments has been set at a higher value of 2.2 to compensate for the reduced removal rate of larger molecules such as creatinine and vitamin B_{12} (Diaz-Buxo, 1994). As in haemodialysis, higher Kt/V values have been associated with lower mortality and morbidity rates (Churchill *et al.*, 1994).

The gold standard for calculating a patient's average weekly Kt/V involves obtaining a blood sample and separate 24-hour collections of spent dialysate and urine. The weekly urea clearance can be calculated by using equation (13.4) or equation (13.5), substituting the creatinine concentrations for urea concentrations. The patient's residual renal clearance and urea distribution volume can be calculated as previously described in this chapter. Equation (13.6) can then be used to establish the dose of dialysis delivered.

$$\text{Weekly } Kt/V = \frac{\text{Weekly urea clearance (dialysis and residual)}}{\text{Urea distribution volume}} \times 7 \qquad (13.6)$$

The ability of peritoneal dialysis to achieve good clinical outcomes despite lower weekly Kt/V values than are delivered in haemodialysis has led to the development of the peak concentration hypothesis (Keshaviah and Nolph, 1989). This suggests that the success of peritoneal dialysis is due to its continuous steady-state nature compared with the peaks and troughs of solute concentration associated with haemodialysis. If uraemic toxicity is associated with peak urea concentrations rather than time-averaged concentrations the dialysis dose needed for intermittent treatments such as haemodialysis is approximately 50% higher than that for continuous treatments.

Once the initial dialysis prescription has been developed it should be monitored on a regular basis. Whereas haemodialysis dose is usually monitored monthly, the majority of renal units assess peritoneal dialysis dose every 6 months. Adjustments to the prescription may be necessary over time to account for reduced residual renal function, increased body weight, changes in dietary intake or decreased peritoneal membrane function.

Computerized UKM programs

Computer software programs are available to simplify the application of urea kinetic modelling to peritoneal dialysis. As with programs developed for haemodialysis they aid the development and monitoring of individualized dialysis prescriptions by facilitating the comparison of continual and intermittent therapy options. This allows the development of optimum dialysis regimens that best fit the lifestyle of the patient.

UREA KINETIC MODELLING AND NUTRITION

The nutritional management of patients with chronic renal failure is a critical factor that influences their medical treatment and their wellbeing (Bennett, 1981; Lowrie and Lew, 1990). The goal in such patients is to optimize nutrition, maximizing protein and calorie intake while minimizing the extent to which waste products accumulate in the body.

Several methods of nutritional assessment, such as visual assessment, food diaries, anthropometric measurements and biochemical essays, are available but problems can arise with their use with renal patients (Forrest, 1990; Kimura *et al.*, 1988; Levine, 1985). The drawbacks of these methods highlight the need for accurate nutritional assessment measures that are specific for the adult chronic renal failure patient population. It is suggested that the development of UKM has provided such a nutritional assessment tool (Sargent *et al.*, 1978).

UKM provides invaluable nutritional information because it measures the patient's urea generation rate, which has a direct linear correlation with protein catabolic rate (PCR). When a patient is in zero nitrogen balance or a stable state, the protein catabolic rate is equal to dietary protein intake (Garred *et al.*, 1994). Inadequate dietary protein intake was shown in the NCDS to be the second strongest factor associated with patient morbidity and mortality (Laird *et al.*, 1975). The generally accepted target range for **dietary protein intake** (DPI) in patients on either peritoneal dialysis or haemodialysis is 0.8–1.4 g/kg/d with 1.1 g/kg/d commonly adopted as a specific target.

Because dietary protein intake is linked to protein catabolic rate the PCR value obtained from UKM calculations can be used to indicate how well nourished the patient was on a particular dialysis day. If these calculations are repeated regularly a profile can be built up of each patient's ongoing nutritional state.

PCR values are expressed in grams per day but dietary protein intake is usually discussed in grams per kilogram per day. In order to be able to compare like units the normalized protein catabolic rate (nPCR) is used. A patient's nPCR can be obtained from computerized UKM programs or estimated from the patient's urea generation rate using equation (13.7).

$$\text{nPCR} = 149.7 \times \frac{\text{Urea generation rate}}{\text{Urea distribution volume}} + 0.17 \qquad (13.7)$$

The value 1.497 converts urea generation in mmol/l/min to protein catabolic rate in g/kg/d. The value 0.17 represents the amount of protein that is converted to other end products, lost in faeces or sloughed from skin. The urea distribution volume is proportional to the patient's dry weight.

In anuric haemodialysis patients or patients treated with intermittent peritoneal dialysis the urea generation rate is equivalent to the rise in blood

Dietary protein intake and nutritional state

DPI (g/kg/d)	Nutritional state
0.8	Malnourished
0.8–1.4	Well nourished
> 1.4	Likely to develop uraemic symptoms

urea concentrations between dialysis sessions. For patients receiving continuous forms of peritoneal dialysis the urea generation rate can easily be calculated from a 24-hour collection of dialysate and urine.

The PCR values calculated with urea kinetics can identify patients with inadequate or decreasing dietary protein intakes more accurately and at an earlier stage than conventional methods, which are also more time-consuming. Rapid screening of the dialysis population within a hospital, made possible by UKM, allows staff to identify and prioritize patients with compromised nutritional status (Johnson and Schniepp, 1981).

It is important to remember, however, that the information obtained concerning PCR and thus dietary protein intake can only be considered accurate for stable patients. Results calculated for patients who are either anabolic or catabolic, such as patients with acute renal failure or chronic patients with infections, need to be interpreted with great care (Forrest, 1990).

UREA KINETIC MODELLING AND QUALITY ASSURANCE

An example of a standard statement for treatment dose in haemodialysis

- All patients will receive individualized dialysis prescriptions calculated using UKM
- Kt/V to exceed 1.2 in thrice-weekly patients and 1.9 in twice-weekly patients
- Kt/V to be adjusted for treatments less than 4 hours or a dual-pool model used
- Kt/V to be audited monthly and prescriptions recalculated as necessary

Predetermined, explicit **standards** may be used by nephrology staff to define and agree the quality of service that their activities are directed towards achieving (DTNF, 1993). In order to identify clearly whether or not a standard has been achieved it should be closely monitored and evaluated using an appropriate audit tool. It is widely recognized that UKM facilitates the setting of standards for dialysis dose and provides a way of assessing whether or not these standards are being delivered (EDTNA/ERCA, 1995; Renal Association, 1995).

If discrepancies are found when a standard is audited action should be taken to remedy the problem. In such a situation recent treatment-related data could be used to redefine a patient's treatment prescription. Alternatively, clinical procedures might need to be assessed and staff reminded of the need for accuracy and precision regarding all parameters of the treatment regimen. The process of setting and monitoring standards in order to improve quality should be ongoing and cyclic in nature.

ADVANTAGES AND LIMITATIONS OF UREA KINETIC MODELLING

Advantages

UKM provides an orderly, quantitative method for assessing, evaluating and modifying individualized dialysis prescriptions in response to changing patient needs. It also permits a critical review of the conditions of a particular dialysis session and enables each renal unit to audit its performance, guiding systematic improvements in therapy.

Individualization of dialysis therapy can be of significant benefit to both patients and staff. Each patient can be provided with the most effective dialysis prescription for their specific biochemical, physiological and nutritional parameters. Such individual prescriptions have been shown to decrease the incidence of dialysis-related complications and patient morbidity, and improve patient mortality rates (Hakim *et al.*, 1994; Hornberger, 1993a; Parker *et al.*, 1994).

> **Key reference:** Parker, T., Husni, L., Huang, W., Lew, N. and Lowrie, E. (1994) Survival of haemodialysis patients in the United States is improved with a greater quantity of dialysis. *American Journal of Kidney Diseases* 23(5): 670–680.

Rapid screening of the dialysis population within a hospital, made possible by UKM, allows the renal team to identify and prioritize patients with compromised nutritional status and dialysis adequacy (Goldstein and Frederico, 1987). This enables staff to maximize their time efficiently by spending more time with patients who need extra attention. This, in conjunction with alterations in dialysis times, reduced patient complications and improved patient compliance, can contribute to cost savings (Hornberger, 1993b).

> **Key reference:** Goldstein, D. and Frederico, C. (1987) The effect of urea kinetic modelling on the nutrition management of haemodialysis patients. *Journal of American Dietetic Association* 87(4): 474–479.

Limitations

UKM should be carefully applied and its limitations appreciated. Every effort should be made not to apply the method where its basic mathematical assumptions are not valid. For example, great care should be taken when interpreting nutritional information gained from patients who are not in a stable nutritional state and when prescribing ultrashort haemodialysis therapy without the aid of an advanced dual-pool model.

It should be remembered that UKM deals only with urea and cannot give a full picture regarding the molecular aetiology of uraemia. There is still very little understanding of the relationship between uraemia and specified solute concentrations so the extension of this modelling technique to include other components of the dialysis prescription is being considered (Berlo, 1989).

It is vital that nephrology staff understand that although UKM offers several advantages other, more traditional, methods of assessing patient wellbeing are still valid and have an important role to play. UKM was not developed to replace all other methods but rather to complement them. Every resource available should be used appropriately in order to ensure that renal patients receive the best care possible.

UREA KINETIC MODELLING IN THE FUTURE

In years to come it is likely that more emphasis will be placed on the patient's clearance and patient Kt/V rather than on the current definition of Kt/V as dialyser clearance multiplied by dialysis duration divided by urea volume. Patient clearance is a measure of the patient's response to dialysis rather than the amount of dialysis delivered to the patient (Depner, 1994). To measure this it is likely that in the near future there will be more application of modelling methods based on dialysate sampling.

Real-time monitoring of UKM during haemodialysis facilitated by on-line urea sensing devices is another exciting development. Haemodialysis machines introduced during the next few years are likely to be able to offer complete automation of the monitoring application of UKM free from any need for blood or dialysate sampling (Garred *et al.*, 1994).

CONCLUSION

Inadequate dialysis is easier to define and recognize than adequate dialysis. Defining inadequate dialysis is thus the first step and allows the establishment of a minimum acceptable dose of dialysis that is compatible with short-term wellbeing and the absence of uraemic symptoms. An optimal dialysis dose is harder to define but should include such factors as the patient's clinical symptomology, nutritional status and achievement of a fully active, rehabilitated life.

REVIEW QUESTIONS

- What is urea kinetic modelling?
- Why is dialysis adequacy important?
- How can UKM contribute to the nutritional management of patients with CRF?
- What is urea rebound and why is it important?
- How could you apply the information in this chapter to your clinical practice?

REFERENCES

Aldridge, C. and Greenwood, R. (1990) Introduction to UKM, in *Urea Kinetic Modelling*, (ed. F. Filpot), EDTNA–ERCA Series vol. 4, European Dialysis and Transplant Nurses Association–European Renal Care Association, Ghent.

Avram, M., Mittman, N., Bonomini, L. *et al.* (1995) Markers for survival in dialysis: a seven-year prospective study. *American Journal of Kidney Diseases*, **26**, 209–219.

Bennett, N. (1981) Urea kinetics: a dieticians tool in the nutritional management of patients with end stage renal disease. *Dialysis and Transplantation*, **10**(4), 333–334; 350.

Berlo, A. (1989) Urea kinetic modelling. *Journal of the European Dialysis and Transplant Nurses Association–European Renal Care Association*, **10**, 15–21.

Churchill, D., Thorpe, K., Taylor, D. and Keshaviah, P. (1994) Adequacy of peritoneal dialysis. *Journal of the American Society of Nephrology*, **5**(3), 439.

Collins, A., Keshaviah, P., Ma, J. and Umen, A. (1992) Comparison of haemodialysis survival in URDS patients vs. regional kidney disease program patients. *Journal of the American Society of Nephrology*, **3**, 359.

Daugirdas, J. (1994) Chronic haemodialysis prescription: a urea kinetic approach, in *Handbook of Dialysis*, 2nd edn, (eds J. T. Daugirdas and T. S. Ing), Little, Brown & Co, Boston, MA.

Daugirdas, J. and Depner, T. (1994) A nomogram approach to haemodialysis urea modelling. *American Journal of Kidney Diseases*, **23**, 33–40.

Depner, T. A. (1994) Assessing adequacy of haemodialysis: urea kinetic modelling. *Kidney International*, **45**, 1522–1535.

Diaz-Buxo, J. (1994) Chronic peritoneal dialysis prescription, in *Handbook of Dialysis*, 2nd edn, (eds J. T. Daugirdas and T. S. Ing), Little, Brown & Co, Boston, MA.

DTNF (1993) *Standards for Renal Nursing Care*, Royal College of Nursing, London.

EDTNA/ERCA (1995) *European Standards for Nephrology Nursing Practice*, European Dialysis and Transplant Nurses Association–European Renal Care Association, Lucerne.

Forrest, C. (1990) The use of urea kinetic modelling in the renal dietician's quality assurance programme. British Renal Symposium Paper. *Artery Magazine*, **Dec.**, 3–7.

Garred, L., Canaud, B. and McCready, W. (1994) Optimal haemodialysis – the role of quantification. *Seminars in Dialysis*, **7**(4), 236–245.

Goldstein, D. and Frederico, C. (1987) The effect of urea kinetic modelling on the nutrition management of haemodialysis patients. *Journal of the American Dietetic Association*, **87**(4), 474–479.

Gotch, F. and Sargent, J. (1985) A mechanistic analysis of the National Cooperative Dialysis Study (NCDS). *Kidney International*, **28**, 526–534.

Hakim, R., Breyer, J., Ismail, N. and Schulman, G. (1994) Effects of dose of dialysis on mortality and morbidity. *American Journal of Kidney Diseases*, **23**(5), 661–669.

Haraldsson B (1995) Higher *Kt/V* is needed for adequate dialysis if treatment time is reduced. *Nephrology, Dialysis and Transplantation*, **10**, 1845–1851.

Held, P., Levin, N., Bovbjerg, R. *et al.* (1991) Mortality and duration of treatment. *Journal of the American Medical Association*, **265**, 871–875.

Hornberger, J. (1993a) The haemodialysis prescription and quality-adjusted life expectancy. *Journal of the American Society of Nephrology*, **4**(4), 1004–1020.

Hornberger, J. (1993b) The haemodialysis prescription and cost effectiveness. *Journal of the American Society of Nephrology*, **4**(4), 1021–1027.

Johnson, W. and Schniepp, B. (1981) Comparison of urea kinetic modelling with other approaches to dialysis prescription. *Dialysis and Transplantation*, **10**(4), 280–284.

Keshaviah, P. and Nolph, K. (1989) The peak concentration hypothesis: a urea kinetic approach to comparing the adequacy of CAPD and haemodialysis. *Peritoneal Dialysis International*, **9**, 257–260.

Khanna, R., Nolph, C. and Oreopoulos, D. (1993) *The Essentials of Peritoneal Dialysis*, Kluwer Academic Publishers, London.

Kimura, G., Kojima, S., Saito, F. *et al*. (1988) Quantitative estimation of dietary intake in patients on haemodialysis. *International Journal of Artificial Organs*, **11**(3), 161–168.

Kramer, P., Broyer, M., Brunner, F. and Brynger, H. (1982) Combined report of regular dialysis and transplantation in Europe XII 1981. *Proceedings of the European Dialysis and Transplantation Association*, **19**, 4–59.

Laird, N., Berkley, C. and Lowrie, E. (1975) Modeling success or failure of dialysis therapy: the National Co-operative Dialysis Study. *Kidney International*, **7**, 2–15.

Levine, S. (1985) Pitfalls of nutritional assessment in end stage renal disease: a case approach. *Dialysis and Transplantation*, **14**, 612.

Lopot, F. (1990) Evolution of the mathematical methods for the assessment of dialysis adequacy, in *Urea Kinetic Modelling*, (ed. F. Filpot), EDTNA–ERCA Series vol. 4, European Dialysis and Transplant Nurses Association–European Renal Care Association, Ghent.

Lowrie, E. and Laird, N. (1983) National Cooperative Dialysis Study. *Kidney International*, **23**(11), 51–122.

Lowrie, E. and Lew, N. (1990) Death risk in haemodialysis patients: the predictive value of commonly measured variables and an evaluation of death rate differences between facilities. *American Journal of Kidney Diseases*, **15**, 458–482.

Mailloux, L. (1992) More dialysis leads to better survival: a point of view. *Seminars in Dialysis*, **5**(3), 224–226.

Owen, W., Lew, N., Liu, Y. *et al.* (1993) The urea reduction ratio and serum albumin concentration as predictors of mortality in patients undergoing haemodialysis. *New England Journal of Medicine*, **329**, 1001–1006.

Parker, T., Husni, L., Huang, W. *et al.* (1994) Survival of haemodialysis patients in the United States is improved with a greater quantity of dialysis. *American Journal of Kidney Diseases*, **23**(5), 670–680.

Parker, T., Laird, N. and Lowrie, E. (1983) Comparison of the study groups in the National Co-operative Dialysis Study and a description of mortality, morbidity and patient withdrawal. *Kidney International*, **23**(Suppl. 13), 42–49.

Renal Association (1995) *Treatment of Adult Patients with Renal Failure: Recommended Standards and Audit Measures*, Renal Association, London.

Sargent, J., Gotch, F., Boral, M. *et al.* (1978) Urea kinetics: a guide to nutritional management of renal failure. *American Journal of Clinical Nutrition*, **31**, 1696–1702.

Sargent, J. (1990) Shortfalls in the delivery of dialysis. *American Journal of Kidney Diseases*, **15**, 500–510.

Smye, S., Dunderdale, E. and Will, E. (1994) Estimation of treatment dose in high efficiency haemodialysis. *Nephron*, **67**, 24–29.

Tattersall, J., Greenwood, R. and Farrington, K. (1995) Urea kinetics and when to commence dialysis. *American Journal of Nephrology*, **15**, 283–289.

Valderrábano, F. (1996) Weekly duration of dialysis treatment – does it matter for survival? *Nephrology, Dialysis and Transplantation*, **11**, 569–572.

Watson, P., Watson, I. and Batt, R. (1980) Total body water volumes for adult males and females estimated from simple anthropometric measurements. *American Journal of Clinical Nutrition*, **31**, 1696–1702.

Wineman, R. (1983) Rationale of the National Cooperative Dialysis Study. *Kidney International*, **23**, 8–11.

14 Community care of the dialysis patient

Victoria Warmington

LEARNING OBJECTIVES

At the end of this chapter the reader should be able to:

- Understand why there has been an increase in the popularity of community nursing care.
- Discuss the main aims of community renal nursing.
- Describe the primary roles and responsibilities of the community renal nurse.
- Discuss the factors involved in home dialysis success.
- Describe the safe disposal of clinical waste in the community.

THE MOVE TO THE COMMUNITY

The provision of care in the community underpins one of the foremost philosophies of the NHS: enabling patients to live longer as independently as possible while enjoying a better quality of life (DoH, 1990). The last 50 years have seen a dramatic development in health-care technology. Improved means of diagnosis and treatment have resulted in longer survival (Caress, 1995). These changes have increased the prevalence of chronic illnesses and fostered an aging population with a high demand for health and social services. There is now an expectation that patients will take a more active role in their treatment, with self-care being the ideal.

Interest in the development of primary and community care and the place of nursing within it has been growing rapidly in the last 10 years. The Cumberledge Report (DHSS, 1986) recommended an expanding role for nurses in these areas. The NHS and Community Care Act 1990 has precipitated many of the changes in structure and function of community nursing. More recently, other health service reforms have strengthened the pressure to transfer substantial elements of health-care from acute and long-stay hospitals to community settings. The increased sophistication of primary and community nursing services means that many more patients with chronic illnesses can be and are being cared for in their own homes (Beardshaw and Robinson, 1990; Walton Spradley, 1991). As the population ages and patients' dependency increases there may be a need to seek alternative forms of care in order for home-based treatment to continue. Residential and nursing homes have become a popular alternative for patients requiring additional help with care.

Key reference: Walton Spradley, B. (Ed) (1991). *Readings in Community Health Nursing*. (4th ed) J.B. Lippincott Co., Philadelphia.

As a result of health-care reforms, community nursing is undergoing rapid expansion and development in both general and specialist areas. Specialist nurse positions have grown in number and popularity in the last 5 years. Structural and financial changes to the NHS have had an enormous impact on the developments and popularity of community health-care (Hunter, 1994). The central aim of the NHS reforms is to provide patients with a wider choice and quality health-care. The change in the nature of the NHS has kept the needs of the patient as fundamental to its philosophy (Hunter, 1994). Nurses are a key resource in this new organization.

The development of CAPD in the late 1970s and its increasing acceptance as an efficient and acceptable alternative to haemodialysis have changed the nature of home dialysis (Brunier and McKeever, 1993). The bulk of dialysis now occurs in the community, with patients being largely self-caring. It should naturally follow that the best environment for their continuing care is at home.

The scenario whereby an increased amount of treatment and care is being shifted out of the traditional hospital setting arises because of the cost of long-term hospital treatment. Marks (1991) argues that home care for dialysis patients is an example of a clinically safe, organizationally feasible and financially viable alternative to hospital care. There is also a desire to minimize disruption to the patient's lifestyle and provide patients with a wider choice of dialysis treatment and location (Marks, 1991; Caress, 1995).

Key reference: Marks, L. (1991) *Home and Hospital Care: Redrawing the Boundaries.* Research Report No 9. Kings Fund Institute. London.

THE NATURE OF COMMUNITY NURSING

Burgess (1983) states that there are a number of skills that are unique to community nursing and do not simply transfer from hospital to the home environment. Community nursing should be seen as a specialized area of practice. This happens at many levels, from individuals through families to community groups (Hyde, 1995; Tinson, 1995).

The attitude that community care is peripheral to inpatient care will change as the need for complex home care gathers momentum (Hyde, 1995). Nurses will have to be innovative and resourceful in their practice (Hyde, 1995), with the consequence that the community nurse's clinical skills will become more extensive and varied.

THE AIM OF THE COMMUNITY RENAL NURSE

Community renal nurses have very specific aims related to problem prevention and reducing the risk of dialysis-associated complications, as well as long-term follow-up and care.

As the incidence of end-stage renal failure rises steeply with age so does the requirement for dialysis services (Renal Standards Subcommittee, 1995). Many dialysis patients, especially those on PD, are elderly and require considerable support from community nurses to enable them to remain in their own homes (Wilkie and Brown, 1994).

Before embarking on any home visits a knowledge of the community in which the patient lives is required. This is an essential prerequisite to planning and implementing effective nursing care (Walton Spradley, 1991). Burgess (1983) suggests that nurses gather information as to the socioeconomic, cultural and environmental factors affecting the lives of people who live in their community. It is also necessary to have a knowledge of local resources and services that patients can use or be referred on to.

Caring for patients at home is complex and requires nurses to consider many factors involving the patient, family and home and to understand how environmental, psychosocial, economic, cultural and personal health are interrelated components affecting the patient's response to having renal failure and requiring dialysis. This broad approach to community renal nursing is the cornerstone of good clinical community nursing practice (Humphrey and Milone-Nuzzo, 1991).

The home is the undisputed territory of the patient (Brindle and Brown, 1991). The visiting nurse must remember that s/he is a guest in the patient's home and abide by the rules of the house, showing due respect for the patient's and family's lifestyle.

Jaffe and Skidmore Roth (1993) argue that home care is primarily concerned with providing for activities of daily living, teaching the patient about self-care for dialysis, diet and fluid restrictions, and preventing complications arising from the treatment. Although these are important elements of community renal nursing, this prescription does fail to acknowledge a role beyond practical tasks. In the current climate of health services demanding value for money, providing patients with choice and encouraging clinical audit it is vital that any renal replacement programme has clearly defined aims as to what a home visiting service should achieve. The following should be considered as the most important.

Key reference: Jaffe, M.S. and Skidmore-Roth, L. (1993) *Home Health Nursing Care Plans* (2nd ed). Mosby. St. Louis.

Admission rates

To reduce admission rates for dialysis-related problems must be the prime aim of any service. Most, if not all, problems when detected early enough can be safely managed by the community renal nurse.

It is vital that patients are encouraged to maintain their motivation for safe, effective and largely unsupervised dialysis at home. Strategies to prevent peritonitis and exit site infections, and to promote and preserve the patient's fistula should be discussed during each home visit.

It is impossible to calculate how much is saved in patient mortality and morbidity, unnecessary stress to the patient's family, time taken off work and financially for the health service in general by nurses preventing these problems. Many authors agree that enhancing the length of time a patient is on dialysis and preventing hospital admission must be the prime aim of any home visiting programme (Naylor, 1992; Miller, 1990; Uttley and Prowant, 1994).

Patient contact

Regular contact with the patient and family is important to those suffering with a chronic illness. Visits and telephone calls can reduce the sense of isolation the patient experiences. They can also enhance the relationship between the patient, the family and the community renal nurse (Brunier and McKeever, 1993).

> **Key reference:** Brunier, G.M. and McKeever, P.T. (1993) The Impact of Home Dialysis on the Family: Literature Review. *ANNA Journal* 20(6): 653–658.

Health potential

To maximize the patient's health potential and minimize the potential complications of dialysis means that care provided should be holistic and not simply dialysis care. Accordingly more time, effort and financial resources must be channelled into health promotion and illness prevention.

Education

Continuing education and training are vital to the success of any home dialysis programme. As some complications of the therapy are potentially life-threatening the initial training period should not be seen as an isolated event but the start of a process. Learning should continue for the length of time a patient remains on dialysis.

This continuing learning is best carried out where the patient normally dialyses, i.e. at home, using familiar equipment and surroundings. This makes the training more applicable to the individual and his/her situation. The amount of work undertaken by nurses in informal education and teaching for problem prevention should not be underestimated (Audit Commission, 1992).

Communication

Communication and liaison have been highlighted as important in the provision of home care (Uttley and Prowant, 1994). By establishing strong lines of communication between the hospital, community and the patient an appropriate package of care can be formulated.

The provision of good-quality support and advice is probably one of the largest aims of a community renal nursing service. Patients will require frequent guidance and support if they are to have a relatively trouble-free dialysis career (Uttley and Prowant, 1994).

THE ROLE OF THE COMMUNITY RENAL NURSE

From the broad aims of a home dialysis programme outlined above it can be seen that the community nurse's role is complex and not simply directed towards solving practical dialysis problems. Brindle and Brown (1991) have highlighted five major roles of specialist nurses, which can be adopted by nurses caring for home dialysis patients.

Symptom control

It is imperative that nurses encourage patients to maintain their motivation and enthusiasm for safe and effective dialysis, thus helping them stay well and symptom-free. This can be difficult for some patients when they are home and in charge of their treatment. It is important that patients and their carers have completed the training programme with enough skills and knowledge as well as confidence to be self-caring and to maintain their health and wellbeing.

During the first home visit baseline observations should be established, including target weight, blood pressure, oedema, urine output, state of hydration and exercise tolerance level. The community renal nurse is well placed to monitor the course of the dialysis and look for signs and symptoms of how well the treatment is progressing.

Patients should always be aware of their target weight and ensuing problems if they exceed or fall short of this goal. Some patients may not feel confident enough to change the strength of the PD fluid or alter their fluid intake without first consulting the community nurse. Patients should always be informed of their vital signs and encouraged to understand the importance of such readings so that in time they may feel reassured and in charge of the treatment. The responsibility for empowering patients to take an active and ongoing role in their treatment and care often falls to the community renal nurse.

During follow-up visits baseline targets set with the patient may need to be revised. When a patient's uraemic symptoms have improved so may their appetite and the taste sensation may return. An increase in flesh weight can be expected and in this situation the target weight will need to be adjusted after accurate assessment. The patient needs to be informed of the new target and offered an explanation as to why the revision was necessary.

Feedback to the hospital renal team is important, as certain signs and symptoms may indicate the need for various tests to be arranged, such as a PET, adequacy studies or UKM. These may be routinely carried out by the renal unit but the community nurse is well placed to inform other staff of their necessity. Another important component of symptom control is to encourage the patient to adhere to the diet advised by the renal dietitian. Reinforcing the importance of this as a fundamental part of dialysis success is a role for the community renal nurse and the patient's diet must be discussed on each home visit. By following the suggested dietary guidelines patients can be taught to control symptoms such as itching. If the patient is experiencing pruritus the community nurse may decide it is appropriate to take blood to ascertain levels of phosphate and calcium. These need to be discussed with medical staff and any action required fed back to the patient. Giving the patient advice as to the correct time to take phosphate binders could improve some of the symptoms.

The anaemia of chronic renal failure has been documented as it affects the patient's exercise tolerance and quality of life (Jaffe and Skidmore-Roth, 1993; Temple, 1994). Anaemia imposes extra restrictions on a patient's ability to perform activities of daily living and self-care. Recombinant human erythropoietin is now widely available and is a cost-effective way to treat and manage renal anaemia. Many patients will be using EPO routinely to control anaemic symptoms. The community renal nurse is well placed to monitor the effectiveness of the EPO and subsequent improvement in activity tolerance and energy levels. The dosage and administration must be managed correctly to minimize any complications for the patient (Ellis and Abbott-Ellis, 1995). It is important to provide information for the patient about when an improvement in symptoms might be expected.

Support and advice

Burgess (1983) highlights the fact that providing supportive counselling for patients is an important role for specialist nurses working in the community. It is probably the foremost yet least tangible of the roles of the community dialysis nurse. It can range from verbal encouragement and reassurance to taking action by talking to other providers, agencies or family members. Uttley and Prowant (1994) point out that home visits are a critical part of follow-up support and patients need to realize that this service is available. Family and carers will also need support at the outset of caring, while they are caring and after the death of the patient (McClure, 1995). Good-quality home support can reduce the number of hospital attendances or in-patient episodes (Naylor, 1992; Uttley and Prowant, 1994).

Predialysis home visiting is an ideal time to commence the supportive role that is so vital to the success of the patient's therapy. These visits serve many purposes. By meeting the patient and family before renal replacement starts both parties can begin to establish a relationship that may continue for many years. Uttley and Prowant (1994) advocate meeting patients prior to commencement of dialysis or as soon as they become known to the community team, as there is often very little time to prepare a patient for what could be a life-long treatment.

The community nurse may well be involved with providing information about the different options available to the patient prior to starting dialysis (Van Waeleghem and Edwards, 1995). Having to choose a treatment that will profoundly affect one's life and that of one's family is a very complex decision to make. This often happens at a time when the patient has symptomatic uraemia, finding it difficult to concentrate and fully understand the implications of the choice. Ewles and Simnett (1985) point out that the process involves:

- weighing up the advantages and disadvantages of peritoneal and haemodialysis;
- considering the implications of pursuing each type of treatment;
- deciding which type of dialysis will suit the patient's lifestyle best.

Having made the choice of the most suitable renal replacement therapy it is important that the patient is supported in his/her decision. Rivetti *et al.* (1993) state that acceptance is more likely if the patient has made the choice of therapy.

Jaffe and Skidmore-Roth (1993) have highlighted 'ineffective family coping' as a problem for dialysis carers. The diagnosis of renal failure and the need for dialysis can alter the dynamics of a family. Patients and their carers will often experience tiredness, fatigue and changes in mood state. The uncertainty of the course of the disease and treatment as well as financial and employment worries can lead to depression. Appropriate referral to a social worker or to counselling for psychological care can help ease the strain on family relations or prevent a situation from reaching crisis point. Caress (1995) argues that nurses should try and understand how regimens affect patients lives and intervene wherever possible to minimize this disruption.

Families have been expected to take an increasingly larger role in dialysis since the rise in popularity of home care treatments. Although the emphasis is on self-care this will have a rebound effect on the family and can cause considerable stress upon them (Brunier and McKeever, 1993). Brunier and McKeever (1993) point out that spouses may be scared, hostile or have aggressive feelings towards the patient. Accurate assessment is essential before treatment starts rather than coping with a crisis afterwards. Carers can experience varying degrees of strain, anxiety and fatigue, as well as a deterioration in family relationships and social contact. Wagner (1996) urges nurses to help family members support each other in the tension of uncertainty that renal failure imposes. Families and carers should be allowed and positively encouraged to express their reactions and fears over their relative's disease. Hull *et al.* (1989) highlight the fact that carer wellbeing is of paramount importance to the patient as well as to the health service.

Caring is acknowledged as causing extra strain and placing a burden on family relationships (Caress, 1995; Wagner, 1996). Many restrictions can be placed on the carer's life, such as being expected to be present during haemodialysis sessions, disposing of PD effluent or performing aspects of physical care. The community renal nurse can introduce a variety of interventions to ease this strain by providing accurate information about the treatment, likely prognosis and outcomes. Hyde (1995) acknowledges that providing information is key in the provision of support to a patient. It is critical that the nurse allows time for the patient and family to ask questions, and for getting answers and clarification. It is often when the patient is discharged home that any fears s/he has over the treatment are verbalized as questions. The community renal nurse may be the most appropriate of the health-care team to answer these (Hyde, 1995). In the relaxed and non-threatening environment of the home more sensitive issues can be discussed (Uttley and Prowant, 1994). The nurse is also perceived as having time to spend and will not be called away to another task.

Stewart (1991) outlines some of the benefits of support in the community.

- The patient's ability to adjust to the rigours of dialysis can be monitored and referrals made as appropriate.
- Family members have the opportunity to discuss and seek answers to physical, emotional and sexual problems away from the hospital environment.
- The sense of isolation that may be felt on being discharged from the hospital training programme and left to 'get on with it' can be reduced.

Patients and relatives can also gain support from each other as they have a greater understanding of how renal failure and dialysis has affected their lives. The community renal nurse can facilitate this self-help by introducing patients to each other.

The ultimate aim of support and advice to dialysis patients and the family is to foster a sense of security, provide accurate information to reduce strain and isolation and give patients autonomy and control over their lives. Wagner (1996) argues that above all patients and families need to have hope and be assured that they are being cared for by competent and caring health-care workers.

Coordinate care

As the number of frail and elderly patients on dialysis increases so do their needs and dependencies. Therefore, a number of health and social agencies will be involved in enabling patients to live as independently as possible in their own homes. The role of care coordinator is a common one for community nurses to undertake (Burgess, 1983).

To coordinate care requires an in-depth knowledge of local services and roles to ensure that the resulting care package is appropriate for the patient's needs. The coordination of care is now complex as technology increases, treatments become more demanding and interdisciplinary collaboration becomes essential (Walton Spradley, 1991). Burgess (1983) states that a familiarity with other service providers is required to fulfil this role.

The community renal nurse should be involved in the preparation for the patient's discharge home. By coordinating with the home training team a sensible and appropriate discharge time and day can be negotiated. This ensures that all parties involved are ready and the patient's requirements are in place. Ideally, the nurse should be present for the first haemodialysis session or PD exchanges. In this way any initial problems can be addressed and corrected. It is vital to do this before there is a deleterious affect on the patient's health and confidence.

As coordinator of services the community nurse is in a key position to keep all members of the multidisciplinary team informed of the patient's progress. Feedback is vital to the hospital team, the GP and the district nursing teams. Wilkie and Brown (1994) regard community renal nurses as the key to liaison with GPs, keeping them informed of the patient's condition, ability to cope with home dialysis and any changes in dialysis prescription. Informing all team members fosters a cohesive approach to the patient's care.

The community renal nurse may be responsible for formulating a care plan that can be used by all home care personnel. Under the current Patients Charter, patients are entitled to a needs assessment, which should include the following:

- patients' own description of their needs and how they can best be met;
- the opportunity to have an advocate present;
- assistance for those whose first language is not English;
- carers' opinions or ideas;
- accurate information-giving;
- interagency coordination to provide comprehensive assessment (DoH, 1994).

The document *A Framework for Local Community Care Charters in England* (DoH, 1994) sets out the entitlements a patient can expect from a care plan.

- It is in writing.
- It is shared with users and carers.
- It covers all services and agencies involved.
- It gives points of contact for the patient.

There should be a statement of when the assessment and care plan will be reviewed to ensure it remains appropriate. The care plan and notes need to remain accessible to all service providers to ensure that the patients receive the individual care they need and are entitled to. The prime aim of well coordinated care is to ensure that the patient receives high-quality seamless health and social care.

Practical aspects

Despite the fact that home dialysis patients are largely self-caring, the community renal nurse does have a practical role in managing and maintaining effective dialysis therapy. Patients need to understand how to start and maintain their self-care activities.

Burgess (1983) states that providing care is one of the most commonly adopted aspects of the community nurses work. Working in patients homes can be challenging and accordingly requires innovation and creativity (Burgess, 1983). Performing clinical tasks at home will invariably require some modification and adaptation. Many of the practical problems and issues caused by this transition can be addressed during predialysis visits. Advice as where and how to store equipment and supplies and the amount of space needed for performing the treatment.

It is important that the community renal nurse observes the patient's exchange technique during the first home visit to ensure that the patient learns to adapt to dialysing in the home environment. On subsequent visits it is a part of continuing care to scrutinize the dialysis method to ensure that the procedure has not become slack over time, as infectious complications can be potentially very serious.

Peritonitis is one of the most serious side-effects of peritoneal dialysis. The community renal nurse has a practical role in the detection and treatment of peritonitis. Having established that the patient has PD peritonitis the community renal nurse can decide whether s/he needs to attend the renal unit for assessment by medical staff. If s/he is well enough to remain at home the nurse can take specimens of the PD effluent and initiate antibiotic therapy according to the renal unit's policy. Depending on the treatment protocol it may be necessary to teach the patient or carer to inject further doses of antibiotic into bags of PD fluid. The community nurse needs to monitor the patient carefully during episodes of peritonitis to ensure that s/he remains well while at home and that the infectious episode is resolving. An important part of follow-up care with respect to infection is observing the technique, pointing out any possible sources of contamination. Advice on aspects of care during peritonitis will be required. The ultrafiltration capacity of the peritoneal membrane will be compromised during infective episodes. The patient needs to be advised that s/he may need to use more hypertonic PD fluid to maintain the correct fluid balance and weight. If district nurses are involved in this aspect of the patient's care this must be documented in the care plan.

Depending on renal unit policy the patient may need to be prescribed sip feeds to combat the protein loss through the peritoneum that occurs during infection.

For PD patients the importance of exit site care is paramount. This needs to be discussed during each visit. If the site becomes red or is discharging it is necessary to take a swab and commence antibiotic therapy prior to the culture and sensitivities being available as this may prevent a tunnel infection and the loss of the catheter. The nurse can demonstrate correct exit site care and immobilization technique and watch the patient do the same, explaining the reasons for the procedure.

Patients on home haemodialysis have different needs to those using PD but the community nurse must be involved in their long-term care. Difficulties with needling may be encountered and the patient will need help to insert the needles correctly or to find new sites on the fistula. This time can be used productively to reinforce the importance of good fistula care as well as to observe the patient's procedure for commencing and completing dialysis. The nurse can offer respite care to the patient's dialysis partner by being present during a haemodialysis session.

Education and training

Education about the disease is the first step in helping patients adjust to the diagnosis. With the change in emphasis for self-care, patients need to be well prepared to cope with complex treatment regimens. Education and training are a traditional role and responsibility for nurses (Burgess, 1983; Priest, 1989; Caress, 1995). They should be regarded as an important role for any home care nurse (Uttley and Prowant (1994). In order to teach patients effectively, their knowledge, skills, motivation and ability to communicate must be accurately assessed so that the teaching can be individually tailored to suit the patient.

Priest (1989) points out that the possession of knowledge and clinical expertise is not enough to ensure that education is effective. With expert knowledge and skills in a specialty the community dialysis nurse is well placed for patient and family education (Priest, 1989). Benner (1984) states that nurses need to know what the illness means to the patient and understand the skills and demands put on the patient at each stage of the disease. In this way patients and carers can be 'coached' through the diagnosis and treatment.

The period of training a patient undergoes should not be viewed as an isolated event. It should be seen as a process and the start of what will be lifelong learning. The community nurse is vital in providing this aspect of care. Education in the community largely involves updating the patient's practical skills and knowledge. As more becomes understood about the treatments for renal failure, the patient needs to be updated on pertinent facts affecting his/her care.

After the training programme the community dialysis nurse needs to assess the patient's level of knowledge and what has been retained from the teaching in hospital. Having established this, knowledge and skills can be built upon to ensure that the patient and carer are equipped to cope with the demands of dialysis. A home visit can be used for educational and teaching purposes using familiar equipment and surroundings.

Teaching must be relevant and interesting to the patient (Webb, 1994). Patients must be actively involved in this process to ensure that the maximum is gained from the experience (Ewles and Simnett, 1985). In order to achieve this a variety of teaching methods and equipment will be required but the overall aim will be independence and the promotion of self-care.

Stewart (1991) points out that any skill and knowledge deficits can be identified and corrected by the community nurse before there is a knock-on effect to the patient and their health suffers.

The community renal nurse will be involved in teaching other members of the caring team. District nurses will need formal and informal training on many aspects of dialysis care, including weight assessments, selection of PD fluid, exit site care and administration of EPO. The provision of up-to-date information and literature is an important aspect of care. Joint visits can be a very productive means of teaching both practical and theoretical aspects of nursing care.

As already discussed, there are a large number of elderly and more dependent patients on home-based therapy. Patients may need to have residential care or move into a nursing home for respite or on a permanent basis. The community renal nurse needs to ensure that staff members are equipped with the knowledge and ability to safely care for, or assist the patient with the dialysis. Even if the patient remains self-caring staff need to be aware of what the treatment involves and action that should be taken if complications arise. A point of contact is necessary for residential and nursing home staff. Regular updates and training also need to be given to ensure nurses are equipped to care for a patient on dialysis.

CULTURAL CONSIDERATIONS IN COMMUNITY CARE

Culture has a profound influence over people's lives (Walton Spradley, 1991). Although there are broad cultural values shared by people who live in the UK there is a huge range of subcultures within each society. It is important that the community renal nurse understands and is sensitive to the needs of patients from different cultures (Walton Spradley, 1991). In order to provide individual nursing care the nurse needs to understand how culture influences a patient's behaviour and the relationship s/he has with family members.

Adapting to the rigours of dialysis requires a change in behaviour. This may be more difficult for a patient from a minority ethnic group to achieve if the nurse is unaware of factors such as family, religion, desire to self-care and how these shape behaviour. Priest (1989) maintains that the nurse first needs to establish credibility. This can be done by addressing the patient's and family's needs specifically and on an individual basis (Elliott, 1994). Nursing has an obligation to provide meaningful care that is sensitive to the needs of people from all cultures (Waller, 1996). Building up a community profile will aid the community nurse's awareness of the composition of the population being cared for. This will provide data as to the ethnic make-up of an area, causes of renal failure and any other key health problems. This facilitates an holistic approach to community nursing care.

Difficulties in communication and language may be experienced. Although family members can be used for translation purposes this may not be appropriate, as sensitive and personal issues often need to be discussed. The nurse should not assume that a patient is willing to discuss such details through bilingual family members, who are often children. It should not be assumed that the correct meaning is being translated or that the correct interpretation is given. Some people may find certain subjects 'distasteful'. In this instance a linkworker or interpreting service may be more appropriate. Fuller and Toon (1988) consider that it is desirable that the interpreter:

- is fluent in both languages;
- has training in interpretation;
- has some medical knowledge;
- has a good knowledge of how health services work;
- is available every time the patient is seen;
- is accepted and trusted by the patient and nurse;
- is sensitive to the patient's and nurse's needs;
- will not allow his/her own beliefs to override the patient's;
- puts the patient at ease;
- has a good memory and pays attention to detail;
- can translate fine shades of meaning;
- is able to know when the patient has a problem;
- is aware of the cultural expectations of the patient and nurse;
- is the same sex as the patient;
- is able to carry the responsibility.

Although this list is long and probably rather idealistic it does serve as a reminder to the community renal nurse as how important it is to be aware of cultural diversity and the needs of the patient.

SAFE DISPOSAL OF CLINICAL WASTE IN THE COMMUNITY

As dialysis generates a large amount of clinical waste patients need to be aware of safe disposal methods. After liaison with the patient's local authority the community nurse needs to reinforce the nature of the risks that can arise from unsafe refuse disposal. Hazards to public health or the environment need to be prevented or dealt with correctly should they occur (DoE, 1990). Local authorities have a duty to collect clinical waste so there should be no need for nurses to transport refuse.

The community nurse needs to ensure that patients are aware of the following requirements laid down by the Department of the Environment (1990).

- All dialysis waste should be placed in a yellow clinical waste bag and sealed properly with a tie to prevent leakage.
- Until collection day the refuse should be kept inside the patient's home. All waste containers should be left outside for the minimum amount of time possible to reduce the risk of infection to others.

CONCLUSION

As health-care technology becomes more complex and there is increasing financial pressure and a demand for better value for money, more care and treatments are being transferred to community settings. Community renal nurses have a responsibility to promote optimum health and provide on-going support, advice and nursing care for the patient and family.

This holistic approach to care can reduce the incidence of dialysis-related complications and hospital admission, one of the key aims of the role of the community renal nurse.

REVIEW QUESTIONS

- What has driven the move to community renal nursing care?
- Why do dialysis patients and their carers need follow-up nursing care in the community?
- How do environmental, psychological and cultural factors impinge on the success of home dialysis?

REFERENCES

Audit Commission (1992) *Homeward Bound: A New Course for Community Health*, HMSO, London.

Beardshaw, V. and Robinson, R. (1990) *New for Old? Prospects for Nursing in the 1990s*, Research Report 8, Kings Fund Institute, London.

Benner, P. (1984) *From Novice to Expert. Excellence and Power in Clinical Nursing Practice*, Addison-Wesley, Redwood City, CA.

Brindle, C. and Brown, K. (1991) *Community Health Care*, Macmillan, Basingstoke.

Brunier, G. M. and McKeever, P. T. (1993) The impact of home dialysis on the family: literature review. *American Nephrology Nurses Association Journal*, **20**(6), 653–658.

Burgess, W. (1983) The nature of community health nursing and the home visit, in *Community Health Nursing. Philosophy, Process, Practice*, (eds W. Burgess and E. Chatterton-Ragland), Appleton-Century-Crofts, Norwalk, CT.

Caress, A.-L. (1995) Management of long term health problems, in *Clinical Nursing Practice in the Community*, (eds M. Kenrick and K. Luker), Blackwell Science, Oxford.

DHSS (1986) *Community Nursing: A Focus for Care*, (the Cumberledge Report), HMSO, London.

DoE (1990) *Environmental Protection Act 1990. Waste Management. The Duty of Care. A Code of Practice*, HMSO, London.

DoH (1990) *The Health Service. The NHS Reforms and You*, HMSO, London.

DoH (1994) *A Framework for Local Community Care Charters in England*, HMSO, London.

Elliott, O. (1994) Working with black and minority ethnic groups, in *Health Promotion and Patient Education. A Professional's Guide*, (ed. P. Webb), Chapman & Hall, London.

Ellis, P. and Abbott-Ellis, J. (1995) The use of erythropoietin to treat anaemia in end stage renal disease. *Professional Nurse*, **10**(7), 448–450.

Ewles, L. and Simnett, I. (1985) *Promoting Health. A Practical Guide To Health Education*, John Wiley & Sons, Chichester.

Fuller, F. H. S. and Toon, P. D. (1988) *Medical Practice in a Multicultural Society*, Heinemann Medical, Oxford.

Hull, R., Ellis, M., and Sargent, V. (1989) *Teamwork in Palliative Care*, Radcliffe Medical Press, Oxford.

Humphrey, C. and Milone-Nuzzo, P. (1991) *Home Care Nursing. An Orientation to Practice*, Appleton & Lange, Norwalk, CT.

Hunter, D. (1994) The impact of the NHS reforms on community care, in *Caring for People in the Community. The New Welfare*, (ed. M. Titterton), Jessica Kingsley, London.

Hyde, V. (1995) Community nursing: a unified discipline?, in *Community Nursing. Dimensions and Dilemmas*, (eds P. Cain, V. Hyde and E. Howkins), Edward Arnold, London.

Jaffe, M. S. and Skidmore-Roth, L. (1993) *Home Health Nursing Care Plans*, 2nd edn, C. V. Mosby, St Louis, MO.

McClure, L. (1995) Community nursing and carers: what price support and partnership?, in *Community Nursing. Dimensions and Dilemmas*, (eds P. Cain, V. Hyde and E. Howkins), Edward Arnold, London.

Marks, L. (1991) *Home and Hospital Care: Redrawing the Boundaries*, Research Report 9, Kings Fund Institute, London.

Miller, L. A. (1990) At home help for the CAPD patient. *Registered Nurse*, **Aug.**, 77–80.

Naylor, M. (1992) Home is best. *Nursing Times*, **88**(26), 36–38.

Priest, A-R. (1989) The CNS as educator, in *The Clinical Nurse Specialist in Theory and Practice*, 2nd edn, (eds A. B. Hamric and J. A. Spross), W. B. Saunders, Philadelphia, PA.

Renal Association Standards Subcommittee (1995) *Treatment of Adult Patients with Renal Failure. Recommended Standards and Audit Measures*, Royal College of Physicians of London, London.

Rivetti, M., Servetti, L., Cotto, M. *et al.* (1993) The choice of dialytic treatment. *Journal of the European Dialysis and Transplant Nurses Association–European Renal Care Association*, **19**(3), 25–26.

Stewart, G. (1991) The renal nurse consultant: perspectives on a new role. Approaches to cost effective, quality care for the renal patient. *Journal of the European Dialysis and Transplant Nurses Association–European Renal Care Association*, **16**(1), 2–4.

Temple, M. (1994) Use of epoietin in the management of renal anaemia. *Hospital Update*, **Mar.**, 165–171.

Tinson, S. (1995) Assessing health need: a community perspective, in *Community Nursing. Dimensions and Dilemmas*, (eds P. Cain, V. Hyde and E. Howkins), Edward Arnold, London.

Uttley, L. and Prowant, B. (1994) Organization of the peritoneal dialysis program – the nurse's role, in *Textbook of Peritoneal Dialysis*, (eds R. Gokal and K. Nolph), Kluwer Academic Publishers, Dordrecht.

Van Waeleghem, J. P. and Edwards, P. (eds) (1995) *European Standards for Nephrology Nursing Practice*, European Dialysis and Transplant Nurses Association–European Renal Care Association, Lucerne.

Wagner, C. D (1996) Family needs of chronic haemodialysis patients: a comparison of perceptions of nurses and families. *American Nephrology Nurses Association Journal*, **23**(1), 19–26.

Waller, A. (1996) Bringing the cultural perspective into patient care. *Royal College of Nursing Dialysis and Transplant Nursing Forum Newsletter*, **2**.

Walton Spradley, B. (ed.) (1991) *Readings in Community Health Nursing*, 4th edn, J. B. Lippincott, Philadelphia, PA.

Webb, P. (ed.) (1994) *Health Promotion and Patient Education. A Professional's Guide*, Chapman & Hall, London.

Wilkie, M. and Brown, C. (1994) Sharing the management of patients on CAPD. *Prescriber*, **5**(23), 61–65.

15 Nursing care of the renal transplant patient

Josie Digioa and Anne Frankton

LEARNING OBJECTIVES

At the end of this chapter the reader should be able to:

- Identify the risk factors when assessing a patient's suitability for transplantation.
- Describe the nurse's role in the pre- and postoperative care of the transplant patient.
- List the common causes of early graft dysfunction and common surgical complications.
- Describe the nurse's role in preparing the patient for discharge, outlining the advice that should be given.

INTRODUCTION

Renal transplantation is the treatment of choice for most patients with end-stage renal failure. A successful renal transplant not only offers freedom from dialysis and dietary restrictions but will increase wellbeing and quality of life. It is the most cost-effective treatment for kidney disease and will potentially allow the recipient to return to work.

RECIPIENT ASSESSMENT FOR KIDNEY TRANSPLANTATION

It is important to remember that, although transplantation is the treatment of choice for most patients with end-stage renal failure, it is an option that has risks as well as benefits. The most important considerations when assessing patients for transplantation are to identify and evaluate conditions that may later cause complications or unacceptable risk to the patient or graft.

Counselling

Recipient counselling should include information on the operation, results of transplantation, drug side-effects, and potential complications such as delayed graft function, rejection and even death. The chance of readmission and frequent outpatient visits during the early months should also be made clear. It is also important to establish at this stage what the patient's wishes are and to allow time for discussion and questions. Ideally this type of counselling and information-giving is carried out by the surgeon and a senior transplant nurse or coordinator.

Age

Improved patient and graft survival, combined with better health care, and an aging dialysis population has led most transplant centres to relax age limits when assessing potential recipients. Evidence suggests that, although older patients are less likely to reject, they are more likely to die of cardiovascular complications (Briggs, 1995).

PRIMARY RENAL DISEASE

The primary cause of renal disease in the recipient should be established whenever possible. Certain diseases, e.g. focal segmental glomerulosclerosis and type II mesangiocapillary glomerulonephritis, recur rapidly in the graft and careful consideration needs to be given as to whether transplantation is appropriate (Briggs, 1995).

Medical history

Cardiovascular disease is the most common cause of death in transplant recipients and is greater than in the general population (Brown, 1995). Dialysis-dependent patients often present with left ventricle failure and it is important that it is treated. Active tuberculosis should be excluded and prophylactic drugs given to patients with a previous history of the disease or considered at risk.

Screening for viral infections should also form part of the pretransplant assessment. Patients who are hepatitis-B- or hepatitis-C-positive are not necessarily unsuitable; transplantation is only contraindicated when there is evidence of active hepatic disease. However, there may be an increased risk of progressive hepatic disease due to immunosuppressive therapy in the long term (Pereira, 1995).

In patients who test HIV-positive transplantation is contraindicated because of the associated risk of immunosuppression. All potential recipients are screened for Cytomegalovirus (CMV) prior to transplantation. CMV is an opportunist virus that may be fatal in the immunocompromised patient. Problems may arise when CMV-positive kidneys are transplanted into CMV-negative recipients who are subsequently immunosuppressed.

As it is not always possible to avoid giving CMV-positive kidneys to CMV-negative recipients (it is thought that approximately 40% of the general population is CMV-positive) prophylaxis in the form of acyclovir or ganciclovir is given at the time of transplantation in some centres. Clinically significant CMV infection has been associated with increased patient mortality and graft loss (Newstead, 1995).

Careful review of biochemical markers such as alkaline phosphatase, calcium, phosphate and parathyroid hormone is essential in the assessment of renal bone disease, the control of which can help in the prevention of steroid-induced osteoporosis, which may affect as many as 50% of patients (Brown, 1995).

Malignancy

Although immunosuppressed transplant recipients are known to be predisposed to malignant disease, malignancy is not a contraindication to transplantation. It has been shown that recurrence of malignant disease following transplantation is related to the time interval between treatment of the cancer and transplantation. It is therefore accepted practice that transplantation is delayed for at least 2 years following successful treatment of a tumour. The exception to this general rule are non-melanotic skin tumours, which can be treated just as effectively after transplantation as before (Sheil, 1994).

Psychological issues and other factors

Psychological stability must be considered when assessing the patient's suitability for transplantation and this should involve full use of the renal multiprofessional team. This may include the involvement of the renal social worker, psychologist or counsellor. Patients' needs vary but the opportunity for counselling and other support such as home visits and more detailed family assessment should be available. Poor compliance while on dialysis may indicate future problems of compliance with drug regimens. Obesity prior to transplantation will usually be exacerbated by postoperative steroid therapy, and weight reduction should be advised, together with stopping smoking where indicated, to reduce anaesthetic risks and long-term cardiovascular problems.

Tissue typing and immunological status

The major histocompatibility complex (MHC) is a group of genes located on chromosome 6 that is involved in the immune response, particularly graft rejection.

The simplest form of tissue typing is ABO blood grouping, which was discovered in the early 1900s. In the 1940s a more sensitive set of antigens of importance in transplantation were discovered. These were described as histocompatibility antigens and were discovered on leucocytes. The human leucocyte antigen system (HLA system) is the human MHC and forms the basis of tissue typing.

There are six gene sites or loci, which have been identified as DP, DQ, DR, B, C and A and are found on the short arm of chromosome 6. These sites express different antigens, and each site may consist of one or many different gene forms or alleles. Each individual has two antigens at every locus: half of each pair is inherited from each parent as a complete set. The complex of genes inherited from each parent is known as a haplotype and we all have two haplotypes. The antigens coded for by the A, B and C loci are referred to as class I antigens and those coded for the DR, DQ and DP loci as class II antigens. Class I and class II antigens are categorized as such by the type of immune response the antigens evoke.

Today there are well over 100 identified antigens. Most kidney transplant centres in the UK tend to match organs at the HLA-A, HLA-B and HLA-DR loci as well as ABO matching. Although six-antigen-matched transplants have been shown to have a better graft survival than transplants with a lesser degree of match (Dyer *et al.*, 1995), many studies have shown very good graft survival rates with partially HLA-matched grafts, especially at the DR loci or DR and B loci. The reason behind this is that there is a ranking order in the histocompatibility strengths of the different loci. The HLA-DR antigens are the strongest, followed by DQ and B and then A, C and DP (Ting and Welsh, 1994).

Cytotoxic antibodies

Antibodies are immunoglobulins secreted by B lymphocytes and plasma cells into the serum of an individual. They are produced in response to stimulation of the immune system by an antigen.

Cytotoxic antibodies are capable of killing the cells of the transplanted kidney by reacting with HLA antigens. Cytotoxic antibodies are developed as a result of being exposed to foreign HLA antigens by either blood transfusion, pregnancy or a previous transplant. If the individual is exposed to the same antigen(s) through transplantation the result may be hyperacute rejection of the graft.

Regular screening for cytotoxic antibodies is carried out on all potential recipients to detect specific antigens against which antibodies have been formed, thereby reducing the risk of rejection (Brostoff and Male, 1994). All patients undergo blood testing preoperatively for crossmatching against donor cells. A positive result indicates the presence of specific antibodies against the donor antigens and would usually result in cancellation of the transplant operation because of the high risk of hyperacute rejection.

TRANSPLANT PROCEDURE

The kidney transplant is usually placed extraperitoneally in the left or right iliac fossa. Many surgeons prefer the right as it is easier to access the recipient's blood vessels. However, previous surgery, pulse status and which kidney is used will influence the decision. The advantages of placing the kidney extraperitoneally in the iliac fossa are as follows.

- The peritoneal cavity is not entered and therefore it is less painful.
- There is less risk of postoperative paralytic ileus.
- The graft is easily accessed for assessment by palpation, auscultation and biopsy.
- Siting the kidney close to the blood vessels and the bladder makes vascular and ureteral anastomosis easier.
- The distal ureteric blood supply is vulnerable and a short length of ureter is of benefit.

The renal artery is usually anastomosed to the external iliac artery, but the internal iliac, common iliac artery or aorta may be used. The renal vein is anastomosed to the external or common iliac vein or inferior vena cava.

PREOPERATIVE CARE

From the moment the potential recipient is asked to attend the transplant centre psychological care and support are very important. Most patients will experience anxiety, fear and hope. It is usual for the recipients of cadaveric kidneys to attend the transplant centre and undergo preoperative preparation while the donor–recipient crossmatch is being performed. Potential recipients are told that the transplant operation will not go ahead if the result of the crossmatch is positive. Although not ideal, preparing the patient for operation while awaiting the crossmatch result is often necessary to reduce or limit the cold ischaemic time of the cadaver kidney. It has been shown that cold ischaemic times of less than 24 hours are favourable and improve success rates (Marshall *et al.*, 1994). For those patients who are highly sensitized or have had previous positive antibodies the result of the crossmatch may be positive and the disappointment is often difficult to cope with.

Recent studies have shown that not all lymphocytotoxic antibodies are graft-damaging. Most tissue typing laboratories are able to specify whether it is the recipient's T or B cells that have reacted to the donor cells, and can give a value to indicate the strength of the response. Positive T-cell crossmatches are always contraindicated as they indicate a high degree of recipient sensitization and the graft will inevitably reject. A weak positive B-cell crossmatch is not necessarily a contraindication to transplant if a review of recipient history does not indicate any major risk factors. The new and more sensitive flow cytometric crossmatch can be used to help in the assessment of graft suitability (Brostoff and Male, 1994).

Although time is limited psychological preparation is still a very important factor. Fears of rejection and surgical complications are often major concerns (Nakahara *et al.*, 1993). Patients may have misconceived ideas about what rejection is, how it affects them and how it affects the transplant; it is therefore important to allow time for discussion so that fears can be allayed.

Immediately preoperatively it is essential to assess carefully the recipient's biochemistry and fluid status and to look for any potential sources of infection that would contraindicate transplantation. Optimally the patient should be well dialysed, with particular emphasis on achieving a serum potassium within the normal range, and adequately hydrated, i.e. approximately 1 kg above their dry or target weight. The well-dialysed patient should not require immediate postoperative dialysis with its associated risks of heparinization, and ensuring that the patient is adequately hydrated should facilitate the maintenance of appropriate intravascular volume, which is essential to perfusion of the graft (Allen and Chapman, 1994). It is important to note albumin levels at this stage as a low serum albumin may affect subsequent management of intravascular volume. During this time the recipient should be informed that when s/he wakes from the anaesthetic s/he will have a number of catheters and lines *in situ*. These will probably include a urethral catheter, a central venous catheter, a wound drain and one or two peripheral intravenous lines.

It is usual to begin immunosuppressive therapy either before or during the transplant procedure (Allen and Chapman, 1994). This is to ensure that there is an adequate level of immunosuppression before exposure to donor antigens. The use of antibiotic prophylaxis is common practice, and a broad-spectrum antibiotic is usually given for 24 hours following the operation. Intravenous mannitol and frusemide are often given in the operative period to encourage early graft function. Mannitol also acts as a free radical scavenger and may help to reduce the ischaemia reperfusion injury. Many centres prescribe subcutaneous heparin to reduce the risk of venous thrombosis (Allen and Chapman, 1994). Recipients who are CMV-negative and are receiving a CMV-positive kidney may be given prophylaxis such as oral acyclovir (Goodwin, 1992).

POSTOPERATIVE MANAGEMENT

Fluid balance

One of the most important aspects of the postoperative nursing care of a renal transplant recipient is monitoring fluid balance to ensure that the patient is adequately hydrated (Allen and Chapman, 1994). Most centres will use measurements of central venous pressure (CVP), hourly urine output, blood pressure and weight in order to assess fluid requirement and prescription of an appropriate fluid replacement regimen. Optimally the patient should be kept well hydrated with a CVP between 10 and 15 cmH$_2$O. It is not unusual during the first few days for grafts to diurese large amounts of urine. Occasionally this can be up to 1000 ml/h. Most centres will usually take the previous hour's urine output as a basis from which to calculate the following hour's fluid requirement. Replacement fluid is usually normal saline but colloids may need to be given.

Low central venous pressures are usually a result of hypovolaemia and may cause poor graft perfusion and oliguria. Prompt treatment is essential and in these circumstances fluid boluses may be given in amounts of 250–500 ml. Between 1 and 2 litres may be given but caution should be exercised as too much fluid may result in pulmonary oedema, requiring urgent dialysis. When treating hypovolaemia the use of albumin should be considered as this will effectively draw interstitial fluid back into the intravascular space, thereby quickly expanding intravascular volume.

Urine output from the graft should become normal within 24–72 hours. Once this has happened and the patient is able to take adequate amounts of fluid orally the intravenous infusions can be discontinued and normal thirst mechanisms can be relied on for fluid replacement. Assessment of the patient's fluid state should still be carried out once or twice daily, using weight, review of fluid intake and output, blood pressure and clinical examination.

Electrolyte balance

Careful monitoring of serum electrolytes is essential, especially potassium. It is prudent to measure electrolytes on the patient's return from theatre, firstly to ensure they are within safe limits and secondly so there is a baseline to judge future results against (Allen and Chapman, 1994). A second measurement should be made 4–6 hours later regardless of urine output (the patient with ATN may be anuric or oliguric and so may produce some urine but with little clearance of urea and electrolytes). In the event of a non-functioning kidney serum potassium may rise suddenly as a result of cell lysis secondary to surgical dissection and intraoperative blood transfusion. A serum potassium greater than 6.0 mEq/l should always be treated promptly. To reduce serum potassium concentrations quickly the use of intravenous dextrose and insulin or bicarbonate may be considered. These agents will quickly lower serum potassium by driving the potassium back into the cells. Unfortunately, the effects are fairly short-lived as the total amount of potassium in the body is not reduced. Resonium enemas will slowly reduce serum potassium by reducing total body potassium and may be used in conjunction with the intravenous therapies. If rising serum potassium cannot be managed by these measures, haemodialysis with a minimal or tight heparin regimen should be initiated.

Eating and drinking

Oral diet and fluids can be commenced postoperatively when the patient wishes. Although the transplant is placed extraperitoneally recipients can develop postoperative paralytic ileus. Oral intake should be deferred in this situation until there is evidence of the return of bowel function.

Analgesia

Postoperative analgesia should be titrated according to patient demand. Most centres will have their own protocols for postoperative pain management and patient-controlled analgesia is commonly used. The choice of drugs must be carefully considered as there is usually an accumulation of active metabolites of most narcotic drugs in patients with no renal function.

Care of wounds and drains

The usual protocols are used when caring for incision wounds and wound drains. In the immunosuppressed patient consideration should always be given to the increased risk of hospital-acquired infections (Allen and Chapman, 1994). Urethral catheters are usually kept *in situ* for approximately 5 days to safeguard the ureteral anastomosis.

Getting back to normal

After about 3 days most of the drains and infusion lines will have been removed and the patient should be fully mobile. Once this has been achieved the heparin is discontinued. The use of heparin and prophylactic aspirin has been shown to significantly reduce the incidence of cardiovascular complications, especially renal vein thrombosis. Monitoring of graft function is by daily weight and fluid intake and output recordings. These will give an indication of the patient's hydration in relation to the amount of urine being produced. Daily or twice-daily measurements of urea, creatinine and electrolytes are performed. Creatinine is usually used as the main guide to graft function, as other biochemical markers may be influenced by diet or medications.

Most transplant centres will use a combination of cyclosporin, azathioprine and steroids as the basis for their immunosuppressive regimens. During the early days drug dosages are frequently changed as they are titrated against blood levels and full blood counts. Nursing care of the transplant recipient must include monitoring for side-effects of the immunosuppressive agents. It is important that supervision of immunosuppressive regimens is done by staff experienced in their use so that a balance between adequate immunosuppression and minimal side-effects is achieved.

Early graft dysfunction

A decrease or a total lack of urine output during the postoperative period can be the result of a number of conditions. Common causes are hypovolaemia and blood clot retention in the urethral catheter. Hypovolaemia is treated by restoring fluid volume and blood clot retention is easily remedied by irrigating the bladder with normal saline *via* the urethral catheter. If the urine output remains poor, further investigation would include ultrasound, biochemistry, isotope scan and biopsy as well as clinical assessment of the patient.

Acute tubular necrosis (ATN)

Most frequently, ATN-induced anuria occurs immediately; although occasionally anuria may develop after a few hours of initial diuresis. It is the major cause of early graft dysfunction in cadaveric kidneys. Factors associated with ATN are prolonged warm or cold ischaemic times or technical problems with vessel anastomosis before the graft is revascularized. The diagnosis of ATN is usually only made by eliminating all other causes of early graft dysfunction.

The duration of ATN in transplanted kidneys may be days or as long as 3 months. During this time the patient will need regular dialysis and reinforcement of dietary and fluid restriction. If the period of ATN is prolonged, regular biopsies and imaging may be performed to rule out concurrent rejection or other causes of early graft dysfunction. ATN significantly complicates postoperative management and usually results in longer hospitalization for the patient. Psychological support during this time is very important as the patient tires and becomes depressed by a lengthy hospital admission.

COMMON SURGICAL COMPLICATIONS

Urinary leak

Urinary leak is usually caused by distal ureteral necrosis resulting from damage to the ureteral blood supply during donor nephrectomy or implantation. If the wound drain is still *in situ* there may be an increase in drainage. The signs and symptoms are not unlike those of rejection, with fever, graft tenderness, back pain, reduced urine output and a rise in serum creatinine. Diagnosis may be made using biochemical analysis of the drain fluid, ultrasound, isotope scan and antegrade pyelography (see Patient scenario). Treatment may be radiological or surgical. A percutaneous nephrostomy tube can be inserted to allow the leak to heal without the need for surgical reimplantation. Surgical reimplantation may be the initial treatment or when percutaneous nephrostomy has failed. Care of the patient's skin around the drains is important as is teaching the patient to care for them. Again, infection should be a major consideration in these patients.

Patient scenario

A 28-year-old man received a renal transplant and made a good postoperative recovery. There was immediate graft function with no problems for the first week. At day 5 there was a sudden decrease in urine output, fever, abdominal pain and rising creatinine. High-dose oral steroids were commenced following a biopsy that showed mild parenchymal acute rejection. Kidney function did not improve and the patient became dialysis-dependent. A second biopsy was performed on day 9, which showed ongoing rejection, and antilymphocyte globulin (ALG) treatment was started. As the patient remained dialysis-dependent an isotope scan was performed on day 12, which indicated a possible urinary leak. A third biopsy on day 17 showed mild rejection and ultrasound demonstrated the presence of fluid in the pelvis, but on the opposite side to the transplant. An antegrade pyelogram confirmed the diagnosis of a urinary leak and surgical reimplantation of the ureter was performed, resulting in restored electrolyte and fluid balance.

Ureteric obstruction

In the immediate postoperative period ureteric obstruction may be due to oedema around the vesico-ureteric anastomosis. Usually, ureteric stenosis appears weeks or months later and causes slowly deteriorating graft function. The cause is usually an ischaemic stricture at the vesico-ureteric junction and diagnosis is often by ultrasonic evidence of dilatation of the collecting system. Treatment is by percutaneous nephrostomy with stent insertion. Surgical reconstruction is occasionally indicated and often a stent will be left in place to protect the anastomosis. Regular screening and monitoring for infection should be part of the nursing follow-up.

Vascular thrombosis

With improved surgical techniques, renal vein or arterial thrombosis occurs in less than 5% of transplants. Risk factors include hypovolaemia or hypotension, poor surgical technique, multiple vessels, atherosclerosis in the donor or recipient and a history of a previous thrombotic event. A fall in urine output and rise in serum creatinine will indicate a problem but diagnosis is usually by isotope scan, which will demonstrate blood flow through the vessels and the graft. Vascular thrombosis of the graft is rarely recoverable and nephrectomy is usual.

REJECTION

Rejection is defined as hyperacute, acute or chronic depending on time of onset and appearances on biopsy. Hyperacute rejection is very rarely seen today as a result of improved laboratory crossmatching techniques and the routine use of donor–recipient crossmatching by transplant centres. It is immediate in its onset, occurring because of preformed antibodies in the recipient, and usually necessitates removal of the graft.

Acute rejection

This occurs in 30–50% of transplant recipients, usually in the first 3 months after transplantation as a result of sensitization to donor antigens. It can be antibody- or T-cell-mediated, or both (Brostoff and Male, 1994). Prompt diagnosis and treatment are essential to limit graft damage (Allen and Chapman, 1994). Signs and symptoms of rejection include fever, decrease in urine output and graft tenderness, although a rise in serum creatinine may be all that is noticed. As the onset can be sudden, nursing observation and monitoring is vital in ensuring prompt action is taken. Definitive diagnosis can only be made by means of a transplant biopsy. Biopsy results will also give an indication of the severity of the rejection and whether it is cellular or vascular in origin. Most centres will have their own rejection protocols, which may include the use of several immunosuppressive agents. The usual treatment is high-dose steroids but severe episodes which are steroid resistant or vascular in origin may require tacrolimus or an antibody preparation, e.g. ATG, OKT3.

Infection is the major side-effect of these drugs and usual complications may include CMV infection, oral candidiasis, urinary and respiratory tract infections. Although it is not always necessary to nurse these patients in isolation, measures should be taken to prevent hospital-acquired infections, especially strict hand-washing by all health-care professionals.

Psychological care and support during this time is paramount. The patient will experience anxiety and fear regarding potential loss of the graft (Dowsett, 1996). Longer than anticipated hospital admissions are a usual consequence of antirejection therapies and will also influence the patient's state of mind.

Chronic rejection

This may occur months or years following transplantation. Its impact will be discussed later.

RETURNING HOME

Discharge

The role of the nurse in preparing the patient for discharge by providing consistent and clear information is vital to ensure the patient understands the need for frequent monitoring and self-care and adapts well to his/her new treatment. An honest and informative approach by both medical and nursing staff and encouragement of the patient to ask questions during his/her postoperative recovery helps the recipient to develop confidence and establishes an understanding of the need for continual investigation and treatment from an early stage.

Preparation for discharge should begin as early as possible; an appropriate time to start teaching would be once the patient is well enough to assimilate the information and this should be an integral part of nursing care. It is important to remember that individual patients will vary in their request for information as well as in the extent of their existing knowledge and preconceived ideas. Teaching is a process that should not be rushed; some patients will take longer than others to absorb information and act upon it, and for the transplant recipient the process should continue indefinitely following discharge with the aim of promoting health and long-term graft function.

Verbal advice should be reinforced by written information and a structured approach to teaching and discharge procedure has been shown to be effective (Milligan, 1994).

Medication

The transplant recipient will be discharged home with a combination of drugs, most of which will be completely new to him/her. Those given prior to the transplant, such as phosphate binders, vitamin supplements and erythropoietin, are usually discontinued as a functioning transplant returns electrolyte and hormonal imbalances to normal. Antihypertensive medications are introduced again as necessary once fluid balance is stable. The patient will need detailed explanation of the immunosuppressive drugs, including timing of doses and side-effects, particularly the risk of infection. Immunosuppressive drug regimens vary from centre to centre and patient to patient, according to previous transplant history, degree of sensitization and individual tolerance. It is therefore important that patients receive information that is relevant to them and that this is adapted according to any changes made in their treatment. Time should be taken to explain the reasons for other drugs given, for example: those that inhibit gastric acid production (cimetidine, ranitidine, omeprazole) to counteract the irritation caused by prednisolone; prophylactic antibiotics; or antiviral agents. It is useful to provide a written list of medication for the patient to bring back to follow-up appointments. This ensures that both patient and staff remain up to date with dose changes, which are likely to be variable in the early weeks following discharge.

Diet

The need for dietary and fluid restrictions is almost always eliminated following successful transplantation and returning to a 'normal' diet is an important factor in improving the patient's quality of life. This freedom, however, together with an improved sense of wellbeing and the influence of prednisolone in increasing the appetite, can result in considerable weight gain, which patients often find difficult to reverse (Przygrodzka *et al.*, 1992). Dietary advice in the postoperative period and frequent monitoring by the dietitian following discharge helps to prevent excessive weight gain and reduce the risk of associated long-term effects on the patient's health, including hypertension, coronary artery disease and hyperlipidaemia (Patel, 1995). Patients are advised to follow a low-fat, low-salt, high-fibre diet and are actively encouraged to eat the fresh fruit, salad and vegetables that they were previously denied because of their high potassium content.

Activity

Physical rehabilitation varies from a few weeks to months, depending on the patient's state of health prior to the transplant. Transplant recipients usually have more energy and are more active than dialysis patients, although they should be advised that they are likely to feel tired easily in the early weeks following discharge.

Restrictions on activity should be suggested on an individual basis; for example, driving should be attempted only when the patient is comfortable and alert enough to do so. Returning to work depends on the type of job

– manual workers are likely to need a longer recovery time and consideration should be given to those working in an environment likely to increase the risk of infection, e.g. teachers, health-care workers or those in contact with animals. Patients should be encouraged to participate in sports but to avoid contact sports such as rugby, wrestling and judo because of the risk of injury to the kidney.

Infection

The main complication of immunosuppression is the risk of infection, both in the postoperative period and in the long term. High doses (or large combinations) of immunosuppressive drugs can increase this risk.

Bacterial infections are more common during the first few weeks following transplantation. Following discharge, urinary tract infection is most common and patients should be taught how to recognize early signs and symptoms, particularly dysuria, frequency and cloudy urine, remembering that for many patients micturition has ceased during their time on dialysis. Reporting these symptoms promptly ensures early diagnosis and treatment with oral antibiotics and reduces the risk of damage to the transplant, or the need for hospital admission for intravenous therapy. Later infections, up to about 6 months after transplantation, tend to be fungal or viral in origin, commonly candidiasis or herpes simplex. Despite the use of prophylactic acyclovir, CMV infection can occur during the first year of transplantation. Treatment includes intravenous ganciclovir and may necessitate reduction or discontinuation of immunosuppression to prevent systemic effects, particularly on the gastrointestinal tract, lungs, kidney and liver.

Rejection

For many transplant recipients, postoperative recovery is short and they are discharged home within 10 days of surgery. Acute rejection may be a problem they have yet to experience and it is important that they are prepared for this prior to going home. They should be aware of the signs and symptoms, although it should be reinforced that many patients do not experience any signs other than being informed of a rising creatinine level and a need for a biopsy to confirm the diagnosis. The different reasons for a rising creatinine level should be explained, together with the process of investigating these to establish the cause. Urinary tract infection, dehydration, obstruction and cyclosporin toxicity can all have the same effect on kidney function and these causes should be eliminated prior to biopsy. Frequent outpatient visits allow the appropriate investigations to be done promptly; urine is sent for culture, fluid balance is assessed, cyclosporin levels are measured and ultrasound scans are performed. If these tests fail to establish the reason for the deterioration in kidney function a transplant biopsy will confirm the diagnosis of acute rejection. The patient should be reassured that prompt diagnosis and early treatment should ensure that acute rejection is reversed and kidney function restored.

Follow-up appointments

The importance of attending follow-up appointments to monitor both graft function and general health as well as to try and minimize side-effects of drugs needs to be stressed to the patient prior to discharge and a plan should be made to ensure s/he is aware of the frequency of visits and the routine to be followed. Once explained, most patients see this routine as being far more acceptable than that enforced by dialysis and are reassured by their attendances, in the knowledge that problems will be discussed and addressed promptly and kidney function closely monitored.

Outpatient appointments become less frequent as the months go by and graft function stabilizes, although the patient will continue to require lifelong follow-up care by the transplant centre, or by returning to the referring renal unit.

TRANSPLANT FOLLOW-UP: THE FIRST 3 MONTHS

It may be considered that the first 3 months are the most intensive in terms of follow-up appointments, investigations and dose changes, as well as being the most stressful because of the uncertainty of the future (Bergstrom, 1993).

During this time the provision of consistent information and advice is essential to maintain the patient's confidence and compliance, and the role of an experienced transplant nurse in providing this and ensuring a smooth transition from inpatient to outpatient care is recognized as being an important part of a successful transplant programme.

Follow-up visits are used to reinforce information given prior to discharge and to provide a natural progression in the development of the patient's knowledge by answering questions as they arise and ensuring that relevant information is given at appropriate times. This would include explaining the need for using high-factor sun creams during the summer or when taking holidays abroad because of the increased risk of skin cancer from immunosuppressive treatment, or reminding patients about the recommendation for flu vaccines at the appropriate time of the year. During the first 3 months the avoidance of infection is most important as immunosuppressive drug doses are at their highest level. Patients should be advised to adopt a high standard of personal hygiene and a sensible attitude towards contact with others. Avoidance of crowded public places, e.g. pubs and restaurants at busy times, Saturday shopping and public transport should be advised – although not to the extent that patients do not allow themselves to return to a normal lifestyle.

Swimming should be discouraged until immunosuppressive doses start to be reduced and, in CAPD patients, until after the catheter has been removed and the wound healed.

Advice should be given to increase activity appropriately as general health improves. Sexual activity can be resumed once the patient feels comfortable, and discussion of sexuality should include ensuring patients understand the likelihood that they will become fertile again following transplantation. Contraceptive advice is important and relevant to both sexes and women should be advised that pregnancy should be avoided at least for the first year following transplantation to allow time for kidney function and drug doses to be stabilized (Davison, 1995). It should be stressed that fertility can return before the first menstrual period starts and barrier methods of contraception should be used until the menstrual cycle is established. The risk of infection should also be discussed and the use of barrier methods of contraception encouraged in both sexes to reduce the risk of sexually transmitted disease, particularly *Chlamydia* and HIV. The use of hormonal contraception should always be discussed with the renal physician and risk factors such as hypertension and thrombosis considered before starting this method. Women should be advised to have yearly cervical smears because of their increased risk of malignancy from immunosuppressive treatment, particularly if they are premenopausal (Brunner *et al.*, 1995).

Changes in appearance are common following transplantation as a result of immunosuppressive treatment. The patient should be reassured that these changes are usually temporary and associated with the higher doses of prednisolone and cyclosporin given in the first few months following transplantation. Female patients become particularly concerned about changes in body image associated with a cushingoid appearance, increased hair growth and acne, and a sensitive but realistic approach by the nurse helps to restore confidence and ensure that practical advice is well-received.

Gum hypertrophy is a common side-effect of cyclosporin, particularly in patients who take nifedipine for hypertension. Regular dental checks and 3-monthly visits to the hygienist should be advised to minimize the risk of infection. In severe cases substituting a different antihypertensive drug should be considered and the dentist may consider trimming of the gums.

Patient scenario

Darren, a 30-year-old single man, received a live donor transplant from his brother and had an uneventful postoperative recovery. He returned to work within 2 months of his transplant and was soon enjoying an active social life. By 3 months post-transplant Darren had developed a cushingoid appearance and acne that were starting to concern him, although he was reassured that recent high cyclosporin levels and steroids would have exacerbated this. He also revealed that he had recently developed sore, inflamed gums. As well as cyclosporin, he was taking nifedipine for hypertension, which is known to potentiate the effect of cyclosporin on the gums. The dose of nifedipine was therefore reduced and an alternative hypertensive drug was introduced, while maintaining the cyclosporin level within the low range and encouraging regular visits to the dental hygienist. Within 2 months Darren's dental hypertrophy had subsided and dental surgery had been avoided.

THE PSYCHOLOGICAL IMPACT OF TRANSPLANTATION

To the general public, influenced by media attention, a kidney transplant is the optimum solution to the many problems experienced by dialysis patients. In reality, however, it can take many weeks or months for life to improve following a kidney transplant and for some patients the psychological problems caused by long-term uncertainty and drug side-effects can out-weigh the benefits, or at least affect their quality of life. Careful preparation of the patient for the changes s/he is likely to experience, as described earlier, helps to ensure that the psychological impact of transplantation is a positive one and allows the patient to adapt more easily to his/her new lifestyle (Dowsett, 1996).

The attitudes of other people, including family, friends and employers or work colleagues can also influence the patient's ability to return to normal. Overprotective family members, particularly those who had an active role in caring for the patient while s/he was dependent on dialysis, can inadvertently prevent the patient from regaining independence and confidence in his/her abilities. Others may see the patient as being cured and have no understanding of the insecurities of unstable kidney function, particularly in the early days.

Employment is a recurring problem among people with kidney failure, irrespective of the treatment (Jerrum and Blundell, 1995). Transplant recipients frequently experience lack of understanding by their employers, who see continual hospital visits as a reason to declare the patient unfit for work. This may be reasonable in the short term, but in the long term the patient is likely to become far more employable than he ever was on dialysis. The uncertainty of the future can also hinder unemployed trans-plant recipients in their search for a job – a frequent dilemma is whether to declare the fact that they have had a transplant, fearing that this may result in discrimination. Pretransplant employment is an important predic-tor of returning to work post-transplant (Matas, 1996) and every effort should be made to encourage the patient to return to work where appro-priate, as this is a significant way in which quality of life can be improved.

LONG-TERM PROBLEMS

About 90% of first cadaveric kidney transplants are still functioning after 1 year, 60–70% after 5 years and approximately 50% after 10 years (UKTSSA, 1995). The commonest causes of graft failure after the first year are chronic rejection or death with a functioning transplant.

For those patients whose transplants continue to function there are a number of problems that may be experienced as a result of long-term immunosuppression (Table 15.1). Severe joint pains, particularly in the knees and hips, may indicate osteoporosis or avascular necrosis of the hip. Transplant recipients have an increased risk of malignancy, particularly lymphoproliferative disease, skin cancers and cervical cancer (Brunner *et al.*, 1995).

Minimizing the risks of cardiovascular disease is an important part of transplant follow-up care and the role of the nurse in health promotion in conjunction with the dietitian, transplant physician and general practitioner should not be underestimated. Continued advice on healthy eating to assist in cholesterol reduction and weight control, limiting alcohol intake and stopping smoking, as well as strict control of hypertension, are all important

Table 15.1 Oral immunosuppressive drugs, their actions and side-effects

Drug	Action	Common side-effects
Prednisolone	Reduction in circulating lymphocytes Anti-inflammatory effect	Increased appetite, indigestion, sodium and water retention, muscle wasting, acne, mood changes, alteration of fat deposition – cushingoid appearance, osteoporosis, glucose intolerance, decreased wound healing, cataracts
Cyclosporin	Specifically acts on T lymphocytes, suppressing production of interleukin-2, preventing maturation of cytotoxic T cells, thus causing immunosuppression without inhibiting neutrophils	Nephrotoxicity, hepatotoxicity, gum hypertrophy, tremor, drug interactions, hypertrichosis, hyperlipidaemia, gout
Azathioprine	Inhibits DNA and RNA production, reducing lymphocyte proliferation and impairing antibody production	Bone marrow suppression – neutropenia, increased risk of infection, increased risk of malignancy, liver disease
Tacrolimus	Suppresses T-cell activation and lymphokine formation More potent than cyclosporin	Increased risk of infection, tremor, headache, paraesthesia, gastrointestinal problems, nephrotoxicity
Mycophenolate mofetil	Selective for T and B lymphocytes activated against the graft	Digestive disturbances

elements in helping to prevent cardiovascular complications. Lipid abnormalities are common following transplantation and may be partly attributed to steroid and cyclosporin therapy (Raine, 1994). Dietary measures alone have not proved effective in reducing hyperlipidaemia in transplant recipients, and research is currently being undertaken to ascertain the effect of lipid-lowering agents in patients on cyclosporin.

The fear of rejection remains for many patients the overriding cause of anxiety following transplantation in both the short term and the long term. Whereas acute rejection can usually be reversed if diagnosed and treated promptly, chronic rejection is more difficult to treat and is characterized by a gradual deterioration in graft function, usually over months or years. Despite extensive research, the mechanism of chronic rejection remains essentially unclear (Allen and Chapman, 1994), and the appearance of chronic changes on a transplant biopsy would suggest that the patient needs to be prepared for the gradual deterioration in graft function and inevitable return to dialysis. At this stage, following what may have been years of freedom and a normal life, the patient starts to experience the insecurity associated with unstable kidney function and the prospect of returning to a life of restriction and dependence. Careful monitoring of both kidney function and control of symptoms such as loss of appetite, breathlessness, oedema and lethargy associated with anaemia should ensure that dialysis is started at an appropriate time with the minimum detriment to the patient's wellbeing.

Losing a transplant as a result of chronic rejection is a risk that all transplant patients should be made aware of but this should nevertheless be kept in perspective. Although the risk of recurrent disease must be considered for some patients, re-transplantation is a realistic option for most patients losing their first or second graft and the success rates are similar (UKTSSA, 1995): 45% of first transplants and 43% of second transplants are still functioning after 10 years. The risks increase with third or subsequent grafts, although 34% are still functioning after 10 years, proving that re-transplantation in most cases is a worthwhile consideration.

REVIEW QUESTIONS

- List the risk factors that are considered during pretransplant assessment.
- What information would you give the patient while preparing him/her for transplantation?
- Describe the nurse's role in the prevention of infection in the immunocompromised patient.
- What are the main considerations when preparing a patient for discharge?
- List the three most commonly used immunosuppressive drugs and their main side-effects, explaining the nurse's role in minimizing these side-effects.
- Describe some of the long-term problems associated with transplantation and immunosuppression.

REFERENCES

Allen, R. D. M. and Chapman, J. R. (1994) *A Manual of Renal Transplantation*, Edward Arnold, London.

Bergstrom, C. E. (1993) Do I feel better now after the transplantation? *Journal of the European Dialysis and Transplant Nurses Association–European Renal Care Association*, **19**(3), 18–19.

Briggs, J. D. (1995) Patient selection for renal transplantation. *Nephrology Dialysis Transplantation*, **10**(Suppl. 1), 10–13.

Brostoff, J. and Male, D. K. (1994) *Clinical Immunology: An illustrated outline*, C. V. Mosby, St Louis, MO.

Brown, J. H. (1995) Pre-transplant management: cardiovascular and bone disease. *Nephrology, Dialysis and Transplantation*, **10**(Suppl. 1), 14–19.

Brunner, F. P., Landais, P., and Selwood, N. H. (1995) Malignancies after renal transplantation: the EDTA–ERA Registry experience. *Nephrology, Dialysis and Transplantation*, **10**(Suppl. 1), 74–80.

Davison, J. M. (1995) Towards long-term graft survival in renal transplantation: pregnancy. *Nephrology, Dialysis and Transplantation*, **10**(Suppl. 1), 85–89.

Dowsett, D. A. (1996) Psychological needs of adult patients following renal transplantation and implications for care. *Journal of the European Dialysis and Transplant Nurses Association–European Renal Care Association*, **22**(2), 2–6.

Dyer, P. A., Martin, S. and Sinnot P. (1995) Histocompatability testing for kidney transplantation: an update. *Nephrology, Dialysis and Transplantation,* **10**(Suppl. 1), 23–27.

Goodwin, C. (1992) Prophylactic acyclovir: Study of its use in renal allograft recipients. *Journal of the European Dialysis and Transplant Nurses Association– European Renal Care Association,* **18**(2), 29–30.

Jerrum C. D., Blundell L. (1995) Employment and dialysis: investigative study of patients and employers. *Journal of the European Dialysis and Transplant Nurses Association–European Renal Care Association,* **21**(3), 33–36.

Marshall, V. C., Jablonski, P. and Scott, D. F. (1994) Renal preservation, in *Kidney Transplantation Principles and Practice,* 4th edn, (ed. P. Morris), W. B. Saunders, Philadelphia, PA.

Matas A. J. *et al.* (1996) Employment patterns after successful kidney transplantation. *Transplantation,* **61**(5), 729–733.

Milligan, C. (1994) Discharge: outpatient services provided for renal transplant recipients. *Journal of the European Dialysis and Transplant Nurses Association– European Renal Care Association,* **20**(3), 36–38.

Nakahara, N., Harima, M., Nakatani, T. *et al.* (1993) A study of patient teaching on kidney transplantation in a dialysis facility. *Journal of the European Dialysis and Transplant Nurses Association–European Renal Care Association,* **19**(3, 20–22.

Newstead, C. G. (1995) Cytomegalovirus disease in renal transplantation. *Nephrology, Dialysis and Transplantation,* **10**(Suppl. 1), 68–73.

Patel, M. G. (1995) The impact of dietary advice in newly transplanted patients. *Journal of the European Dialysis and Transplant Nurses Association–European Renal Care Association,* **21**(Suppl. 1).

Pereira, B. J. G. (1995) Hepatitis C infection and post transplantation liver disease. *Nephrology, Dialysis and Transplantation,* **10**(Suppl. 1), 58–67.

Przygrodzka, F., Rayner, H. C., Morgan, A. G. and Burden, R. P. (1992) Changes in nutritional status after successful renal transplantation. *Journal of Renal Nutrition,* **23**(Suppl. 1), 18–20.

Raine, A. E. G. (1994) Cardiovascular complications after renal transplantation, in *Kidney Transplantation Principles and Practice,* 4th edn, (ed. P. Morris), W. B. Saunders, Philadelphia, PA.

Sheil, A. G. R. (1994) Cancer in dialysis and transplant patients, in *Kidney Transplantation Principles and Practice,* 4th edn, (ed. P. Morris), W. B. Saunders, London.

Ting, A. and Welsh K. (1994) HLA matching and crossmatching in renal transplantation, in *Kidney Transplantation Principles and Practice,* 4th edn, (ed. P. Morris), W. B. Saunders, Philadelphia, PA.

UKTSSA (1995) *Annual Report,* United Kingdon Transplant Support Service Authority, Bristol.

Patient education  16

Nicola Thomas

LEARNING OBJECTIVES

At the end of this chapter the reader should be able to:

- Assess how far an individual wishes to be self-caring.
- Discuss the potential barriers to learning.
- Understand how to facilitate patient empowerment with respect to patient teaching.
- Explain the main implementation strategies of a patient education programme in a renal care setting.
- Be familiar with the use of a teaching audit tool.

INTRODUCTION

Health education is an integral part of the nephrology nurse's role (Kuentzle and Thomas, 1995). Teaching occurs in a variety of settings. On a small scale, the nurse is involved in educating the patient about taking immunosuppressive therapy, while a lengthy training programme over a number of months allows an individual on haemodialysis to become self-caring at home.

This chapter will be divided into four sections: the assessment of the patient's learning needs; the planning of educational goals; the implementation of the teaching programme; and finally how the patient's learning may be evaluated and how the nurse's teaching skills may be assessed.

ASSESSMENT OF LEARNING NEEDS

It is vital that any patient education programme is individualized to each patient. It could even be argued that some patients fail to become proficient at self-care dialysis because all patients, (regardless of age, gender, social status or culture) are subjected to similar training programmes.

The first stage in any patient education programme has therefore to be the assessment stage. This first section will consider the assessment of self-care abilities and learning styles. It will also help the nurse to identify any potential barriers to learning.

Self-care abilities

A number of influences exist that may affect an individual's ability to self-care. These influences (sometimes called self-care determinants) may be physical, social or psychological. However very little literature exists that specifically examines self-care determinants of individuals receiving dialysis; it is generally accepted that those variables that influence readiness for self-care are poorly understood (Baker and Stern, 1994).

> **Key reference:** Baker, C. and Stern, P.N. (1994) Finding meaning in chronic illness as the key to self-care. *Canadian Journal of Nursing Research* 25(2): 23–36.

Locus of control

Some authors believe that the concept of personal control may be useful in predicting how well an individual might cope with a self-care therapy such as CAPD. 'Locus of control' (LoC) refers to the extent to which individuals believe that people have control over their own destiny (Rotter, 1954). Individuals who are internally controlled believe that what happens to them is primarily due to their own actions or attributes. When events are perceived by an individual to be the result of fate, luck, chance or the influence of powerful others, such individuals are termed externally controlled (Berger, 1972).

Research into locus of control often tends to focus on those who are required to carry out self-care therapies, e.g. individuals who have diabetes mellitus or those who are maintained on dialysis (Christensen *et al.*, 1990; Lowery and Ducette, 1976). The assumption is that it is beneficial for all patients who are self-caring to have control, yet the questions of whether all patients want this control and whether giving patients control is always advantageous is not always addressed.

However it appears important to discuss with the patient at the start of any education programme how much responsibility s/he wishes to take for his/her health. If the patient appears to be internally controlled, then it may be beneficial to teach the patient about all aspects of his/her care. If s/he tends towards being externally controlled, and needs to learn CAPD, for example, then it may be better if s/he is taught just to perform bag changes while other persons such as a relative/district nurse take on responsibilities such as exit site care or blood sugar monitoring.

Readiness for self-care

A patient's readiness for self-care may also be important. Readiness for self-care may be defined in terms of motivation and attitude. How patients see themselves in relation to their illness also appears to be a critical factor in their receptivity to self-care teachings. If an individual has been very debilitated by acute renal failure that has resulted in end-stage renal failure, s/he may not be ready for a self-care therapy until his/her physical health has improved.

A number of authors have described the process of psychosocial adaptation to illness and its effects on receptivity to teaching (Redman, 1993). For example an individual who is still in the denial stage of his/her illness ('This couldn't happen to me') is possibly more likely to suppress and distort information relating to self-care. In later stages of the adaptation, it is considered that people become better able to understand the illness, to hear facts about it and to participate in their own care. The length of time between the diagnosis of end-stage renal failure and the commencement of CAPD training therefore appears important, so if a patient appears to be still in the denial stage it is better to delay the start of training.

Health beliefs

There is evidence to suggest that health beliefs may play an important part in determining whether or not an individual will undertake a recommended health action. The health belief model (Rosenstock, 1974), affirms that an individual's likelihood of undertaking a health action may be affected by the person's susceptibility to the disease, the vulnerability s/he has to the side-effects, the severity of the disease and beliefs about the efficacy of the treatment. This model was originally formulated to explain why people would or would not undertake health actions, and it has later been applied to predict a level of compliance with prescribed therapies.

For example if a patient's parent had died of renal failure caused by diabetes mellitus, the patient may be much more likely to listen to health advice concerning his/her blood pressure control. If another patient does not believe s/he has ESRF because he/she simply does not have symptoms (such as lethargy, itchy skin or nausea), then he/she may be much less likely to learn about fluid allowance effectively.

Social influences – family support

It has been suggested that the amount and quality of social support an individual receives may have an influence upon how well s/he copes with a self-care therapy. As Welch (1994) suggests, simple indicators of social resources such as marital status and number of social contacts are strong predictors of mortality and morbidity. Recent reviews have identified three distinct areas that may be important. These areas are the structural aspects of the individual's social network, such as its size and number; the functional aspects such as the overall ratings of satisfaction with these supports; and the individual's functioning in social roles as a parent, worker, friend (Guadagnoli and Mor, 1990).

Because social support variables that influence coping with self-care may be very complex, it could be argued that the findings of research that attempts to measure the effect of social support may be flawed. Indeed, as Welch (1994) explains, a weakness of generic, multidimensional measures of health status is that they provide a few broad items covering social resources, and important information, such as the type of social network available, may be missed.

However the suggestion that social support is important in coping with home CAPD has not been clearly substantiated. A literature review on this topic found no evidence to suggest that those with strong family support did better than those who lived alone. However it must also be recognized that a daily visit from a district nurse could replace the support given by one or two family members living at home. The effects of social support on coping remain unclear.

Language and culture

If a patient has difficulties in understanding and speaking the English language, it is possible that an incomplete understanding of the self-care philosophy and potential social isolation from other patients might lead to difficulties in coping with dialysis. However there appears to be little literature that examines the effect of culture on health attitudes and behaviour (Dickinson and Bhatt, 1994).

Dickinson and Bhatt (1994) investigated this further and found that Chinese men and south Asian women showed a slight tendency to believe that health was a matter of luck. Interestingly, among the south Asian population there was also a view that suffering caused by ill-health sometimes had a divine purpose, although this was much less believed among Urdu speakers. These results are supported in a study by Howlett *et al.* (1992), who found that higher proportions of Asians and African-Caribbeans than matched respondents saw health as a matter of luck. It appears important to consider the effect of culture on self-care practices prior to the commencement of any patient education programme.

A qualitative study by Anderson (1991) examined the experience of chronic illness of 30 immigrant women in Canada. This author concluded that multiple factors influence the ability to manage illness, although one of the most important factors could be the sense of self that is constructed during the course of a chronic illness. For the immigrant woman, the difficulties of living with a chronic illness are exacerbated by the experience of being uprooted from her home land and resettling in a new country. She must deal with her marginality, social isolation and alienation in a foreign culture.

In the assessment stage, the nurse must examine how far the patient understands spoken/written English. Although the use of professional interpreters is not always practicable in a hospital setting, the ethical dimension of using a family member for interpretation must be considered.

Age

It is difficult to conclude whether the age of an individual is an important variable. There is evidence to suggest that older people consult health-care professionals more than younger people (Reid, 1992), yet in this study it was also found that the older age group reported higher levels of self-management. Kalfoss (1990) found that, as individuals became older, they were more likely to believe that doctors controlled their health. Older adults often appear to lack confidence in learning self-care therapies such as CAPD, but once the training period has been successfully completed it could be argued that older individuals do well if they are aware that they can consult an on-call nurse 24 hours a day. The stereotype of an older adult being more reluctant to take on self-care therapies may be misguided.

Physical difficulties

Barriers to learning CAPD that have been identified by Wild (1994) include physical barriers such as poor vision or manual dexterity. However it is also not clear whether difficulty in manipulating the practical skills required for CAPD has any long-term deleterious effects on the patient's ability to cope.

The severity of uraemic symptoms may also play a part in being a barrier to learning, as severe uraemia may result in lowered mental alertness (Teschan *et al.*, 1979) and memory deficits (Osberg *et al.*, 1982). Although there is evidence that renal disease may affect patients' abilities to concentrate (Schira, 1994), the resultant poor concentration span and memory retention during a training period may not necessarily have any long-term effects.

Summary

This section has examined the psychological, social, demographic and physical influences that need to be considered in the assessment phase of a patient education programme. It appears that the degree of responsibility an individual wishes to take for his/her health needs to be considered, along with his/her motivation and health beliefs. The amount and type of social support a patient receives appears to influence how well s/he copes with a self-care therapy, as long as the complexities of the potential support available are recognized.

It is important to consider the effect that an individual's culture has on the ability to self-care, in terms of language and health beliefs. There appears to be no conclusive evidence that either age or gender has an influence upon self-care practices. Although many nurses assume that there are potential barriers to learning a skill (such as CAPD exchanges) that have a physical basis, there does not appear to be any substantive

Table 16.1 Pre-education assessment

Influence on learning	Examples of questions to be asked
Psychological	
Locus of control	'Do you like to take decisions regarding your illness or do you prefer to leave decisions to the doctor/nurse?'
Motivation	'Do you feel ready to learn about your dialysis?' 'How much do you know about the dialysis already?'
Health beliefs	'Do you worry that the kidney failure may take over your life?'
Social	
Amount/type of social support	'How far does your partner/family wish to be involved in the dialysis?'
Language	'Do you have any difficulties in understanding what I'm saying?'
Age	'Do you think that your age may affect how easily you learn to do the dialysis?'
Physical	
Uraemic symptoms	'How tired are you feeling at the moment?' 'How good do you think your concentration span is at the moment?' 'Do you feel better in the morning or the afternoon?'
Physical ability	'Do you have any difficulties in keeping your hands steady?' 'How good is your eyesight?'

evidence to support the theory that these difficulties will affect the outcome in the longer term.

Table 16.1 shows some pertinent questions that nurses could ask in the assessment of a patient prior to the commencement of CAPD or haemodialysis training.

PLANNING OF EDUCATIONAL GOALS

Following assessment, the nurse needs to negotiate the learning goals with the patient and his/her family. If the assessment has been comprehensive the nurse should now be able to plan the education programme, bearing in mind the needs of the adult learner. This section will consider the educational approach that the nurse may use and will discuss other important areas to consider in the planning process, such as the timing of the educational programme, the learning environment and the inclusion of the patient's family.

Principles of adult learning

It is not possible within the scope of this chapter to discuss in detail the concept of adult learning (andragogy), so the reader is referred to the standard text on this subject (Knowles, 1970). It is also important to recognize that individuals learn in different ways (Kolb, 1976), so the patient educator needs to be aware that some patients may prefer doing while others may prefer watching or thinking.

Patient empowerment

Empowerment has been defined as 'the process of helping people to assert control over the factors which affect their lives' (Gibson, 1991). The EDTNA/ERCA philosophy (Kuentzle and Thomas, 1995) supports the notion of empowerment by stating: 'Partnership in care will be developed between patient, his/her family and nephrology nurse, to stimulate patients' independence, self-care and rehabilitation' (p. 14).

In order that nephrology nurses are able to facilitate empowerment, they must first consider whether they treat patients as true partners in health-care. Indeed, Molzahn (1996) believes that it is hardly likely that patients in nephrology settings can consider themselves empowered, as the research literature abounds in articles describing feeling of helplessness, powerlessness, lack of control and lack of compliance among individuals with ESRF.

Key reference: Molzahn, A.E. (1996) Changing to a caring paradigm for teaching and learning. *American Nephrology Nurses Association Journal* (23)1: 13–18.

Loreno and Drick (1990) believe that nurses' personal beliefs about health may influence the ways in which they act as patient educators. There may also be a tension between the concepts of caring and empowerment, as Malin and Teasdale (1991) suggest. If renal nurses are truly to facilitate patient empowerment with respect to education, then they must help patients realize that they have power and they must educate them about how to exercise that power (Molzahn, 1996).

Molzahn (1996) has suggested that, in order to facilitate empowerment, nurses must reconsider the whole teaching/learning strategy in health education. She states that an important element in this is to be aware that health-care providers do not hold the answers to all problems. She also recommends the importance of self-reflection. Once individuals reflect on topics and identify personal meanings for those topics, they will be more motivated to learn. This could be done by journal writing, discussion with others and allocating time to think in relaxing environments.

Timing of the teaching programme

A common mistake made by health professionals is that of trying to teach too much during a short period of time (Rankin and Duffy, 1983). It is therefore very important to tailor each session to the individual patient's needs.

Consideration needs to be given to the time of day and the length of each session. Some patients may learn better in the morning, while some may only have a concentration span of 10 minutes. It has been suggested that the ideal length of a patient training session is only 15 minutes (Haggard, 1989).

> **Key reference:** Haggard, A. (1989) *Handbook of patient education.* Maryland, Aspen Publishers.

Environment

Ideally the area set aside for patient education should be quiet and away from the busy ward environment. As Wild (1995) suggests, the area suitable for CAPD training could be made to look non-clinical by the use of easy chairs, a coffee table, pictures and bookshelves.

Webb (1985) describes how 'learned roles' may inhibit learning. By this she means that nurses have knowledge that gives them power, they use jargon and they have a certain prestige or status. Conversely patients may have a lack of knowledge, they are possibly inarticulate with respect to their treatment and they feel vulnerable. These concepts may lead to a 'social distance' between patient and nurse, which in turn stops learning taking place. It could be argued that by attempting to train patients in a hospital setting, we are simply perpetuating this social distance. Clearly, training for CAPD in the patient's home should be considered.

How far should the patient's partner/family be involved?

Although some renal units believe that an individual should be solely responsible for carrying out his/her self-care dialysis, the needs of each patient should be considered. If his female partner has completely cared for the patient since he became ill, then it may be appropriate for her to continue to do so. This may include carrying out the CAPD exchange for her husband/partner. The role of the patient's family in his/her care should be discussed in the assessment stage. It is not appropriate that nursing staff should inflict their personal values and beliefs on patients.

Summary

Negotiation of learning goals should always be discussed with the patient and his/her carers. The nurse should always consider the way in which the individual might learn best. If the aim is to safely self-care for a Tenckhoff catheter exit site, the nurse should ask the patient how s/he wishes to achieve this. Options could include observing the skill on a number of occasions, attempting the skill under supervision or watching a video that explains how to carry out the procedure.

Whenever any learning is being planned, the nurse must consider the effect of the length of the teaching programme and the corresponding concentration span of the patient. Health-care providers should always plan an education programme that is patient-centred.

IMPLEMENTATION OF THE LEARNING PROGRAMME

This section considers how the nurse may carry out the educational process and includes:

- principles of teaching;
- learning activities;
- educational media (audio-visual aids);
- possible topics to be included in a CAPD education programme;
- difficulties in teaching older patients.

Principles

Principles that could be used to plan a teaching session are shown in Table 16.2 (adapted from Ewles and Simnett, 1992), which also illustrates how these principles could be applied in educating a patient about his/her fluid allowance.

Learning activities

A number of differing learning activities allow the nurse to individualize education to the patient's needs.

One-to-one teaching

This is an ideal method for teaching the patient a technical skill, such as self-cannulation of arteriovenous fistula or CAPD exchange. As Rankin and Duffy (1983) describe, the advantages of this method include an active

---

Table 16.2 Principles of patient education

- Say important things first
  'It is important that you keep to the fluid allowance as much as possible.'

- Stress and repeat key point
  'A build-up of fluid may cause swelling in the legs.'

- Give specific, precise advice
  'Your allowance is 800 millilitres a day – the equivalent of four teacups.'

- Structure information into categories
  – The signs of fluid overload
  – The signs of dehydration

- Avoid jargon
  Explain what 'going low' on dialysis means

- Use a variety of educational media (e.g. visual aids)
  Use a measuring jug to demonstrate 800 ml

- Get feedback from the patient to ensure that s/he understands
  Ask how s/he might plan to take the fluid during the day, e.g. tea/water for tablets/milk on cereal

---

learner role (which may increase patient's confidence in self-care), an opportunity for consistent and frequent feedback and the flexibility to create an unstructured, informal atmosphere. The main disadvantages of this method is a lack of sharing of the experience with patients in a similar situation.

Group teaching

The advantage of group teaching is that it helps the patient to learn about other people's experiences, which in turn allows the patient to understand that s/he is not suffering from the effects of renal failure in isolation. Possible areas for group discussion include the side-effects of immunosuppression for those who are recently transplanted, explanation of blood results for those on haemodialysis or the importance of good protein intake for those on CAPD.

In large groups it may be difficult for the nurse to evaluate whether individual learning goals have been met, and it is possible that some patients may feel unable to contribute to the discussion because of lack of self-confidence or difficulties with language.

Self-study

A variety of materials have been specifically written to inform patients about renal replacement therapies. Although the majority are written in English and are therefore not always suitable for those who do not have English as their first language, this method of learning allows the patient to go at his/her own pace. However the nurse must ensure that if essential topics are to be learnt this way (such as how to recognize signs of graft rejection), there are sound methods in place to test patient knowledge following the period of self-study.

Computer-assisted learning

Wild (1994) describes the use of a computer-assisted learning package, which was developed by Luker and Caress (1991). She has found that patients find the package both simple and fun to use, and that it is one of the most popular educational aids that her patient group have access to.

Key reference: Wild, J. (1994) 'Education for self-care: a CAPD training programme' in McGee, H. and Bradley, C. (eds) (1994) *Quality of life following renal failure*. Harwood Academic Publishers, Switzerland.

It is disappointing that there are few of these packages available at present for renal patients, but it is possible that many more will be developed in the near future.

Educational media (audio-visual aids)

As patients only remember approximately 7–30% of verbal information (Haggard, 1989) it is recommended that the training programme uses a variety of audio-visual aids. Examples of these are:

- Slides
- Flipchart
- Posters
- Overhead projector
- Videos
- Games (e.g. Robinson *et al.*, 1988)
- Plastic torso (to show position of Tenckhoff catheter).

An example of a CAPD education programme

Table 16.3 shows an example of the topics that might be included in a CAPD education programme. It is useful if all of this information is supplemented with a patient training manual. It is also recommended that the manual be available in other languages than English to cater for the needs of differing ethnic groups.

Table 16.3 An example of a CAPD training programme (Source: adapted from the CAPD training manual of the Royal Hospitals Trust, London)

Healthy kidneys and kidney failure
- Position of kidneys/ureter/bladder
- Kidney function and kidney disease

What is CAPD?
- Explanation of dialysis and what CAPD means
- Exchange procedure and cleanliness

Fluid balance
- Weight and blood pressure control
- Explanation of desired weight/blood pressure/fluid allowance
- Identification of dehydration and fluid overload
- Use of different-strength bags

Care of exit site
- Advice on bathing/showering
- Cleaning site and applying dressing
- Anchorage

Possible complications
– identification and action
- Peritonitis
- Exit site infection
- Leakage of fluid from exit site
- Disconnected/cracked line
- Blood in bag
- Fibrin in bag
- Constipation

Daily activities
- Work
- Sex, fertility and contraception
- Exercise, including simple exercises to strengthen leg and stomach muscles
- Holidays

Diet

Medication
- Phosphate binders and vitamin D supplements
- Laxatives
- Blood pressure controlling agents
- Erythropoietin and iron supplements

Delivery of supplies
- How to reorder
- Collection of waste
- Holiday deliveries

Advice on follow-up
- Clinics
- Blood tests, including information of adequacy
- Home visits
- Line change

Table 16.4 Teaching older patients

Areas to consider	Action
Manual dexterity	Assess which type of CAPD system is most appropriate by use of simulated equipment
Visual loss	Ensure eyesight has been tested and glasses are correct prescription
Hearing loss	Check hearing aid is working Speak towards ear that is less deaf Adjust pitch of voice as required
Concentration span	Use short sessions (less than 10 min) with rest Frequently assess level of tiredness
Short-term memory deficit	Ensure presentation is logical Use reinforcement and repetition
Lack of self-confidence in learning situation	Assess how patient may learn best, e.g. video/computer may not be appropriate Be particularly encouraging and give positive feedback Be realistic about how much patient can achieve Use other health professionals, e.g. district nurse, to aid self-care

Teaching older patients

As there have been a large increase in the number of elderly and frail patients receiving renal replacement therapy over the past years (Will and Johnson, 1994), many of these individuals have to learn to be self-caring on dialysis. It is therefore important to be aware of the very specific educational needs of this group. Table 16.4 shows some areas which need to be considered.

Summary

When carrying out the teaching programme it is important to consider a variety of learning methods in order to sustain patient attention and motivation. All teaching strategies should be individualized to patient need in terms of type of learning activity, educational media used and content of programme. The nurse should be positive and encouraging at every stage of the learning process and be aware of the effect of his/her attitude on the patient's confidence.

EVALUATION OF LEARNING

It is important that patients' learning is assessed at the end of the teaching programme, although sadly it is often a component of the education programme that is neglected.

Rankin and Duffy (1983) have indicated that the evaluation process should include the following steps:

- measuring the extent to which the patient has met his/her learning objectives;
- indicating when there is a need to clarify, correct or review information;
- noting objectives that are unclear;
- pointing out shortcomings in the patient-teaching interventions, specifically addressing content, format, activities and educational media.

Coles (1994) suggests that health-care professionals must learn to assess their own performance and progress. This assessment should include identification of their strengths and weaknesses with respect to the education they have facilitated for the patient.

Haggard (1989) has included an audit document for evaluating how well the nurse has executed the patient education programme. An adapted version of their evaluation form is shown in Table 16.5.

Table 16.5 Teacher evaluation form

	Achieved?	Not achieved?	Comments
RAPPORT			
Introduces self to patient			
Has friendly nature			
Enquires about patient's wellbeing			
ASSESSMENT			
Uses open-ended questions to assess			
• readiness for self-care			
• health beliefs			
• social support			
• physical barriers to learning			
• existing knowledge			
PLANNING			
Sets realistic goals with patient/family			
Communicates goals to rest of health-care team			
IMPLEMENTATION			
Uses adult learning principles			
States objectives to be accomplished			
Uses variety of teaching methods			
Uses appropriate language			
Encourages questions and answers simply			
Allows for rest periods			
Gives positive feedback and encouragement			
Communicates patient progress verbally and in writing			
EVALUATION			
Frequently assesses patient learning			
Ensures that patient is safe to self-care			
Arranges short- and long-term follow-up care			

Summary

This chapter has explored some of the pertinent issues that face renal nurses in their role as patient educators. It is important for nurses to individualize training programmes to patient need and to be aware that assessment of a patient's self-care abilities is a fundamental aspect of successful patient education. Nurses also need to assess their own performance and to be conscious of the effect of their own values and beliefs on the learning process. Carers should be included in any patient education programme and health-care professionals must ensure that a variety of teaching and learning methods are included in order to maintain interest. As Wild (1994) has commented, 'Teaching and learning should be simple and fun'.

REVIEW QUESTIONS

- What are the possible psychological, social and physical influences that may affect learning?
- How might renal nurses facilitate patient empowerment when planning and implementing a patient teaching session?
- What are the different types of educational media that could be used in educating a patient about care of an arteriovenous fistula?
- What criteria might be used to evaluate teaching?

REFERENCES

Anderson, J. M. (1991) Immigrant women speak of chronic illness: the social construction of the devalued self. *Journal of Advanced Nursing*, **16**, 710–717.

Baker, C. and Stern, P. N. (1994) Finding meaning in chronic illness as the key to self-care. *Canadian Journal of Nursing Research*, **25**(2), 23–36.

Berger, S. M. (1972) Locus of control and the effectiveness of direct and vicarious reinforcement. *Psychonomic Science*, **26**, 345–346.

Christensen, A. J., Smith, T. W., Turner, C. W. *et al.* (1990) Type of haemodialysis and preference for behavioural involvement: interactive effects on adherence in end-stage renal disease. *Health Psychology*, **9**(2), 225–236.

Coles, C. (1994) Optimising long-term care of renal patients through the education of health professionals, in *Quality of Life Following Renal Failure* (eds H. McGee and C. Bradley), Harwood Academic Publishers, Chur, Switzerland.

Dickinson, R. and Bhatt, A. (1994) Ethnicity, health and control: results from an exploratory study of ethnic minority communities' attitudes to health. *Health Education Journal*, **53**, 421–429.

Ewles, L. and Simnett, I. (1992) *Promoting Health – A Practical Guide*, Scutari Press, Oxford.

Gibson, C. H. (1991) A concept analysis of empowerment. *Journal of Advanced Nursing*, **16**, 354–361.

Guadagnoli, E. and Mor, V. (1990) Social interaction tests and scales, in *Quality of Life Assessments in Clinical Trials*, (ed. B. Spilker), Raven Press, New York, pp. 85–94.

Haggard, A. (1989) *Handbook of Patient Education*, Aspen Publishers, Rockville, MD.

Howlett, B. C., Ahmad, W. I. U. and Murray, R. (1992) An exploration of white, Asian and Afro-Caribbean people's concepts of health and illness causation. *New Community*, **18**(2), 281–292.

Kalfoss, MH. (1990) Factors in appraisal in chronic illness. *Nursing Times*, **86**(16), 55.

Knowles, M. S. (1970) *The Modern Practice of Adult Education*, Association Press, New York.

Kolb, D. A. (1976) *The Learning Style Inventory: Technical Manual*, McBer, Boston, MA.

Kuentzle, W. and Thomas, N. (1995) *European Curriculum for Nephrology Nursing*. F-Twee, Ghent.

Loreno, P. and Drick, C. A. (1990) Self-care identity formation – a nursing education perspective. *Holistic Nursing Practice*, **4**(2), 79–86.

Lowery, B. J. and Ducette, J. P. (1976) Disease related learning and disease control in diabetics as a function of locus of control. *Nursing Research*, **25**(5), 358–362.

Luker, K. and Caress, A. (1991) The development and evaluation of computer assisted learning for patients on CAPD. *Computers in Nursing*, **9**, 15–21.

Malin, N. and Teasdale, K. (1991) Caring versus empowerment: considerations for nursing practice. *Journal of Advanced Nursing*, **16**, 657–662.

Molzahn, A. E. (1996) Changing to a caring paradigm for teaching and learning. *American Nephrology Nurses Association Journal*, **23**(1), 13–18.

Osberg, J. W., Meares, G. J., McKee, D. C. and Burnett, G. B. (1982) Intellectual functioning in renal failure and chronic dialysis. *Journal of Chronic Diseases*, **35**, 445–457.

Rankin, S. H. and Duffy, K. L. (1983) *Patient Education: Issues, Principles and Guidelines*, J. B. Lippincott, Philadelphia, PA.

Redman, B. K. (1993) *The Process of Patient Education*, 7th edn, Mosby/Year Book, St Louis, MO.

Reid, B. V. (1992) 'It's like you're down on a bed of affliction': aging and diabetes among black Americans. *Social Science and Medicine*, **34**(12),1317–1323.

Robinson, J. A., Robinson, K. J. and Lewis, D. J. (1988) Games: a motivational educational strategy. *American Nephrology Nurses Association Journal*, **15**, 277–279.

Rosenstock, I. M. (1974) Historical origins of the health belief model. *Health Education Monograph*, **2**, 328–335.

Rotter, J. (1954) *Social Learning and Clinical Psychology*, Prentice Hall, Englewood Cliffs, NJ.

Schira, M. G. (1994) The role of cognitive function in educating patients with ESRD. *Nephrology Nursing Today*, **4** (3), 1–2, in *American Nephrology Nurses Association Update*, **24**(3), insert.

Teschan, P. E., Ginn, H. E., Bourne, J. R. *et al.* (1979) Quantitative indices of clinical uraemia. *Kidney International*, **15**, 676–697.

Webb, P. (1985) Getting it right – patient teaching. *Nursing*, **2**(38), 1125–1127.

Welch, P. (1994) Assessment of quality of life following renal failure, in *Quality of Life Following Renal Failure* (eds H. McGee and C. Bradley), Harwood Academic Publishers, Chur, Switzerland.

Wild, J. (1994) Education for self-care: a CAPD training programme, in *Quality of Life Following Renal Failure* (eds H. McGee and C. Bradley), Harwood Academic Publishers, Chur, Switzerland.

Will, E. and Johnson, J. (1994) Options in the medical management of end-stage renal failure, in *Quality of Life Following Renal Failure* (eds H. McGee and C. Bradley), Harwood Academic Publishers, Chur, Switzerland.

Organ donation 17

Pam Buckley

LEARNING OBJECTIVES

At the end of this chapter the reader should be able to:

- Understand the mechanisms for identification, referral and management of the potential organ donor and his family.
- Appreciate the tests performed to confirm brain-stem death.
- Discuss the ethical issues in organ donation and transplantation.

INTRODUCTION

Renal transplantation has become the treatment of choice for many patients suffering from end-stage renal failure. With developments in immunosuppressive therapy regimens, tissue typing and crossmatching techniques graft survival is currently 84% at 1 year and 70% at 5 years (UKTSSA, 1995).

The major problem facing renal transplant units is a shortage of donor organs. In the UK kidney transplant waiting lists have increased from 3468 in 1986 (UKTSA, 1987) to 5150 in 1996 (UKTSSA, 1996). Improving the supply of donor organs is imperative if all patients selected for renal transplantation are to be offered this opportunity.

UK PRACTICE IN OBTAINING ORGANS FOR TRANSPLANTATION

Organ transplantation is dependent on the goodwill of the public, who decide to donate their organs and tissues after death. The donor card scheme was introduced into the UK in 1971 but despite all efforts to encourage the public to carry donor cards only around 25% of the population actually do so.

It has become the practice in most intensive care units (ICUs) to make a request for organ donation to relatives whose family member has become brain-stem dead. The confidential audit of intensive care unit deaths (Gore *et al.*, 1992) found that only one in 10 deaths occurring in ICUs was confirmed as brain-stem death and that only half of these resulted in organ donation from the deceased. This same study discovered that 30% of families to whom the request for organ donation was made refused this request. A further study (UKTCA/BACCN/MORI, 1995) discovered that 26% of families who were asked refused the request for organ donation. Of the donations that took place one in four had come about following an offer from the relatives. Requests to relatives are usually made by a senior doctor, supported by the nursing staff caring for the patient.

Key reference: UKTCA, BACCN and MORI Health Research (1995) *Report of a Two Year Study into the Reasons for Relatives' Refusal of Organ Donation.* Department of Health, London.

The request for organ donation has often to be made when the family are suffering from immense grief and shock due to the diagnosis of brain-stem death in their loved one. At this time it is difficult for many to make any decision, particularly when the wishes of their relative regarding organ donation are not known.

Whether further public education will improve organ donation rates is questionable. However, any prompt to discuss this topic where rational decisions can be taken will only be a good thing. Families can then make an informed response when asked about the wishes of their deceased relative.

OTHER SYSTEMS FOR OBTAINING ORGANS FOR TRANSPLANTATION

Presumed consent/opting out

This is a system whereby citizens either register their wish not to donate organs after death or are automatically removed, if required, for transplantation. Several European countries (Austria, Spain, Belgium, France) have adopted this system. High levels of organ procurement in these countries are attributable to many factors, including the rate of road-traffic deaths and the provision of intensive care beds.

Road-traffic deaths in the UK are among the lowest in the EU (Office for National Statistics, 1997), with 7.42 adult deaths per 100 000 of the population. For Spain, Austria and Belgium, the figures are 16.23, 19.44 and 19.53 respectively.

Required request/required referral

Required request or required referral obliges doctors caring for potential donors either to make the request for donation or to refer the potential donor to the transplant team, in order that the Transplant Coordinator can approach the family. Some states in the USA have adopted this system and failure to comply may bring a penalty.

Opting-in

In the UK, where organ donation is considered to be an altruistic gesture, a system of opting-in is the practice. Citizens opt-in by carrying a donor card, making a verbal statement to their family or registering on the National Donor Register.

The donor register was set up in 1994 in an attempt to improve organ donation rates. Those wishing to register as a donor complete and return an application form. The details of the request are held on a database. To preserve confidentiality, the database can only be accessed by nominated personnel. As a matter of courtesy the relatives are asked for their agreement for the deceased's wishes to be carried out, even if their registration has been confirmed. The National Donor Register is currently located within the premises of the UK Transplant Support Service Authority (UKTSSA) in Bristol.

BRAIN-STEM DEATH

Brain-stem death is the tragic consequence of severe and irreversible injury to the brain stem, which occurs following a major intracranial catastrophe or prolonged cerebral anoxia. Death of the brain stem leads to failure of brain-stem reflexes, including the corneal reflex, gag reflex and cough reflex. The patient is comatose and unable to make any respiratory effort. These patients therefore require full support of the respiratory and cardio-vascular system by artificial ventilation. The application of brain-stem death criteria to confirm brain-stem death in a patient is undertaken by clinicians in intensive care units as part of the management of the patient and not for the purpose of transplantation. Confirmation of brain-stem death facilitates the retrieval of organs for transplantation as these can be retrieved with minimal warm ischaemia.

What tests are applied to confirm brain-stem death

The patient must be in coma and requiring ventilatory support because spontaneous respiration has become inadequate or ceased. The coma must be due to irremediable structural brain damage.

Prior to application of the brain-stem death tests, the two doctors who will perform the tests must satisfy themselves that the patient is not in apnoeic coma due to:

- the influence of depressant or sedative drugs;
- metabolic or endocrine disturbance;
- primary hypothermia.

Diagnosis of brain-stem death

- Patient in apnoeic coma
- Confirmation of irreversible structural brain damage
- Exclusion of reversible cause of coma:
  - Hypothermia
  - Drugs
  - Metabolic or endocrine disturbance
- Absent brain-stem reflexes
- Apnoea confirmed

The **diagnostic tests** for the confirmation of brain-stem death are described in the UK Code of Practice (Department of Health Working Party, 1983). All brain-stem reflexes are absent:

- The pupils do not respond to light.
- There is no corneal reflex.
- The vestibulo-ocular reflex is absent.
- There are no motor responses within the cranial nerve distribution when stimuli are applied to any of the somatic areas.
- There is no gag reflex or reflex response to bronchial stimulation by a suction catheter passed down the trachea.
- No respiratory movements occur when the patient is disconnected from the ventilator for long enough to ensure that the arterial carbon dioxide tension rises above the threshold for stimulation of respiration.

The tests should only be applied when the patient has been in coma for a minimum of 6 hours, unless the primary cause of the coma was a cardiac arrest, when 24 hours should elapse before testing.

The medical staff performing the tests should have expertise in carrying out neurological examinations but need not be neurologists or neurosurgeons. The two doctors must not be part of the transplant team. It is usual for one to be the consultant of the patient and the other a consultant or senior registrar who is clinically independent of the first. The tests are usually applied twice and although there is no specific instruction in the code of practice, it is usual in many intensive care units to wait 1–8 hours between the first and second testing. Repetition of the tests is to confirm the observations that have been made and it is imperative that the relatives are counselled appropriately to avoid misunderstanding and false hope. The British Paediatric Society recommends that it is rarely possible to confidently diagnose brain-stem death in babies between 37 weeks gestation and 2 months of age (British Paediatric Association, 1991).

Following the second set of tests, the patient is declared dead and the ventilatory support is withdrawn, unless organ donation is taking place, when full ventilatory and circulatory support should continue until organ retrieval takes place. At this point, it may be necessary to make some changes to the management of the deceased to ensure optimum function of the organs to be transplanted and this is referred to as 'donor management'. It is important to note that a death certificate may be issued upon completion of the second set of brain-stem death criteria and before organ retrieval, unless this is precluded by the requirement to refer investigation of the of the death to the Coroner or Procurator Fiscal.

REFERRAL OF THE POTENTIAL DONOR TO THE TRANSPLANT TEAM

Any patient who is brain-stem dead should be considered for **potential organ donation**. The contraindications to donation are that the patient is:

Sequence of events for cadaveric organ donation

Patient suffers brain injury
↓
Treatment in Intensive Care
↓
1st set brain-stem death tests
↓
Request for donation/Referral to transplant coordinator
↓
2nd set brain-stem death tests and confirmation of death
↓
Donor maintenance
↓
Organ retrieval

- aged over 75 years;
- suffering from gross and untreated sepsis;
- suffering from a malignancy outside the central nervous system;
- HIV-, Hepatitis-B- or Hepatitis-C-positive, or has any other transmissible virus;
- suffering from certain neurological disorders, including Creutzfeldt–Jakob disease.

The referral of a potential donor is usually made to the transplant coordinator. S/he will attend the intensive care unit to facilitate the process of organ donation. Assessment of the past medical history and current status will ascertain which organs are suitable for transplantation.

For kidney donation areas of interest are:

- **Past medical history**
  - a history of long-standing untreated or poorly controlled hypertension;
  - a history of diabetes mellitus where there is renovascular disease;
  - repeated urinary tract infections that may have caused scarring to the kidneys;
  - the presence of renal calculi, haematuria or abnormal anatomy of the urinary tract that may either make the kidney unsuitable for transplantation or make the transplant technically more difficult;
  - a family history of adult polycystic kidney disease or other hereditary renal disease that may also affect the potential donor.
- **Current status**
  - blood pressure;
  - urine output;
  - urea and electrolyte estimations;
  - presence of any urinary or other infection;
  - any injury to the abdomen, pelvis or urinary tract.

To encourage immediate function of the kidney following transplantation, the donor should have medical management to optimize renal function by:

- maintenance of a systolic blood pressure of over 90 mmHg; inotropic support, usually low-dose dopamine, may be prescribed to improve renal function if hypertension persists despite adequate hydration;
- optimizing urinary output to 1–3 ml/kg. body weight/h; desmopressin may be prescribed as an intravenous or intramuscular injection to treat diabetes insipidus, which can lead to electrolyte imbalance and cardiovascular instability.

Samples of urine should be sent to the microbiology laboratory for culture.

Multiorgan donation, where the liver and thoracic organs may also be transplanted, demands attention to the instigation of other donor management manoeuvres appropriate to these organs.

Blood samples are taken from the donor for tissue typing and virological screening once relatives' consent for donation has been obtained.

Requirements for the virological screening of all organs and tissue donors have been laid down (NHS Executive, 1996). Current screening tests are to detect HIV antibody, Hepatitis B surface antigen and antibody to Hepatitis C. It has also become the practice in many units to ascertain the Cytomegalovirus antibody status of the donor.

TISSUE TYPING

All human tissue transplants from one individual to another are at risk of rejection. The extent of the risk depends on the differences in genetic products between the donor and the recipient. One of the most important factors is matching for the HLA system genes. The HLA antigens, first identified on leukocytes, are now recognized on all nucleated cells within the body.

The genes of the major histocompatibility complex (MHC-HLA) are divided into loci, with the main HLA loci considered in solid organ transplantation being HLA-A, HLA-B and HLA–DR. The MHC is highly polymorphic; hence there are many alleles at each locus, making exact matching very difficult.

Each individual has two HLA alleles at each loci, one inherited from each parent. An example of an individual's tissue type would be A2, A11, B7, B44, DR4, DR7, the A2, B44, DR7 haplotype being inherited from one parent and the A11, B7, DR4 haplotype from the other. Certain tissue types are found more frequently in certain populations, allowing calculation of the chance of a well-matched kidney and the probable waiting time for each patient. For example, the alleles A2, B44 and DR4 are common within the white British population. When matching a donor kidney to a possible recipient it is usual to give a figure for the number of mismatches at the A, B and DR loci, recording how many alleles the donor has that the recipient has not. Examples of mismatch grading between donor and recipient are shown in Table 17.1. In the first example, where the mismatch grade is 101, this gives an indication that there is one mismatch at each of the A and DR loci, i.e. the donor has two alleles, A25 and DR15, that the recipient does not possess. The recipient is then likely to develop antibodies against these, increasing the chances for rejection if not adequately controlled. The third example identifies a total of five alleles that the donor possesses and the recipient does not, two HLA-A alleles (A30, A5), two B alleles (B50 and B60) and one DR allele (DR17).

Table 17.1 Examples of mismatch grading between donor and recipient

Donor type	Recipient type	Mismatch grade HLA A, B, DR
A2, A3, B7, B8, DR1, DR17	A25, A3, B7, B8, DR17, DR15	101
A28, A31, B44, B45, DR13, DR15	A31, A32, B41, B44, DR13, DR15	110
A2, A29, B37, B57, DR8, DR18	A5, A30, B50, B60, DR8, DR17	221

The practice in the UK is to treat mismatches 100, 110 and 010 as preferentially matched, as matches at the DR locus give a much higher graft survival rate. Unfortunately, because of the scarcity of donor organs, even to give a DR match in all cases is not possible; hence kidneys are matched first by blood group. This practice ensures that everyone on the waiting list has a fair chance of receiving a transplant, especially group O recipients, who would otherwise be disadvantaged, as group O organs can be transplanted to anyone, although the above matching criteria still apply.

ORGAN ALLOCATION

Patients selected for renal transplantation are registered by their local transplant unit with the UK Transplant Support Service Authority (UKTSSA), whose base is in Bristol. At UKTSSA, all patients are entered into a national database that holds data on all patients awaiting transplantation in England, Scotland, Wales, Northern Ireland and Eire. When a kidney becomes available, the tissue typing details are entered into the database and the computer selects the patients with the least antigen mismatches to it. Should there be several patients who are equally matched, then the kidney is offered to the centre that is in the most credit with the national sharing scheme. On each occasion that a kidney is exported from the centre that retrieved it for use in another centre, one credit point is awarded to the retrieving centre. On acceptance of a kidney from another centre, a unit loses a point. This creates a 'balance of trade' between all units participating in the sharing scheme.

Other factors taken into consideration when allocating kidneys are the panel reactive antibody status of the recipient and clinical urgency. On a local basis, each transplant unit is allowed to select its recipient for a kidney by its own criteria. Antigen mismatching is usually considered to be very important but the duration of dialysis treatment, efficacy of dialysis and age-matching between the donor and recipient are also taken into account by many units.

Final allocation depends upon the lymphocytotoxic crossmatch test, which is performed between lymphocytes taken from the donor, the source of which is usually the spleen, and serum from the potential recipient. A positive crossmatch, particularly in respect of T cells, usually precludes transplantation. Some units are also using flow cytometric crossmatching, which is said to be more sensitive than the conventional lymphocytotoxic technique.

ORGAN RETRIEVAL

Organs are retrieved by the donor transplant team from the local transplant unit. The team usually comprises two surgeons, a theatre nurse and a perfusionist. The donor will be transferred from the ICU to the operating theatre. An anaesthetist will be responsible for the ventilatory and circulatory support management of the donor until these are withdrawn just prior to vascular clamping and perfusion of the organs.

The operation is performed to normal standards of theatre practice and asepsis although there is no necessity to do a swab count. The technique of kidney retrieval from a cadaveric donor is well described in many surgical textbooks. The surgeon mobilizes the kidneys, arterial and venous blood supply, and ureters. After this dissection, but prior to removal, the kidneys are preserved *in situ* by the placement of an aortic cannula through which cold kidney preservation fluid is flushed into the renal arteries. The effluent is drained by a cannula placed into the inferior vena cava. This flushing is commenced immediately after discontinuation of ventilation and minimizes warm ischaemia to the kidneys. Once cool and flushed, the kidneys can then be carefully removed from the donor.

The kidneys can be removed *en bloc* or singly depending upon the preference of the surgeon but great care must be taken to preserve the vasculature and ureters. Each kidney is transported double-bagged in sterile polythene bags containing preservation fluid and surrounded by an ice–water mixture in an insulated box to achieve a temperature of 4°C. The kidney is then transported to the potential recipient as quickly as possible to reduce the cold ischaemia time. Methods of transportation currently in use are road, rail and air. It is imperative that the method of transport chosen is quick, reliable and cost-effective. Transplantation of the kidney should ideally take place within 24 hours but a recent study on the outcomes of 17 937 kidney transplants (Peters *et al.*, 1995) reported that there was no adverse result from longer cold ischaemic times. However, many units are unwilling to transplant kidneys with 48 hours or more of cold ischaemia.

The surgical technique of renal transplantation is well described. The renal artery is usually anastomosed to the internal, external or common iliac artery of the recipient and the renal vein to the external iliac vein. The ureter is implanted into the bladder to re-establish the urinary tract, although in some patients with bladder or urethral problems an ileal conduit will have been fashioned in preparation for transplantation.

OBTAINING CONSENT FOR ORGAN DONATION

Counselling relatives about the impending death of a loved one is a task undertaken regularly by staff working in ICU. The requirement to make a request, when appropriate, for organ donation is viewed by some as an extra burden but also by many as an opportunity to offer the family something positive in what is otherwise a very negative situation. Staff should be trained in how to make this approach and how to handle the responses and questions that may ensue.

The transplant coordinator is always willing to make the approach to the relatives. A survey in the UK (UKTCA/BACCN/MORI, 1995) discovered that the approach is most commonly made by a senior doctor. Further information is usually given by the transplant coordinator once consent has been obtained. The person making the request for donation should have a positive attitude towards transplantation. Any negative feelings that s/he displays will be transmitted to the relatives. The request should be made in an unhurried fashion in a quiet room where relatives can be allowed to discuss their response. In many ICUs, the request is made between the first and second set of brain-stem death tests. It is preferable not to apply any time limits as to when a reply has to be made but, for practical reasons to do with the management of the patient, a decision should ideally be reached just prior to, or within a short space of time after, the second set of brain-stem death tests.

Information given to the relatives as part of the request should include:

- the need for the deceased to be transferred to the operating theatre while still having ventilatory support;
- reassurance that the operation will be carried out by skilled surgeons with due care and respect for their relative;
- the information that the wound will be sutured at the end of the operation and dressings applied;
- the necessity to screen the patient for certain viruses, including HIV.

Many relatives will ask about the timing of the release of the body from the hospital and if organ donation will hold up their organization of the funeral. Reassurance can be given that organ donation will not delay the funeral but the requirement for a post-mortem on behalf of the Coroner may do so. This would be the case even if donation did not take place.

Should the relatives agree to donation they should be thanked and, although there is no requirement to obtain written consent, this is good practice. There should be clarity about which organs and tissues the relatives have agreed to donate. The relatives should be offered the opportunity to remain in the ICU with their relative until s/he is transferred to the operating theatre.

Within a few days of the donation the transplant coordinator will contact the family to offer thanks for allowing donation and also to give them some information on the outcome of the transplants that have been performed, if they would like this. Most families are keen to hear about the welfare of the recipients. It is important to be honest and sadly, on occasions, this means giving news of the failure of a transplant operation.

Recipients of organ transplants often ask about their donor and can be offered the opportunity, if they so wish, to write a short letter to their donor's family, given that this would also be welcomed by them. Anonymity is preserved by the use of Christian names only and by all correspondence being handled through the transplant coordinator.

INITIATIVES TO IMPROVE ORGAN DONATION RATES

Public education

Public awareness campaigns have been undertaken on a national basis primarily by the Department of Health but there is also an organization called Transplants In Mind (TIME), which is made up of representatives from the various transplant charities. TIME organizes an annual event called National Transplant Week that aims to bring to the notice of the public the current shortage of organs and the successes of transplantation. The Department of Health have centred their campaigns on the donor card scheme and in the more recent past the donor register. The use of television advertising by the various agencies has been limited by the high cost of 'prime-time' TV.

The portrayal of issues surrounding organ donation and transplantation, as story lines in major television drama series or soap operas that are watched by millions is helpful in initiating discussion within families.

Continued public education must continue in order to reduce the number of refusals given by relatives because they do not know the wishes of their loved one. Information should be targeted at young people in schools and colleges if donation is to become an accepted part of death.

Professional education

The transplant coordinator is responsible for dissemination of information on organ donation and transplantation to health-care professionals. The target groups are medical and nursing staff working in critical care areas. These staff will identify potential organ and tissue donors. Education of medical and nursing students is undertaken to ensure support from the next generation of carers.

The education programme will provide the basis for the development of solid working relationships between the transplant team and staff in hospitals that provide donors. These relationships are the cornerstone of any successful organ donation programme.

LIVE DONATION

Live donor transplantation accounts for only 5–10% of all kidney transplants performed annually in the UK. This level of activity compares poorly with Norway, where 40% of all kidney transplants performed since 1969 were from live donors (Jakobsen, 1995). Reasons for the low rate in the UK are not known but one factor may be the increasing age of patients registered for transplantation. Many of these will not have a suitable donor among their siblings or elderly parents. It has not become common practice in the UK to transplant a kidney from a son or daughter to a parent but spouse to spouse transplants have been performed in several units. The ethics of a friend to friend transplant are under debate. All live donor transplants are required to comply with the Human Organ Transplant Act 1989 (HOTA). Part of the Act requires the surgeon to establish the genetic relationship between the donor and recipient. Where they are not related, the surgeon must apply to the Unrelated Live Transplant Regulatory Authority (ULTRA) for permission to perform the transplant.

Key reference: Human Organ Transplant Act (1989) Chapter 31. Her Majesty's Stationery Office, London.

Non-heart-beating donation (NHBD)

Prior to the acceptance of brain-stem death criteria, kidneys were retrieved on asystole. The warm ischaemia time between cardiac arrest and flushing of the kidneys led to delayed graft function in many of these kidneys. Some kidneys never functioned at all when retrieved in this way. Consequently, the advent of the acceptance of brain-stem death criteria and opportunity to retrieve kidneys from the heart-beating cadaveric donor was heralded as major progress in organ retrieval. Warm ischaemia was markedly reduced, with subsequent benefits in both immediate graft function and long-term graft survival.

A technique of *in situ* preservation of the kidneys in NHBD has revived interest in the use of a selected group of patients who die in the Accident and Emergency Department or hospital wards. On certification of death by cessation of respiration and cardiac output, a double-balloon, triple-umen catheter is introduced into the aorta *via* a small incision in the femoral artery. Once the catheter is in position, the two balloons are inflated, isolating the segment of the aorta from which the orifices of the renal arteries arise. Cold kidney perfusion solution is then rapidly infused. This flushes through the kidneys and the effluent is drained from the vena cava by the placement of second catheter *via* the femoral vein. The perfusion of the kidneys must take place as soon as possible after death and certainly within 45 minutes. Not all attempts at kidney retrieval by this method are successful. Misplacement of the aortic catheter with subsequent poor perfusion of the kidneys is an acknowledged problem. The Maastricht group (Wijnen *et al.*, 1995) report that 60% of NHBD kidneys suffer from delayed graft function. The requirement for immediate attendance at the site of the donor's death restricts the use of this technique to hospitals within a limited geographical radius of the base of the transplant unit. Despite some early encouraging results in Leicester, where they have adopted this technique, there has not been widespread interest in the UK.

Elective or interventional ventilation

Elective or interventional ventilation for the purpose of organ donation was first described by a team from Exeter (Feest *et al.*, 1990), who implemented a protocol drawn up by the transplant team and intensive care clinicians. Patients suffering from intracranial haemorrhage who fulfilled certain neurological criteria were considered for transfer to the ICU. The criteria were:

- characteristic mode of onset – sudden, with rapid development of coma;
- progressive decline in conscious level;
- deep coma – lack of withdrawal response to painful stimuli;
- intracranial vascular accident confirmed by computed tomography desirable.

Ventilatory support was instigated and death was confirmed by brain-stem death criteria, after which, with relatives' consent, organ donation

> **Key reference:** Feest, T. G., Read, H. N., Collins, C. H., Golby, M. G. S., Nicholls, A. J. and Hamond, S. N. (1990) Protocol for increasing organ donation after cerebro vascular deaths in a distinct general hospital. *Lancet* 335, 1133–1135.

took place. Despite the local success of the protocol, it was withdrawn on the instructions of the Department of Health following legal advice that the use of elective ventilation prior to brain-stem death constitutes a battery (an assault) in law.

ETHICAL ISSUES IN TRANSPLANTATION

The possibility of the restoration of health and preservation of life by the transplantation of organs from one human being to another became a reality in 1954 with the first successful kidney transplant in man. Earlier attempts at such a procedure had resulted in some very short-term success, which inevitably ended in the death of the recipient. Much of the success in the mid 1950s was due to improved knowledge of immunology and tissue rejection.

As with any major advances in medical treatment, transplantation has brought ethical problems that must be debated and resolved if the public are to have confidence in a mode of treatment that has an impact on the rights of the other human beings and other creatures.

Consent for donation

The Human Tissue Act 1961 allowed the removal of parts of the body for medical purposes provided that the deceased had not objected to this and that the surviving spouse or any surviving relative of the deceased do not object to this. This puts the onus on the relatives to decide, in cases where there has been no expression of a wish by the deceased, whether or not organ donation should take place. The relatives can override an expressed wish by the deceased to become a donor by refusing consent. Many object to this on the grounds that the deceased's stated wish, i.e. the carrying of a donor card, can be thwarted by any relative, including a long-lost, distant one. One way around this problem would be to have a family member who acted as a 'proxy' when his/her relative was unable to make a decision because of illness or death (see Patient scenario).

Patient scenario

A 48-year-old female suffered an intracranial haemorrhage and was declared brain-stem dead. Her family were asked about her wishes on organ donation. Her mother and sister stated that she had declared to them that she would wish to be a donor. The husband, who had not been present during this conversation, refused the request for donation on the grounds that he did not know what her wishes were. The organs were not removed.

Live donation

Live-donor transplantation raises many ethical issues. Coercion of potential donors by family pressure, financial reward, reduction of prison sentences and other incentives has thrust live donation into the world media and brought this form of transplantation into disrepute. In the UK, live donor transplantation has been supervised by the HOTA, which among its legislation ensures that transplantation occurs within clearly defined regulations. However, in the Third World the sale of kidneys continues, usually by the poor to the rich with the ethical decisions being made by transplant surgeons and others who benefit financially from such practices.

Xenotransplantation

Animals have been used for many years in medical therapies and research. There have always been those who felt that this was inappropriate and formed animal rights movements. The use of animals as organ donors, as in the early days of cardiac transplantation and the more recent advances towards the use of genetically engineered pigs as kidney donors, continues the debate. Concerns about the transmission of viruses and other diseases from the animal population to humans have been fired by the development of BSE in cattle and its transferral through the food chain.

> REVIEW QUESTIONS
>
> - What are the medicolegal requirements for organ donation to take place from a brain-stem-dead donor?
> - How are cadaveric kidneys allocated to recipients?
> - How can the number of kidney transplants performed be increased?

REFERENCES

British Paediatric Association (1991) *Diagnosis of Brain Stem Death in Infants and Children – A Working Party Report*, British Paediatric Association, London.

Department of Health Working Party (1983) *Cadaveric Organs for Transplantation A Code of Practice Including the Diagnosis of Brain Death*. Report of a Working Party on behalf of the Health Department of Great Britain and Northern Ireland, HMSO, London

Feest, T. G., Riad, H. N., Collins, C. H. *et al.* (1990) Protocol for increasing organ donation after cerebrovascular deaths in a district general hospital. *Lancet*, **335**, 1133–1135.

Gore, S. M., Cable, D. J. and Holland, A. J. (1992) Organ donation from intensive care units in England and Wales and two year confidential audit of deaths in intensive care. *British Medical Journal*, **304**, 349–355.

Human Organ Transplant Act (1989) *Human Organ Transplant Act 1989*, HMSO, London, ch. 31.

Human Tissue Act (1961) *Human Tissue Act 1961*, HMSO, London, ch. 54.

Jakobsen, A. (1995) *Transplantation '95. The Outlook for Transplantation Towards 2000*, (ed. R. W. G. Johnson), International Congress and Symposium Series 211, Royal Society of Medicine, London.

Office for National Statistics (1997) *Social Trends 27*, Government Statistical Services Publication, HMSO, London

Peters, T. G., Shaver, T. R., Ames, J. E. *et al.* (1995) Cold ischaemia and outcome in 17 937 cadaveric kidney transplants. *Transplantation*, **59**(2), 191–196.

NHS Executive (1996) *Guidance on the Microbiological Safety of Human Tissues and Organs Used in Transplantation*, Department of Health, London.

UKTCA/BACCN/MORI (1995) *Report of a Two Year Study into the Reasons for Relatives' Refusal of Organ Donation*, Department of Health, London.

UKTSSA (1995) *Renal Transplant Audit 1984–93*, United Kingdom Transplant Support Service Authority, Bristol.

UKTSA (1987) *Annual Report*, United Kingdom Transplant Service, Bristol.

UKTSSA (1996) *Monthly Bulletin*, United Kingdom Transplant Support Service Authority, Bristol.

Wijnen, R. M. H., Bouster, M. H., Stubenitsky, B. M. *et al.* (1995) Outcome of transplantation of non-heart beating donor kidneys. *Lancet*, **345**, 1067–1070.

FURTHER READING

Allen, R. D. M. and Chapman, J. R. (1994) *A Manual of Renal Transplantation*, Edward Arnold, London.

Pallis, C. and Harley, D. H. (1996) *ABC of Brain Stem Death*, 2nd edn, BMJ Publishing Group, London.

New, B., Salamon, M., Dingwall, R. and McHale, J. (1994) *A Question of Give and Take – Improving the Supply of Organs for Transplantation*, Kings Fund Research Report 18, Kings Fund Institute, London.

Wood, R. F. M. (1983) *Renal Transplantation – A Clinical Handbook*, Baillière Tindall, London.

Renal failure in childhood and adolescence

18

Marcelle de Sousa and Geraldine Ward

LEARNING OBJECTIVES

At the end of this chapter the reader should be able to:

- Describe the physical and emotional differences between children and adults.
- Understand the importance of the family in the care of the child with chronic renal failure.
- Identify main causes of chronic renal failure and its incidence in childhood.
- Recognize that children's dialysis requirements differ from those of adults.
- Be able to calculate BSA, FV and circulating blood volume for children requiring dialysis.
- Identify potential problems for the child on dialysis or after transplantation.
- Be aware of the psychological and emotional effects of treatment on child and family.

INTRODUCTION

Childhood and adolescence are unique periods of life in which many physical and emotional changes occur. Nurses caring for this group of patients must understand the social, psychological and developmental influences that may affect them and be able to plan their care to meet their needs appropriately. Chronic illness in childhood or adolescence may interfere with the maturation process and predispose to long-term problems affecting psychosocial adjustment to adult life.

When renal replacement therapy (RRT) first became available, many health-care professionals pondered on whether it was right that it should be offered to children. Treatment was traumatic and the efficacy and long-term

results were unpredictable (Riley, 1964). In spite of these misgivings, paren
tal pressure and the willingness of some physicians and surgeons to take risk
meant that paediatric RRT programmes did develop and children, b
surviving, showed that they could withstand the rigours of treatment. RR′
is now a widely accepted form of treatment for children in renal failure.

INCIDENCE OF CHRONIC RENAL FAILURE IN CHILDHOOD AND ADOLESCENCE

Chronic renal failure (CRF) in childhood is rare and numbers of patient
are small when compared with adults. Figures from the British Associatio
for Paediatric Nephrology (BAPN) give UK acceptance rates of nev
patients (aged less than 15 years) in 1993 to all treatment modalities (i.e
conservative, dialysis and transplantation) as 53 per million child popula
tion (p.m.c.p.), with 9.7 p.m.c.p. starting RRT (i.e. dialysis or pre-emptive
transplantation) in the same year. Although numbers of children may be
small they are best cared for in specialist paediatric renal units, which car
provide a child and family-orientated service (BAPN, 1995).

CAUSES OF CRF IN CHILDHOOD

Table 18.1 shows the main causes of CRF in childhood. 60% children wil
have a congenital or inherited renal disorder and some of these may have
a syndrome of problems of which renal failure is just one component. Such
children will require management by more than one specialist team, e.g
ophthalmology for the retinitis pigmentosa associated with nephronophthisis in Senior–Loken syndrome. It is important that other disabilities
are given appropriate attention and are not overshadowed by the renal
disorder.

Table 18.1 Common causes of CRF in childhood

- Dysplasia/hypoplasia
- Reflux nephropathy
- Obstructive uropathy
- Prune belly syndrome
- Cystinosis
- Henoch–Schönlein nephritis
- Infantile polycystic disease
- Alport's syndrome
- Nephronophthisis (medullary cystic disease)
- Haemolytic uraemic syndrome

THE CHILD, THE FAMILY AND THE NURSE

The child is vulnerable and dependent on others to nurture it until it reaches
maturity. For most children the family provides the ideal environment in

which growth and development can take place. Within the family the child feels secure but illness requiring hospitalization may threaten that security. Family-centred care (Casey, 1988), in which both the child and his/her parents are fully involved in the therapeutic programme, is vital in any paediatric renal unit. The nature of CRF is such that much of a child's treatment will be carried out by parents at home and the need for nurses to develop an effective, educative and supportive partnership with them is of prime importance. Children require explanations appropriate to their level of understanding (Douglas, 1993) and a knowledge of normal cognitive development will assist in this process.

Paediatric nurses are well aware that opportunities for play (not just the provision of toys) under the auspices of a qualified hospital play specialist are very important in helping children of all ages to develop strategies for coping with their treatment and in providing stimulating activity to promote normal development. Access to hospital schoolteachers is also vital to ensure that educational continuity is maintained.

PHYSIOLOGICAL DIFFERENCES BETWEEN CHILDREN AND ADULTS

At birth the process of development is incomplete: the healthy term infant has sufficient major organ function to live but the immaturity of these organs makes them vulnerable to insult. Infants and small children have fewer reserves and will in consequence decompensate more quickly than adults (Hadzinski, 1992). Growth is a dynamic process that differentiates childhood and adolescence from adulthood, which marks its completion. It is in infancy and again at puberty that statural growth occurs at a rapid rate. During the first year of life a baby grows approximately 25 cm, achieving 85% of its ultimate head circumference measurement. By 2 years of age a child should have reached 50% of its final adult height. Accurate measurements of height, weight and head circumference (in infants) should be carried out at regular intervals to detect abnormalities.

Although nephrogenesis is complete by 34 weeks gestation the glomeruli continue to grow to more than double their diameter by adulthood. Glomerular filtration rate (GFR) increases with age but only becomes proportional to body surface area (BSA) at about 3 years of age (Taylor, 1994). The term infant has a GFR of approximately 25 ml/min/1.73 m^2 BSA, which increases 50–100% in the first week of life. The relative immaturity of the kidneys at birth must be borne in mind when assessing renal function in the neonatal period. As the kidneys mature, even in the presence of CRF, it is possible for renal function to improve considerably after birth. Water comprises 80% total body weight in healthy neonates and falls to adult levels of between 45% and 60% by 1 year of age. Infants with CRF are often polyuric, lacking the ability to concentrate their urine, and in consequence may dehydrate rapidly: signs such as weight loss, reduced skin turgor, depression of the anterior fontanelle and skin mottling may occur.

Blood pressure (BP) rises with age so that normal adult values are higher than those expected in childhood. Size and gender have an effect on BP, so children of the same age may have a variation in normal levels. Measuring BP in infants and small children may be difficult and the interpretation of the results problematic if a child is distressed and uncooperative during the procedure. An appropriate size cuff, i.e. one whose bladder covers two thirds of the arm circumference, should be used to obtain an accurate reading (Dillon, 1994) and every effort should be made to ensure the child is as relaxed as possible during the procedure. This may mean waiting until the child is asleep or using distraction such as toys. Recordings that are high should be repeated (possibly several times) to ensure an accurate measurement is obtained. In paediatric renal units a selection of different cuff sizes should be available, as well as Doppler instruments, which provide a more accurate recording of systolic BP in infants in whom auscultation methods are unsuitable. Hypertension is rare in childhood and adolescence, between 1% and 3% of the child population being affected. Of this group 80–90% have underlying renal disease (Dillon, 1994). Control of BP is important in preventing decline in renal function and consequences such as encephalopathy and seizures.

PRESENTATION OF CRF IN CHILDHOOD AND INFANCY

CRF may manifest itself at any stage from the antenatal period onwards. Congenital causes of CRF are frequently detected during pregnancy, a factor which, in some cases, may result in termination. Where the parents choose to continue the pregnancy immediate referral to a paediatric renal unit should be made after delivery so that the baby can be assessed and appropriate treatment started as soon possible. Chronic dialysis from birth is rarely a treatment of choice and should be commenced only after appropriate discussion since it can be extremely difficult to obtain and maintain access. Biochemical abnormalities that do not require dialysis can cause neurological damage if left untreated and may compromise future quality of life; hence the need for appropriate treatment to be initiated as soon as possible so that if the child survives s/he will do so with minimal disability. The signs and symptoms of CRF are shown in Table 18.2.

One of the most noticeable signs of renal failure during childhood is failure to thrive, i.e. growth and development less than expected for age. The child with CRF often presents as a small, poorly nourished individual who is uninterested in food, may vomit frequently and appears lethargic and irritable.

Ill-health in childhood may be accompanied by many non-specific symptoms, which can make diagnosis difficult. A child's inability to say exactly where a pain is or to give a detailed history, coupled with what may be perceived as naughtiness, can lead to delays in parents or professionals recognizing that something is really wrong. Infants and small children in particular require thorough examination and assessment to exclude serious illness.

Table 18.2 Some signs and symptoms of CRF in childhood and adolescence

Young children	Older children
• Failure to thrive	• Small stature
• Feeding problems/vomiting	• Delayed puberty
• Lethargy/irritability	• Nausea and/or vomiting
• Failure to pass urine	• Anorexia
• Pallor/anaemia	• Pallor/anaemia
• Abdominal mass	• Enuresis/nocturia
• Developmental delay	• Polyuria/polydipsia
	• Tiredness
	• Learning difficulties/poor concentration

The goals of effective treatment of CRF should be to achieve:

- good biochemical balance;
- correction of anaemia;
- optimum nutrition;
- normal growth and development;
- pre-emptive transplantation (where possible).

NUTRITION

The majority of children with CRF have feeding problems, and symptoms such as anorexia, nausea and vomiting are common. Such symptoms may prevent intake of essential nutrients, leading to malnutrition, which in turn exacerbates the eating problem by impairing gastrointestinal motor function (Ravelli, 1995).

Nutritional therapy is one of the cornerstones of treatment since it can modify the effects of CRF by making the child feel better and improving growth. Residual renal function may also be preserved, thus delaying the need for RRT. To achieve the therapeutic goals of dietary management, appropriate and adequate intakes of energy, water, electrolytes, vitamins and minerals are needed. In addition protein and phosphorus intake will need to be regulated (Rigden et al., 1987). These criteria apply to children being treated either conservatively or by dialysis.

Key reference: Rigden, S.P.A., Start, K.M. and Rees, L. (1987) Nutritional management of infants and toddlers with chronic renal failure. *Nutrition and Health* 5(3/4): 163–174.

The benefits of protein restriction (to reduce uraemia) in children with CRF have to be balanced against the risks of protein malnutrition, which may impair growth, so in practice calorie supplementation (in the form of glucose polymers and/or fat emulsions) is the dietary manipulation most often used to restore anabolism (Rigden et al., 1987). Although protein restriction is rarely necessary once calorie intake is optimized, other dietary restrictions will be needed. Reduction of phosphate intake is of particular importance in the prevention of secondary hyperparathyroidism. Low phosphate formula milks are recommended for infants and young children for whom milk is an important fluid source and these can be fortified with calorie supplements. Calcium carbonate is the phosphate binder of choice since aluminium hydroxide is associated with neurological and skeletal toxicity in children (Andreoli et al., 1984). Restriction of sodium and potassium intake are only usually necessary when renal function is very poor or the child has become dialysis-dependent.

Most infants and small children with CRF require enteral feeding (nasogastric or gastrostomy) to achieve the desired intake of nutrients since they are usually reluctant to eat and may vomit frequently. Feeding such children orally may take several hours and the introduction of enteral feeding can make this a much easier process. (Parents are taught to carry out this process at home.) Enteral feeding may be necessary for many years and may be discontinued when the conservatively managed child starts school, since at this stage s/he can manage to drink the calorie supplements, including high-calorie commercially available drinks. Small children on dialysis may require tube feeding for much longer.

The principles of dietary management for children and adolescents on dialysis is the same as for CRF with the exception of fluid allowance. Some children continue to produce large quantities of urine even when being dialysed but for those who don't it must be remembered that fluid allowance will include a calorie supplement and compliance with this restriction can be difficult to enforce. Trying to interest anorexic children in food can be an uphill task. However, allowing them occasional treats and encouraging them to be aware of how they can control their own biochemistry can improve their cooperation.

After transplantation the emphasis changes from encouraging a high calorie intake to aiming for a nutritionally balanced diet. This can cause problems, particularly for older children and parents. Children whose appetite is stimulated by steroids and for whom food has suddenly become interesting can eat non-stop if allowed. Parents, thrilled that their child is at last showing an interest in food, may be reluctant to restrict his/her food consumption. This situation can soon lead to obesity, with its attendant problems both physical and psychological. By contrast, it is the authors' experience that younger children (particularly those who were being enterally fed immediately prior to transplant) may take some time to establish a normal eating pattern and rarely have problems with overeating.

Recombinant human growth hormone, an expensive and for some a painful treatment, has been used with varying success to improve statural growth.

TREATMENT MODALITIES

Treatment for children with CRF can be divided into three categories:

- conservative management;

- dialysis – peritoneal or haemo;
- transplantation.

Most children will experience a combination of treatment modalities during their lifetime.

Conservative management

Conservative management is usually necessary when the GFR falls below 50 ml/min/1.73 m^2, since below this level the metabolic consequences of impaired kidney function become apparent (Rigden et al., 1987). Conservative management should achieve the treatment aims mentioned earlier, which may slow the progression to ESRF. To meet these goals the child and family will require constant support from the multidisciplinary team. Delaying RRT is only worthwhile if the child feels well, is growing and is able to undertake normal activity.

Many paediatric centres aim to transplant children without prior dialysis (Rigden et al., 1990; Nevins and Davidson, 1991) since it can expose them to potential problems (Flom et al., 1992) and is associated with higher stress levels in children and their families (Reynolds et al., 1988).

Transplantation

Renal transplantation offers the best chance of a normal life to the child with CRF. Pre-emptive transplantation is favoured in many paediatric centres in order to avoid the negative effects of dialysis. However this is not possible for every child. Children with congenital nephrotic syndrome or some forms of focal segmental sclerosis will usually require bilateral nephrectomy and at least a 3-month period on dialysis to normalize their body composition, which will have been compromised by huge urinary protein losses.

Successful renal transplantation has been carried out in very young children but poorer outcome is associated with either a donor or recipient aged less than 6 years (Arbus et al., 1991). Survival figures of 100% for patients and 57% for cadaveric grafts at 1 year have been reported (Fitzpatrick et al., 1992), compared with an 82% rate for recipients older than 5 years. Technical problems associated with the vascular anastomosis (leading to thrombosis) account for many of the graft failures. Older children and adolescents have graft survival figures similar to those of adults. Children are suitable candidates for either cadaveric or living-relative donation. Cadaveric kidneys for children tend to be from paediatric donors over 6 years of age; related donors are usually parents, since siblings may be too young to consent to surgery. The size of donor parent and recipient child should be considered in the planning phase. The psychosocial implications of live donation must be carefully assessed prior to surgery.

Preparation of the paediatric transplant recipient

This covers both physical and psychosocial elements and should be carried out in an ordered fashion to ensure that nothing that might compromise

Table 18.3 Transplant 'work-up'

- Tissue typing
- Infectious disease history
- Immunization history and completion of schedule, including BCG, HBV and Varicella
- Bladder assessment – surgery if needed to correct abnormalities
- Dental assessment and hygiene advice
- Ultrasound of IVC – to check patency
- Information – written, verbal and through play
- Meeting staff who will be involved in care
- Preparation for dialysis – it may be needed for some

Estimation of GFR (Morris et al., 1982)

GFR (ml/min/1.73 m^2) = 40 × height (cm) ÷ Pcr (plasma creatinine in mol/l)

future graft function is omitted. Most things can be done on an outpatient basis and in the authors' unit it is the practice to start this preparation in conservatively managed patients when the **estimated GFR** falls to 15 ml/min/1.73 m^2 (see margin). Table 18.3 shows the main aspects of the transplant 'work-up'. Children should complete the normal recommended immunization schedule and it is important to be aware of their immunity status, especially to those viruses associated with significant morbidity post-transplant, e.g. CMV, Epstein–Barr virus and Varicella (chickenpox).

Children, especially the very young, are less likely to have been exposed to the full range of infectious diseases than adults. The complication rate of common childhood diseases is high in immunocompromised individuals. Varicella vaccine is available on a named-patient basis and the Department of Health recommends its administration to those with negative antibody status prior to transplantation. Abnormalities such as the small, thick-walled bladder that frequently accompanies posterior urethral valves may require augmentation cystoplasty and the child or parent will need to be trained to carry out intermittent catheterization to ensure that the transplanted kidney is not damaged by a high-pressure system (Churchill *et al.*, 1996). When preparation is complete the child will go 'on call' for a cadaver kidney or a date will be arranged for a live donor transplant. Waiting times for first cadaver transplants can be variable, depending on blood group, tissue type and degree of matching required.

During the transplant work-up period there should be time for child and family to learn more about the treatment ahead and have an opportunity to discuss their fears and anxieties and decide (together with nursing and medical staff) what course of action will be best for them. Children being followed in the CRF clinic can start this preparation when their estimated GFR falls to around 15 ml/min/1.73 m^2.

Transplantation management

The care of children following transplantation is similar to that of adults but meticulous attention in ensuring accurate fluid management is crucial. An adult kidney may sequester between 150 and 250 ml blood (Ettenger *et al.*, 1991) and in the small child this can lead to hypovolaemia and hypotension with consequent delayed graft function. It may be prudent to electively ventilate a very small child for at least the first 12 hours postoperatively, especially when they are receiving an adult kidney, as an increase in intra-abdominal pressure due to the placement of the transplant may cause respiratory distress. Care will involve constant and regular monitoring of central venous pressure, BP and core and peripheral temperatures (Haycock, 1984). Intensive nursing care by paediatric nurses familiar with the significance of even seemingly unimportant changes in vital signs is essential.

Graft dysfunction may occur for all the same reasons as in adult patients but it must be remembered that even a small rise in plasma creatinine may represent a significant diminution in renal function (especially in small children receiving large kidneys; Ettenger *et al.*, 1996), and a rise of 10% above the accepted baseline or the previous reading requires investigation. Opportunistic infections in children, as in adults, are a significant cause of morbidity post-transplantation (see Patient scenario).

Organisms such as Varicella, CMV and *Pneumocystis carinii* may account for over 50% of the relatively few deaths (10%) in this patient group (Harmon, 1991).

Patient scenario

Polly's parents were told at routine antenatal scan that she had small, poorly functioning kidneys and given a gloomy prognosis for her survival. After her birth they were told to take her home to die, but at 5 weeks of age she was still alive and was referred for treatment to a paediatric renal unit. A diagnosis of renal dysplasia and vesico-ureteric reflux was made and at this time Polly had an estimated GFR of 5.44 ml/min/1.73 m^2, which never rose above 7.4 ml/min/1.73 m^2 during conservative management. Her weight was 3.1 kg and nasogastric feeding was commenced along with standard conservative drug therapy. At 15 months of age she underwent a pre-emptive cadaver transplant (7-year-old donor). During the first 6 months Polly experienced seven rejection episodes, which were all treated with high-dose oral prednisolone. At 3 months post-transplant, when Polly was noted to be consistently hypertensive, a renal artery stenosis was diagnosed. Balloon angioplasty at this time was successful but 3 months later the stenosis recurred and two further attempts at angioplasty failed. It was decided to treat Polly's hypertension with medication and at this time she required a combination of four drugs to maintain her BP within acceptable limits for her age. Two years post-transplant Polly contracted chickenpox and was treated in hospital with i.v. acyclovir, suffering no ill effects. Now, 7 years post-transplant, Polly, aged 8, is very well with excellent graft function. She attends mainstream school and is growing normally. Her BP is well controlled with only two antihypertensive drugs.

Medication

Immunosuppressive protocols vary between centres but most are based on triple therapy (prednisolone, azathioprine and cyclosporin), although newer immunosuppressants such as tacrolimus and mycophenalate mofetil (Ettenger, 1996) are being used in some cases. The side-effects of these drugs in both the short and the long term must be considered and whenever possible, the aim should to be achieve effective immunosuppression with the minimum medication possible, e.g. by using an alternate-day steroid regimen once graft function is stable about 12–13 weeks post-transplant (Guy's Hospital, 1996). The physical effects of steroids and cyclosporin can be very distressing for both children and parents (Maynard, 1993) and may result in failure to take medication. Teenagers who experience changes in body image, in particular, are at risk of becoming non-compliant with therapy. Ettenger *et al.* (1991) reported non-compliant behaviour in 64% of patients over the age of 13 years.

Key reference: Ettenger, R.B. (1996) Kidney transplantation in children, in *Handbook of Kidney Transplantation*, 2nd edn (ed. G. M. Danovitch), Little, Brown & Co., Boston, MA.

Liberation from previous dietary restrictions may result in obesity, often worsened by parental delight at seeing a previously anorexic child constantly hungry. Advice on healthy eating should be part of discharge planning and ongoing education.

Activity

There is no limit to the type of activity that can be undertaken post-transplant and all children should be encouraged to participate in sporting activities, both for their benefits to health and for the opportunities for social interaction that they offer. Some centres recommend the wearing of a protective shield to prevent trauma to the transplanted kidney, because of the vulnerability of its position in the abdomen (Burgess, 1982).

Children and adolescents are usually followed very closely after discharge from hospital and the frequency of outpatient visits gradually decreases as renal function stabilizes. As mentioned previously, childhood and adolescence is a time of continuous change, which may be affected by CRF and its treatment, so patients tend to be seen more frequently than in adult clinics to ensure that development is progressing normally. If this is not the case then modifications in therapy may be needed to ensure an acceptable quality of life.

Dialysis

Both peritoneal and haemodialysis are accepted and successful treatment modalities for children with either acute or chronic renal failure. Peritoneal dialysis is the preferred mode of treatment, since this is technically less demanding and less stressful for the child and family. Distance from the centre and social circumstances may be the deciding factor in the choice of treatment for chronic dialysis.

Dialysis disposables (lines, dialysers, filters, etc.) for even the smallest infant are now commercially available, permitting very young children to be treated. When dealing with small children special attention must be given to ensuring that lines and dialysers appropriate to the size of the individual child are used (Knight *et al.*, 1993). Dialysis by whatever method in infants (1 year of age) is associated with mortality rates of 16% (Bunchman, 1995).

Key reference: Knight, F., Gorynski, L., Bentson, M. and Harmon, W.E. (1993) Hemodialysis of the infant and small child with chronic renal failure. *ANNA Journal* 20(3): 315–323.

Haemodialysis and haemofiltration

It must be remembered that circulating blood volume is related to body size (Table 18.4). In order to prevent haemodynamic instability, extracorporeal blood volume (ECBV) should be calculated as 8–10% of circulating blood volume. Choice of dialysers will be determined by body surface area (BSA; equation (18.1)) and that of haemofilters by ECBV.

$$BSA = \sqrt{\frac{Height \times Weight}{3600}} \qquad (18.1)$$

Blood flows achievable for HD will depend on the size of the child: in the smallest (below 10 kg) rates vary from 30 to 75 ml (Knight *et al.* 1993) while those over 40 kg can tolerate flows up to 250 ml (Donckerwolcke *et al.*, 1996).

Children who require chronic dialysis need to attend a paediatric centre thrice weekly for HD and should be cared for by appropriately experienced nursing and medical staff (Bunchman, 1995). In the UK, home HD is no longer considered a suitable treatment modality for children.

Vascular access for HD may present problems in young children because of the small calibre of their blood vessels. When blood vessels are inadequate, synthetic grafts, e.g. Gore-tex®, may be used (Donckerwolcke *et al.*, 1996). Double-lumen central venous catheters are preferable for immediate use and as an alternative to cannulation of an arteriovenous fistula in the severely needle-phobic child. As with adults, clotting and infection are significant problems. The child and parent will require education about the care of his/her access.

Primary nursing in the paediatric HD unit is important in ensuring that the child experiences a consistent standard of care. Provision of an interactive environment in which it is possible for children to carry on with their education and develop as individuals will help to minimize disruption to their daily lives. Adolescent support groups can help to alleviate some of the alienating effect of chronic dialysis (Gorynski and Knight, 1992). The assistance of a play therapist and/or psychologist is sometimes necessary to aid children to overcome their fears about treatment (Knight *et al.*, 1993).

Table 18.4 Calculation of circulating blood volume

Age	Blood volume (ml/kg)
Neonates	85–90
Infants	75–80
Children	70–75
Adults	65–70

Haemofiltration is a popular treatment method for the acutely ill child in the paediatric intensive care unit where peritoneal dialysis is not a viable choice (Donckerwolcke *et al.*, 1996). This treatment may be carried out by suitably trained paediatric intensive care nurses.

Key reference: Donckerwolcke, R., Broyer, M., Chantler, C. and Rizzoni, G. (1996) Renal replacement therapy in children. In Jacobs, C., Kjellstrand, C.M., Koch, K.M., Winchester, J.F. (eds) *Replacement of Renal Function by Dialysis*. 4th Ed. Dordrecht: Kluwer Academic Publishers.

Peritoneal dialysis

In acute renal failure, PD is initiated after the insertion of a temporary peritoneal catheter, which can be inserted (in a heavily sedated child) in the ward treatment room. Continuous cycling peritoneal dialysis (CCPD) allows gentle removal of excess fluids and solutes without the risk of destabilizing the patient. Intensive nutritional therapy should be initiated as soon as possible to reduce catabolism. High calorie feeds may be given *via* a nasogastric tube or as total parenteral nutrition. Continuous fluid removal on CCPD allows greater flexibility in feeding regimens.

Chronic PD carried out in the home after an initial training period in hospital allows children and their families more control over their lives. Automated cycling dialysis machines are preferred to continuous ambulatory peritoneal dialysis (CAPD) in children, as they allow them to attend school full-time and the peritonitis rate is dramatically reduced, obviating the need for frequent hospitalization.

Fill volumes (FV) for PD in children are calculated according to BSA (equation (18.2)).

$$FV = 1.1 \text{ l/m}^2 \tag{18.2}$$

Machines can be programmed to suit individual requirements. Peritoneal equilibration tests enable more accurate dialysis prescription (Twardowski *et al.*, 1987) and have been adapted for children (Hanna *et al.* 1993). Very small infants can be successfully dialysed at home using appropriate lines.

Peritonitis rates vary from centre to centre but are reported to occur more frequently in children (Warady *et al.*, 1996) than in adults, whose overall average rate is approximately 1.1–1.3 episodes per patient per year (Keane, 1996). In the authors' centre during the period January 1995 to December 1996 figures for peritonitis in those treated by APD were 0.85 episodes per patient per year and for CAPD 1.2 episodes per patient per year (Reid and de Sousa, unpublished data), which are similar figures to those reported by other centres (Kuizon *et al.*, 1995). Peritonitis and catheter-related infections remain the most common cause of morbidity and treatment failure in patients on either CAPD or APD (Kuizon *et al.*, 1995). Clinical presentation of peritonitis is similar in children and adults, although Keane noted that infants appear to be less capable of keeping bacterial infections within the peritoneal cavity and often become systemically ill, requiring more extensive treatment.

CONCLUSION

This chapter has attempted to show the major differences in treating children with renal failure. It has hopefully emphasized that these patients must be cared for by paediatric nurses and nephrologists in a specialist unit that has access to other professionals such as play specialists, psychologists and dietitians. To the paediatric team, trying to achieve normality for the child and parents is of the utmost importance. For the child, this entails promoting normal growth, achieving attendance at school and encouraging appropriate social development (Taylor, 1996). Families may require additional support from psychologists and others to help deal with problems such as disturbed siblings and difficulties with family dynamics.

Advances in technology have meant that it has become relatively safer to dialyse and transplant babies but one must not ignore the enormous burden taken on by the family when they decide that their child will be treated. When presenting treatment options to families, death has to be included as a possibility, particularly when dealing with very young infants or severely handicapped children for whom the stress of treatment may be overwhelming. Long-term medical and psychological sequelae may outweigh the benefits of treatment in childhood (Doyal and Henning, 1994). Within the authors' unit there have been teenagers who, on reaching 16 or 18 years of age after years of therapy (including several failed transplants), decided they did not want to have any more treatment and refused dialysis, dying peacefully a few days later.

> **Key reference:** Doyal, L. and Henning. P. (1994) Stopping treatment for end-stage renal failure: the rights of children and adolescents. *Pediatric Nephrology* 8: 768–771.

'Nursing a child with renal failure is a challenge and nurses must be able to focus not only on the child's unique needs, but also enable and encourage them to enjoy as much normality as possible' (Frauman and Gilman, 1985).

Nurses must play their part in helping adolescents to move towards independence, by encouraging them to take responsibility for themselves by assuming control of their medication, appointment-making and interaction with hospital staff (Watson *et al.*, 1996). Achieving such measures of independence will help in the inevitable transition to adult renal units and help them grow to maturity with confidence.

REVIEW QUESTIONS

- In what ways do children and adolescents differ physically from adults?
- What role does the nurse play in helping a child accept treatment?
- How can nurse and parents work together for the benefit of the child?
- Describe the possible signs and symptoms that might be displayed by a 2-year-old child with undiagnosed CRF?
- If called on to haemodialyse a child, how would you calculate a safe ECBV?
- What are the advantages of peritoneal dialysis for children?
- How would you deal with a non-compliant adolescent?

REFERENCES

Andreoli, S. P., Bergstein, J. M. and Sherrard, D. J. (1984) Aluminium intoxication from aluminium-containing phosphate binders in children with azotemia not undergoing dialysis. *New England Journal of Medicine*, **310**, 1079–1084.

Arbus, G. S., Rochon, J. and Thompson, D. (1991) Survival of cadaveric renal transplant grafts from young donors and in young recipients. *Pediatric Nephrology*, **5**, 152–157.

BAPN (1995) *The Provision of Services in the United Kingdom for Children and Adolescents with Renal Disease. Report of a Working Party*, British Association for Paediatric Nephrology, London.

Bunchman, T. E. (1995) Chronic dialysis in the infant less than 1 year of age. *Pediatric Nephrology*, **9**, S18–S22.

Burgess, M. (1982) Protective support for children following renal transplant. *Physiotherapy*, **68**(11), 386.

Casey, A. (1988) A partnership with child and family. *Senior Nurse*, **8**(4), 8–9.

Churchill, B. M., Jayanthi, R. V., McLorie, G. A. and Khoury, A. E. (1996) Pediatric renal transplantation into the abnormal urinary tract. *Pediatric Nephrology*, **10**, 113–120.

Dillon, M. J. (1994) Hypertension, in *Clinical Paediatric Nephrology*, 2nd edn, (ed. R. J. Postlethwaite), Heinemann, Oxford.

Donckerwolcke, R., Broyer, M., Chantler, C. and Rizzoni, G. (1996) Renal replacement therapy in children, in *Replacement of Renal Function by Dialysis*, 4th edn, (eds C. Jacobs, C. M. Kjellstrand, K. M. Koch and J. F. Winchester), Kluwer Academic Publishers, Dordrecht.

Douglas, J. (1993) *Psychology and Nursing Children*, Macmillan, Basingstoke.

Doyal, L. and Henning, P. (1994) Stopping treatment for end-stage renal failure: the rights of children and adolescents. *Pediatric Nephrology*, **8**, 768–771.

Ettenger, R. B. (1996) Kidney transplantation in children, in *Handbook of Kidney Transplantation*, 2nd edn, (ed. G. M. Danovitch), Little, Brown & Co., Boston, MA.

Ettenger, R. B., Rosenthal, J. T., Marik, J. L. *et al.* (1991) Improved cadaveric renal transplant outcome in children. *Pediatric Nephrology*, **5**, 137–142.

Fitzpatrick, M. M., Duffy, P. G., Fernando, O. N. *et al.* (1992) Cadaveric renal transplantation in children under 5 years of age. *Pediatric Nephrology*, **6**, 166–171.

Flom, L. S., Reisman, E. M., Donovan, J. M. *et al.* (1992) Favourable experience with pre-emptive renal transplantation. *Pediatric Nephrology*, **6**, 258–261.

Frauman, A. C. and Gilman, C. (1985) 'Normal life', a goal for the child with chronic renal failure. *American Nephrology Nurses Association Journal*, **12**(3), 192–195.

Gorynski, L. and Knight, F. (1992) A peer support group for adolescent dialysis patients. *American Nephrology Nurses Association Journal*, **19**(3) 262–264.

Hadzinski, M. F. (1992) *Nursing Care of the Critically Ill Child*, 2nd edn, C. V. Mosby, St Louis, MO.

Hanna, J. D., Foreman, J. W., Todd, W. B. G. *et al.* (1993) The peritoneal equilibration test in children. *Pediatric Nephrology*, **7**, 731–734.

Harmon, W. E. (1991) Opportunistic infections in children following renal transplantation. *Pediatric Nephrology*, **5**, 118–125.

Haycock, G. B. (1984) Intraoperative and immediate postoperative care in the management of the paediatric transplant recipient, in *Pediatric Nephrology*, (eds J. Brodehl and J. H. H. Ehrich), Springer-Verlag, Berlin.

Keane, W. F. (1996) *Peritoneal Dialysis Related Peritonitis Treatment Recommendations 1996 Update*, Advisory Committee on Peritonitis Management of the International Society of Peritoneal Dialysis, .

Knight, F., Gorynski, L., Bentson, M. and Harmon, W. E. (1993) Hemodialysis of the infant and small child with chronic renal failure. *American Nephrology Nurses Association Journal*, **20**(3), 315–323.

Kuizon, B., Melocoton, T. L., Holloway, M. *et al.* (1995) Infectious and catheter-related complications in pediatric patients treated with peritoneal dialysis at a single institution. *Pediatric Nephrology*, **9**, S12–S17.

Maynard, L. (1993) Transplantation in children: psychosocial issues. *Paediatric Nursing*, **5**(10), 20–22.

Nevins, T. E. and Davidson, G. (1991) Prior dialysis does not affect the outcome of pediatric renal transplantation. *Pediatric Nephrology*, **5**, 211–214.

Ravelli, A. M. (1995) Gastrointestinal function in chronic renal failure. *Pediatric Nephrology*, **9**, 756–762.

Reynolds, J. M., Garralda, M. E., Jameson, R. A. and Postlethwaite, R. J. (1988) How parents and families cope with chronic renal failure. *Archives of Disease in Childhood*, **63**, 821–826.

Rigden, S. P. A., Rees, L. and Chantler, C. (1990) Growth and endocrine function in children with chronic renal failure. *Acta Paediatrica Scandinavica (Supplement)*, **370**, 20–26.

Rigden, S. P. A., Start, K. M. and Rees, L. (1987) Nutritional management of infants and toddlers with chronic renal failure. *Nutrition and Health*, **5**(3/4), 163–174.

Riley, C. M. (1964) Thoughts about kidney homotransplantation in children. *Journal of Pediatrics*, **65**, 797.

Taylor, C. M. (1994) Assessment of glomerular filtration rate, in *Clinical Paediatric Nephrology*, 2nd edn, (ed. R. J. Postlethwaite), Heinemann, Oxford.

Taylor, J. H. (1996) End stage renal disease in children: diagnosis, management and interventions. *Pediatric Nursing*, **22**(6), 481–490.

Twardowski, Z. J., Nolph, K. D., Khanna, R. *et al.* (1987) Peritoneal equilibration test. *Peritoneal Dialysis Bulletin*, **7**, 138–147.

Warady, B. A., Sullivan, E. K. and Alexander, S. R. (1996) Lessons from the peritoneal dialysis patient data base: a report of the North American Pediatric Renal Transplant Co-operative Study. *Kidney International*, **49**(Suppl. 53), S68–S71.

Watson, A., Phillips, D. and Argles, J. (1996) Transferring adolescents from paediatric to adult renal units. *British Journal of Renal Medicine*, **1**(2), 24–26.

Subject index